GENES, ENZYMES, AND POPULATIONS

BASIC LIFE SCIENCES

Alexander Hollaender, General Editor

Biology Division
Oak Ridge National Laboratory
and The University of Tennessee,
Knoxville

1973: Volume 1 • GENE EXPRESSION AND ITS REGULATION
Edited by F. T. Kenney, B. A. Hamkalo, G. Favelukes,
and J. T. August

Volume 2 • GENES, ENZYMES, AND POPULATIONS
Edited by A. M. Srb

In preparation:

Volume 3 • CONTROL OF TRANSCRIPTION
Edited by B. B. Biswas, R. K. Mandal, A. Stevens,
and W. E. Cohn

• REPRODUCTIVE PHYSIOLOGY AND GENETICS
Edited by F. Fuchs and E. M. Coutinho

A Continuation Order Plan is available for this series. A continuation order will bring delivery of each new volume immediately upon publication. Volumes are billed only upon actual shipment. For further information please contact the publisher.

GENES, ENZYMES, AND POPULATIONS

Edited by
Adrian M. Srb
Section of Genetics, Development, and Physiology
Cornell University
Ithaca, New York

PLENUM PRESS • NEW YORK — LONDON

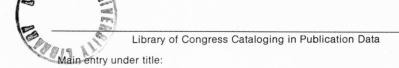

Library of Congress Cataloging in Publication Data

Main entry under title:

Genes, enzymes, and populations.

(Basic life sciences, v. 2)
"Proceedings of the twelfth International Latin-American symposium, held in Cali, Columbia, November 27-December 1, 1972."
Includes bibliographical references.
1. Genetics—Congresses. 2. Plant-breeding—Congresses. 3. Tropical crops—Latin America. I. Srb, Adrian M., ed. II. Title. [DNLM: 1. Animals, Domestic—Congresses. 2. Breeding—Congresses. 3. Plants—Congresses. S494 L357g 1973]

QH426.G46	575.1	73-15867

ISBN 0-306-36502-2

Proceedings of the Twelfth International Latin American Symposium, held in
Cali, Colombia, November 27-December 1, 1972

© 1973 Plenum Press, New York
A Division of Plenum Publishing Corporation
227 West 17th Street, New York, N.Y. 10011

United Kingdom edition published by Plenum Press, London
A Division of Plenum Publishing Company, Ltd.
Davis House (4th Floor), 8 Scrubs Lane, Harlesden, London, NW10 6SE, England

Organizing Committee

Honorary President
Alexander Hollaender, Biology Division, Oak Ridge National Laboratory, Oak Ridge, Tenn.

Alvaro Alegría, Departmento de Ciencias Fisiológicas, Bioquímica, Universidad del Valle, Cali.

Eduardo Alvarez, Centro Internacional de Agricultura Tropical, C.I.A.T., Palmira.

Jorge Allende, Departamento de Bioquímica, Facultad de Ciencias, Universidad de Chile, Santiago.

Rafael Bravo, Instituto Colombiano Agropecuario, I.C.A., Palmira.

Francis Byrnes, Centro Internacional de Agricultura Tropical, C.I.A.T., Palmira.

Nelson Castelar, Facultad de Ciencias Agropecuarias, Universidad Nacional, Palmira.

Gabriel Cerón, Departamento de Morfología, Universidad Nacional, Bogotá.

Alvaro Figueroa, Facultad de Ciencias Agropecuarias, Universidad Nacional, Palmira.

Mario Guimaraes Ferri, Facultade de Filosofía, Ciencias e Letras, Universidade de Sao Paulo.

Hugo Hoenigsberg, Departamento de Biología, Universidad de los Andes, Bogotá.

Adrian Srb, Department of Genetics, Cornell University, Ithaca, N.Y.

Henrique Tono, Bogotá.

General Secretary
Carlos Corredor, Departmento de Ciencias Fisiológicas, Bioquímica, Universidad del Valle, Cali.

Sponsors

Departamento de Ciencias Fisiológicas, Sección Bioquímica, Universidad del Valle, Cali.
Facultad de Ciencias Agropecuarias, Universidad Nacional, Palmira.
Instituto Colombiano Agropecuario (I.C.A.), Palmira.
Centro Internacional de Agricultura Tropical, (C.I.A.T.), Palmira.
Cornell University, Ithaca, N.Y.
National Academy of Sciences (USA), Washington, D.C.
Oak Ridge National Laboratory, Biology Division, Oak Ridge, Tenn.
Panamerican Association of Biochemical Societies (PAABS).
Asociación Colombiana de Ciencias Biológicas.

Supporting Institutions

Universidad del Valle, Cali, Colombia.
Universidad Nacional de Colombia.
Asociación Colombiana para el Avance de la Ciencia (ACEACE).
Fondo Colombiano de Investigaciones Científicas y Proyectos Especiales Francisco José de Caldas' (COLCIENCIAS).
Instituto Colombiano para el Fomento de la Educación Superior, (ICFES).
Organización de Estados Americanos, OEA, Programa Regional de Desarrollo Científico tecnológico.
Ford Foundation (USA).
U.S. Atomic Energy Commission.
U.S. National Science Foundation.
Federación Nacional de Cafeteros, Colombia.

Acknowledgments: The following institutions and companies have extended generous collaboration and assistance:

Federación Nacional de Cafeteros
Laboratorios Bayer
Gobernación del Valle
Secretaría de Fomento y Agricultura
Oficina de Turismo
Carvajal y Cia.
CELA colombiana
Quaker de Colombia
Corporación del Valle del Cauca, (C.V.C.).

Foreword

The present volume includes the large majority of papers given at the symposium entitled "Fundamental Approaches to Plant and Animal Improvement," held at Cali, Colombia, in November, 1972. The primary focal points were on various genetic mechanisms, including gene action and mutation, the development of phenotypic attributes, and on evolution, including that controlled by man for agricultural purposes. In fact, very little referring in any particular way to animal improvement was included, while a great deal of attention was paid to higher plants and to microorganisms. On the other hand, both the population genetics of insects and insect control were considered. Thus *Genes, Enzymes, and Populations,* the title given to this published work, seems to me to represent somewhat more fairly the contents than does the original symposium title.

Given the intent of the symposium, which is expressed in the original title, the published record cannot be expected to be a neatly packaged presentation of some highly defined subject matter. Indeed the diverse subjects represent some, but by no means all, of the varied and dynamic scientific activities that need to be components in the improvement and production of agriculturally significant plants at a time when world populations are rapidly increasing and shortages of food occurring. In any case, the organizers of the symposium wisely decided that considerations of environment as well as of genetics should be introduced into the thinking of the group and that physiology and molecular biology could not be ignored.

One of the aims of the symposium was to foster interactions among representatives of basic and applied science and to establish communication, in reference to common goals, among representatives of scientific fields who generally use rather separate methodologies and manners of thought. How far such aims were met is not easy to evaluate, but certainly they were met in part. The mere presentation of papers found in this volume, excellent as they may be, cannot convey the excitement of certain conversations among participants as these conversations occurred before and after the formal sessions.

Much of the excitement emerged from consideration of the implications of increasing ability to utilize cell culture techniques in order to manipulate higher plants in the ways used by microbial and molecular geneticists. Thus the paper by Rasse-Messenguy and Fink, on yeast, turns out to have close ideological and procedural interrelationships with the paper by Carlson *et al.,* who report work on disease tolerance in tobacco. I have placed these papers in sequence in the published work, because of their interrelationships, and otherwise in ordering the material have taken a few liberties with the sequence followed at the symposium itself.

In any case, a reading of the various papers reveals increasing cross-infusions of technique and of problem orientation among basic and applied scientists. Perhaps eventually something like a continuous spectrum in direction of efforts will emerge, so that gaps in communication will be bridged. Nevertheless, a major challenge to the biology of the future is evident. None should doubt the validity and relevance of efforts so diverse as represented in Ferri's survey of the ecology of Latin America on the one hand or in Skoog's highly molecular treatment of plant growth regulators on the other. How to muster rapidly and effectively this information in reference to agricultural problems in areas of Latin America presents the challenge. And the final paper, by Marquez-Sanchez, makes clear that sociological perceptiveness is an essential ingredient in successfully applied biology.

I myself found satisfying, in the context supplied by the intent of the symposium, that the natural world retains magnificent untapped genetic resources. These emerge dramatically in Rick's fascinating account of wild tomato species whose varied germ plasms appear to have great potential for further improvement of one of our important garden crops.

Adrian M. Srb

Introduction

Cali, Colombia, situated at the head of one of the most fruitful valleys in the country, plays a unique role in the development of strong agricultural research. The location of the Tropical Agricultural Station at Palmira, just outside Cali, and many other aspects of agriculture, suggested that the topic for our 1972 Latin American Symposium, "Fundamental Approaches to Plant and Animal Improvement," would be an excellent opportunity to combine the basic aspects of biochemistry and genetics with the application to the improvement of plants and animals. This twelfth in our series of Latin American Symposia turned out to be most successful, and will surely influence the status of agriculture not only in Colombia and other southern hemisphere countries but worldwide as well. The Proceedings volume will, I am sure, be an important contribution to the literature on new developments in plant and animal breeding. Dr. Adrian Srb of Cornell University has done an outstanding job as editor of these Proceedings.

Early plans for the Symposium were initiated in cooperation with Dr. Henrique Tono, who was Associate Dean of the Medical School at the University of Cali. Dr. Tono later resigned this position, and Dr. Carlos Corredor of the Biochemistry Department of the Medical School took over the organization of the Symposium and did an excellent job under sometimes complicated circumstances.

While travel restrictions in certain countries made it impossible for some individuals to attend the meeting, many scientists were there from various Latin American and other countries.

This Symposium, as previous ones, was supported by special grants from the United States Atomic Energy Commission and the National Science Foundation and by a Ford Foundation grant administered through the United States National Academy of Sciences. The Office of American States and other groups, especially in Colombia, made important contributions. Cornell University was the U. S. university cosponsoring the Symposium with the Pan American

Biochemical Society. I want to thank the various groups that helped so much, often under emergency conditions, to make the Cali Symposium a success; we are most grateful.

A complete list of previous Latin American symposia, with publication information on each, is given below.

1961

International Symposium on Tissue Transplantation—Santiago, Viña del Mar, and Valparaiso, Chile. Published in 1962 by the University of Chile Press, Santiago; edited by A. P. Cristoffanini and Gustavo Hoecker; 269 pp.

1962

International Symposium on Mammalian Cytogenetics and Related Problems in Radiobiology—São Paulo and Rio de Janeiro, Brazil. Published in 1964 by The Macmillan Company, New York, under arrangement with Pergamon Press, Ltd., Oxford; edited by C. Pavan, C. Chagas, O. Frota-Pessoa, and L. R. Caldas; 427 pp.

1963

International Symposium on Control of Cell Division and the Induction of Cancer—Lima, Peru, and Cali, Colombia. Published in 1964 by the U.S. Department of Health, Education, and Welfare as *National Cancer Institute Monograph 14;* edited by C. C. Congdon and Pablo Mori-Chavez; 403 pp.

1964

International Symposium on Genes and Chromosomes, Structure and Function—Buenos Aires, Argentina. Published in 1965 by the U.S. Department of Health, Education, and Welfare as *National Cancer Institute Monograph 18;* edited by J. I. Valencia and Rhoda F. Grell, with the cooperation of Ruby Marie Valencia; 354 pp.

1965

International Symposium on the Nucleolus—Its Structure and Function—Montevideo, Uruguay. Published in 1966 by the U.S. Department of Health, Education, and Welfare as *National Cancer Institute Monograph 23;* edited by W. S. Vincent and O. L. Miller, Jr.; 610 pp.

1966

International Symposium on Enzymatic Aspects of Metabolic Regulation—Mexico City, Mexico. Published in 1967 by the U.S. Department of Health, Education, and Welfare as *National Cancer Institute Monograph 27;* edited by M. P. Stulberg; 343 pp.

1967

International Symposium on Basic Mechanisms in Photochemistry and Photo-biology—Caracas, Venezuela. Published in 1968 by Pergamon Press as Volume 7, No. 6, *Photochemistry and Photobiology;* edited by J. W. Longworth; 326 pp.

1968

International Symposium on Nuclear Physiology and Differentiation—Belo Horizonte, Minas Gerais, Brazil. Published in 1969 by The Genetics Society of America as a supplement to *Genetics,* Volume 61, No. 1; edited by R. P. Wagner; 469 pp.

1969

International Symposium on Fertility of the Sea—São Paulo, Brazil. Published in 1971 by Gordon and Breach Science Publishers, New York; edited by J. D. Costlow; 2 volumes, 622 pp.

1970

International Symposium on Visual Processes in Vertebrates—Santiago, Chile. Published in 1971 by Pergamon Press as Volume 11, Supplement No. 3, *Vision Research;* edited by Thorne Shipley and J. E. Dowling; 477 pp.

1971

International Symposium on Gene Expression and Its Regulation—La Plata, Argentina. Published in 1973 by Plenum Publishing Corporation, New York, as *Vol. 1 Basic Life Sciences Series* (Alexander Hollaender, General Editor); edited by Francis T. Kenney, Barbara A. Hamkalo, Gabriel Favelukes, and J. Thomas August.

Alexander Hollaender
Biology Division
Oak Ridge National Laboratory
Oak Ridge, Tennessee
and
University of Tennessee, Knoxville

Contents

Population Genetics

Applications of Genetics

1

Introductory Address

Carlos Corredor*

Departamento de Ciencias Fisiológicas, Facultad de Medicina
Universidad del Valle
Cali, Colombia

Some 12 years ago, the City of Santiago, in Chile, was host to a group of scientists from all over the hemisphere. The group intended to evaluate what was then known about tissue transplant. It does not really matter whether or not any of the spectacular advances in that field during the past decade had anything to do with that first meeting. The one important fact for us, and our America, is that with that event a series of annual meetings was started. The themes of such Symposia have always dealt with some exciting frontier of science. Their fundamental purpose, which has always been fulfilled, has been to gather the most distinguished scientists in one particular field from all over the world together in some place in Latin America and to allow them to share their individual experiences among themselves and with Latin American students and young scientists who have just been initiated into the difficult art of wresting secrets from nature.

These meetings spring from the ideas and the work of a man, Dr. Alexander Hollaender, who has dedicated these past years to the one purpose of making their objectives a reality renewed once a year and each passing year stronger. The fruition of his initiative has been plainly expressed in the many multinational research and teaching efforts that have resulted from the direct contact between investigators.

It is in the city of Santiago de Cali, which was host to the Third Symposium of this series, where we gather again in order to consider what perhaps is today the most important challenge ever presented to human ingenuity: what steps

* Secretary General and Head of the Biochemistry Department.

1

must man take in order to assure the conservation of the species against a disordered growth of the population in a world with limited natural nutritional resources. Obviously, just as with any other problem, the present challenge must be attacked on different flanks. Educational, religious, political, and scientific solutions should be advanced. We shall be occupied here only with those which may be placed under the heading of scientific solutions. We believe that any recommendations that do not have a firm scientific basis are only blind attempts to change reality. Our work should then present others with objective alternatives which can be utilized to make the right decisions, even if they run counter to political expediency or to ingrained fears and prejudices, fruits of ancestral ignorance.

Our purpose, then, is to consider what is now known about the basic mechanisms that determine and control phenotype and the ways in which it is possible to manipulate it, both at the laboratory bench and in the open field, in order to produce new individuals with certain features of greater value to mankind and a greater resistance against their natural enemies.

In the first conference, the problem is defined and a mark of reference is set against which the following topics will be considered and referred to the area of Latin America. The following talks will make reference to new knowledge about the regulation of expression of eukaryotic genes at the molecular level. The biosynthetic pathways of some amino acids, the extranuclear gene activity and protein synthesis, are taken as examples of such regulation. The action of light on normal biochemical mechanisms in plants will then be taken up, and next, in view of these basic findings, we will consider the way in which molecular changes cause biochemical changes with the end-result that special phenotypes in which one or more particular amino acids appear augmented are produced. Later conferences will evaluate the action of environmental factors on certain plant processes such as seedling morphogenesis, tuber formation, the flowering of coffee trees, and the ecological aspects of the distribution of animal and vegetable life in the Americas. The advances obtained in the selection of vegetable species of economic importance adapted to the particular ecological conditions of the Latin American environment will then be explored. Next, we will hear about the methodology of producing specific mutants and the advances obtained using such methodology to produce new varieties. We will have occasion to evaluate the technique of tissue culture as applied to the study of cell processes *in vitro*. I believe that this methodology opens a new horizon to research and development and holds great promise in obtaining particular varieties of plants in very short periods of time. Finally, we will talk about biological control of plagues. This is a pressing necessity in a world ever endangered by increasing environmental pollution. We will end the meeting at a basic level, and justly so, by considering the advances in knowledge at the molecular level of the phenomenon of reparation of genetic material altered by chemicals and by ionizing radiation.

It was a particular honor for me to have served as Secretary General to this event that gathers the best of the scientific world in the field. I must commend the decisive work of the members of the Coordinating Committee, starting with that of the always dynamic mentor, Alexander Hollaender; of Henrique Tono, first Secretary General of this Symposium; of Gabriel Cerón, of Alvaro Alegría, of Nelson Castellar, and of the great many individuals and institutional groups, both Colombians and from other countries, who made this meeting possible. I would like to emphasize that this is a Pan American Association of Biochemical Societies (PAABS) Symposium and that the Colombian Society of Biological Sciences has collaborated in its organization and promotion.

For those of you to whom my Spanish may have seemed a little bit difficult to understand, I may summarize everything said in one word: WELCOME.

2

Ecological Problems in Latin America

Mario G. Ferri

Departamento de Botanica
Instituto de Biociências
Universidade de São Paulo
São Paulo, Brasil

Ecological problems in Latin America are extremely difficult to discuss for three reasons: first, the subject is too broad; second, the space available is too short; third, my knowledge is too restricted.

When I accepted the invitation to discuss this subject, I made it clear that my personal knowledge of ecological problems was confined to the main types of Brazilian vegetation. I know the vegetation of other Latin American countries only from the literature. Since, however, many types of Brazilian vegetation also occur in many other Latin American countries, under similar environmental conditions, some of my experience may be useful in other parts of Latin America.

INTRODUCTION

I shall first examine the main types of vegetation found in Latin American countries. By "main types of vegetation," I mean the types that cover more extensive areas as well as some types that have very peculiar characteristics.

If we look at a vegetation map of Latin America, such as the map published by Smith and Johnston (58), or de Lemps' maps (14), or Hueck's vegetation map of South America (38), we shall see that all of them agree in their general outlines. They differ in that one is more synthetic or another more detailed. Another map may even show different limits of the various vegetation zones. In all, however, the main types are shown to cover, in general, the same areas, and this fact seems to be a good assurance that, as far as the main points are concerned, there are no very important discrepancies.

If we start with Mexico and work southward, we find first the dense tropical forests which occur also, for instance, in Cuba, San Domingo, Nicaragua, Costa Rica, and Panama. The same type of forest is also to be found in Colombia, Venezuela, the Guianas, Peru, and Brazil. Then we find different types of savanna vegetation in Cuba, Panama, Colombia, Venezuela (*llanos*), the Guianas, and Brazil (*cerrados*). High mountain tropical forests occur in Mexico, the Central American countries, Colombia, Peru, Ecuador, and Bolivia, for instance. Vegetation adapted to warm semiarid conditions is found in Mexico, Venezuela, northeastern Brazil, and the north of Argentina. Clear forests in which a great many palms are mixed with dicotyledons exist in the north of Brazil. There is also clear forest of a different composition in southwestern Brazil, as well as in the *chaco* region of Bolivia, Paraguay, and Argentina. The *pampas* that have their northernmost limit in southern Brazil spread themselves all over Uruguay and northeastern Argentina. Deserts are found in Peru, Chile, and Patagonia. Finally, forests of a temperate character can be found in Chile, Patagonia, and southern Brazil.

These, to my belief, are the main types of vegetation to be considered. A detailed analysis of other types such as *paramos, lomas, puna,* and so on cannot be made here. The mangroves and the vegetation of sand dunes along the shores, so typical and so regular in their floristic composition wherever they occur (and they do occur in many Latin American countries), should not be forgotten.

The types of vegetation presented above can be grouped in the following way:

A. Forests

1. Evergreen rainforest
2. Tropical deciduous forest
3. Palm forest
4. Temperate forest

B. Grasslands and savannas

1. Northern savannas
2. *Cerrados*
3. *Campos*
4. *Pampas*

C. Deserts or semideserts

1. Deserts of South America (Pacific coast)
2. Deserts of Patagonia
3. Semidesertic vegetation

MAIN TYPES OF VEGETATION IN LATIN AMERICA

Evergreen Rainforest

In the Amazon, with high even temperatures and heavy rainfall all year around, we may find *terra firma* forests, which are above flood level and are never (or almost never) flooded; *varzea* forests, which are in the plains and may be temporarily flooded; and *igapos,* which are permanently flooded forests.

In the Guianas, Venezuela, Colombia, Ecuador, Peru, and Bolivia, more or less vast areas are covered by tropical rainforest. In the midst of the forest, however, different types of vegetation can be found. For instance, in the Amazon *campos* of several types and *cerrados* occur. In the upper Rio Negro and also in the upper Solimoes, there are evergreen *caatingas* which are much poorer than the rest of the Amazonian forest.

These *caatingas* are quite different from the northeastern *caatingas* in all respects: they occur under warm and wet climate (high air humidity and heavy rainfall) and on poor wet soil (almost pure sand with perhaps a 10-cm layer of more or less decomposed litter); the big Cactaceae so peculiar to the deciduous *caatingas* are completely absent; floristic composition in general is quite different. The northeastern *caatingas* grow under dry conditions, whereas in the Amazonian *caatingas* yearly rainfall is 3000 mm or more and in northeastern Brazil it is 500 mm or even much less. In the latter area, temperatures are rather high, air humidity is in general low, soils can be fairly rich. Big and small Cactaceae are frequent in the *caatinga.*

The reason such different vegetation types have the same denomination is that the word *caatinga,* of Indian origin, means "whitish, clear forest." The deciduous *caatinga* is clear when it is leafless, and this is the aspect which persists longer, since the dry season lasts 8–9 months or even longer. The evergreen *caatinga* appeared whitish to the Indians in contrast to the compact, dark forest nearby.

Whereas the deciduous *caatinga* is clearly conditioned by the lack of water, the evergreen *caatinga* is conditioned by lack of nutrients in the soil. This aspect will be discussed later.

In Brazil, on the eastern slopes of the mountains, are forests similar to the Amazonian forest. They are not quite so high, but they are compact, have a rich composition, and exhibit a great number of lianas and epiphytes.

Also similar to the Amazonian rainforest are the forests found in Venezuela, on the western slopes of the Andes in Colombia and Ecuador, and in some parts of Central American countries, among other places.

Of course, these forests that have the same general appearance are not similar. On the contrary, they are locally differentiated in many ways, especially floristic composition, the height and diameter of trees, the density of the vegetation, the number of lianas and epiphytes, and so on.

Tropical Deciduous Forest

Tropical deciduous forests are found in areas where there are two distinct seasons: a rainy season in which the leaves turn the vegetation green and a dry season in which the vegetation is leafless.

Tropical deciduous forest occurs in Colombia flanking the *llanos*. The trees of this forest are of moderate height, and the forest itself has been called "subxerophilous" in Venezuela and Colombia. In certain parts of Central America from Panama to Mexico, there are tropical deciduous forests in regions with a distinct dry season. Of course, the vegetation of northeastern Brazil and that of the *chaco* can be placed under this ample denomination.

The deciduous forest called *caatinga* which exists in the dry Brazilian northeast is an open scrub forest. According to Andrade-Lima (3), with whom I agree, *caatinga* should be considered a region rather than a special type of vegetation, since man has interfered with the natural vegetation.

The vegetation of the *chaco* is basically composed of xerophilous forests and savannas, "with many halophytic and swampy associations" (58). In the *chaco*, the dry forest is especially made up of slow-growing hardwood trees (*algarrobos* and *quebrachos*, for instance).

Ecological aspects and problems of the Brazilian deciduous *caatinga* which may apply to other tropical deciduous forests will be discussed later.

Palm Forest

In the northern parts of Brazil, especially in the states of Maranhao and Piaui, there are forests that are called *cocais* (*Orbignya martiana* is the dominant species) and *carnaubais* (*Copernicia cerifera* dominates). Other palms (e.g., *Mauritia* and *Attalea*) are also present but are less frequent. To the northwest, the *cocais* (or *babacuais*) dominate and are confined by the hygrophilous Amazonian forest. To the southeast, the *carnaubais* are predominant and in contact with the deciduous *caatinga* (see refs. 3 and 40).

Evergreen *Araucaria* Forest

The Parana pine (*Araucaria angustifolia*) is the dominant species in the southern states of Brazil: Rio Grande do Sul, Santa Catarina, and Parana. It occurs in association with another gymnosperm (*Podocarpus lambertii*) and with several dicotyledons (e.g., *Ilex paraguariensis* and *Ocotea porosa*). In this region, rains are more uniformly distributed throughout the year. There are two seasons (winter and summer) clearly defined by the variations in maximal and minimal temperatures. This vegetation is also found in lower latitudes, but only at higher altitudes, a fact which indicates that it is conditioned by temperature rather than by any other environmental factor.

Savannas

It seems that the word "savanna" was first used by Oviedo in 1935 in connection with the *llanos* of Venezuela (see refs. 14 and 58). Smith and Johnston state that "if one were to insist upon priority for phytogeographic terms, savanna might well be used only for those grasslands of the northern part of South America which are definitely climatic rather than edaphic in origin." The literature makes it obvious that the term "savanna" has been used so widely to designate so many different types of vegetation that it has become somewhat misleading. In fact, in Africa French botanists employ the term very frequently to designate various kinds of vegetation. Thus it became necessary to establish types of savannas such as *la savane herbeuse* (grass savanna), *la savane arborée* (tree savanna), *la savane à boqueteaux* and *la savane boisée* (savanna woodland). Adding to this the fact that sometimes the so-called savanna is the result of climatic conditions, in other cases it seems to be conditioned by edaphic factors, and in still other instances it is conditioned by anthropic influence (fire is an important factor), we come to the conclusion that this word has become a *nomen ambiguum* (the same is the case with the term "steppe").

While it might be argued that the same is true of the term "forest" because there are deciduous forests, evergreen forests, and rainforests, one element is common to all forests: the tree is dominant. The different types of savannas do not have a single element common to all of them. It is possible, however, to use the word "savanna" in opposition to the term "forest" to designate the vegetation forms in which trees are not dominant. No objection can be made to this use, but there will be examples in which it will be difficult to say if vegetation forms are savannas or forests (e.g., the *cerradao*).

Under the name of "true savanna," we have to consider the *llanos* which are not open prairies (such as those of the United States) or *pampas* (such as found in Uruguay and Argentina). The ground is covered by several grasses (e.g., *Andropogon* and *Trachypogon*). Many trees that belong to genera and even species that are frequent in Brazilian *cerrados* are found there (e.g., *Curatella americana, Bowdichia virgilioides,* and *Byrsonima;* see refs. 38 and 58).

There is a long dry season that lasts 5 months or more. The rainy season is short, but the rains are heavy and large areas of the surface are flooded. Part of the Rio Branco-Rupununi region is covered with similar vegetation. Costa Rica, Surinam, French Guiana, Trinidad, and Cuba also have vegetation with similar physiognomy and floristic composition.

In some places, this vegetation is conditioned, possibly by climatic factors, and in other places it may be conditioned by edaphic factors. Anthropic influences may also have enlarged areas occupied by the so-called savannas. This possibility has been discussed by many authors. The interested reader might look at Schnell's *Introduction à la Phytogeographie des Pays Tropicaux* (55) in which the problem is discussed at length and in which the author gives other bibliographical references.

Cerrados

Cerrado is a savannalike vegetation characterized by a great number of tortuous shrubs and trees which often have thick bark and large simple or compound leaves that are sometimes densely hairy or leathery with a brilliant surface (20–23, 51, 63, 64). (For background information, *cf.* refs. 31 and 32.) *Kielmeyera coriacea, Qualea grandiflora, Stryphnodendron barbatimao, Dimorphandra mollis, Caryocar brasiliense, Curatella americana,* and several species of *Erythroxylum, Annona, Byrsonima,* etc., could be mentioned among the most frequent species. As a rule, Cactaceae, Bromeliaceae, and succulent Euphorbiaceae are not important components of the *cerrado* vegetation.

Cerrados are found over a very large part of the Brazilian territory. In central Brazil alone, the area occupied by *cerrados* is calculated to be 1.5 million km^2 (2). They are not restricted to central Brazil, however, and go as far south as Campo Mourao (state of Parana) at a latitude of 24°S. They are found in the northeast, for instance, in Goiana close to the border between the states of Pernambuco and Paraiba (28) at a latitude of approximately 8°S. In the Amazon, close to the Equator, they also occur as islands of special vegetation surrounded by the exuberant rainforests (7). In the northeast, *cerrados* are only a few kilometers from the sea but go inland as far as the vicinity of Brazil's western border.

With such a large distribution, it is clear that we shall find *cerrado* vegetation growing under the most varied climate and soil conditions.

More often, the *cerrados* are found on flat lands, but they are frequent on soils with steep inclination and in this case may occur on the top or on the lower slopes. In the states of Mato Grosso and Goias, there are examples of *cerrados* in each of these circumstances.

Cerrados may also grow on very sandy soils, on soils that were originally rich in calcareous materials, or on soils resulting from the decomposition of diabase. In Brazil, the last very frequently is the origin of the best type of soil, the so-called *terra roxa*. As a rule, the soils in which the *cerrado* vegetation occurs are very deep. Depths of 20–30 m or even more are not unusual. Sometimes we find in soils covered by *cerrados* an impervious layer (hardpan) that is called *canga* in Brazil. This *canga* may occur at different depths, sometimes at the very surface. Although this situation is not the rule, an example can be found in the *cerrado* of Goiana already mentioned. Even in this case, the soil must be considered deep for the natural vegetation because the layer of *canga* is hardly continuous and the roots of most of the permanent plants pass through this layer and grow very deeply, sometimes as far down as the water table (16–18 m in some cases).

Climatic conditions prevailing in places with *cerrado* vegetation also vary greatly. The yearly rainfall in Campo Mourao is about 1600 mm, and there is not a distinct dry season in the region. In central Brazil, we may have 1300 mm with 3–5 months almost without rains. The Amazon region displays *cerrados* in places with 2000 mm or more of rainfall, where it is hard to find a sequence of only a few days without rains. As to temperatures and relative humidities, it is easy to see that there must be a great variation from places near the Equator to those south of the Tropic of Capricorn and also from places close to the coast to the ones near the western limits of Brazil.

As far as the vegetation is concerned, we should say that there are many different types of *cerrados*. Several authors, for instance, Eiten (16) and Rizzini and Heringer (53), have made important contributions here. Papers by Rawitscher *et al.* (52), Ferri (18, 20), Rachid (50), Rawitscher (51), and Ferri and Coutinho (26) also give information about the different groups of plants. All these papers contain lists of the most characteristic species of the *cerrado* vegetation. Ferri (25) describes about 100 species selected from among those that are more frequent and characteristic in the *cerrado*. Other publications that will give satisfactory indications include Warming's *Lagoa Santa,* published first in Danish (1892) (63) and translated later into Portuguese by Loefgren (1909) (14); Goodland's thesis "An Ecological Study of the Cerrado Vegetation of South-Central Brasil" (31), submitted to the Faculty of Graduate Studies of McGill University (1969); the volumes (1963, second printing 1971; 1966, 1971) containing the papers presented in three *Cerrado* Symposia that took place in Brazil in 1962, 1965, and 1971. The reader will find much valuable information, especially pertaining to taxonomy and ecology, in these publications. Both physiological and sociological studies have been included, but there is very little work in synecology.

The *cerrado* vegetation displays a marked xeromorphy, so much that it used to be called *campo seco* or dry grassland. The *cerrado,* however, cannot be considered a truly xerophytic vegetation since it is never found in really dry habitats. The yearly rainfall in the areas where there are *cerrados* is usually great, more than 1000 mm, although in many of those places there is a dry season of variable duration, sometimes as long as 5 months. In general, the *cerrado* soil has a good water-storing capacity and great reserves of water can be found in it. In fact, Rawitscher *et al.* (52) found in a *cerrado* in Emas near Pirassununga in the state of São Paulo that the water stored in the soil from the surface down to the water table, which is permanent and at an approximate depth of 18 m, was equivalent to the total rains of 3 average years.

The superficial layers of the soil show a pronounced drying during the dry season, but the root systems of the shrubs and trees are in general very deep, even when the tops are small. *Andira humilis*, for instance, has an aerial system of about 30 cm but forms roots which may grow down to the water table. Most plants do not send their roots as deep as that but grow down to a depth of about 10 m. Thus the root systems of the majority of the permanent plants of the *cerrado* are in contact with soil layers which have a high water content throughout the year, since a value of less than 7.5% of the dry weight of the soil was never found 1 m below the surface. From that depth down, the water content increases rapidly.

The level of the water table shows fluctuations which were studied by Schubart (56) and by Schubart and Rawitscher (57) in two wells dug in that *cerrado*. They observed that the highest level occurs during the dry season and the lowest in the rainy period. It takes about 5 months for the water to move from the surface down to the water table.

Anatomical studies have shown that the morphological elements usually connected with dry conditions appear with great frequency in *cerrado* plants. Thus thick cuticle and cuticular layers are found in many species such as *Annona coriacea, Andira humilis, Butia leiospatha, Didymopanax vinosum,* and *Ouratea spectabilis.* Sunken stomata are also frequent in such plants as *Andira humilis, Annona coriacea, Butia leiospatha, Didymopanax vinosum* (18), *Xylopia grandiflora, Bowdichia virgilioides, Stryphnodendron barbatimao,* and *Dimorphandra mollis* (48). A large number of hairs of different types may be found in *Duguetia furfuracea, Didymopanax vinosum* (18), *Dimorphandra mollis, Platypodium elegans, Xylopia grandiflora, Qualea grandiflora, Connarus suberosus, Aspidosperma tomentosum, Strychnos pseudoquina, Curatella americana,* etc. (48). Hypodermis, biseriated epidermis, and colorless parenchyma, which are generally connected with water storage, are found in *Kielmeyera coriacea, Erythroxylum suberosum, E. tortuosum* (18), *Bowdichia virgilioides, Strychnos pseudoquina,* etc. (48). Well-developed mechanical tissues, such as sclerenchyma and stone cells, occur in *Erythroxylum suberosum, Annona coriacea, Ouratea spectabilis* (18), *Qualea grandiflora, Connarus suberosus, Aspidosperma tomentosum, Strychnos pseudoquina,* etc. (48).

OTHER TYPES OF VEGETATION IN LATIN AMERICA

Among the many other types of vegetation in Latin America, we are going to consider only the main types that occur at the littoral, and these only very briefly.

In the littoral, one should consider the rocks, the sand, and the mangroves. In the rocks, associations of algae are to be found at different levels. This association has been studied by specialized phycologists, including Joly (39) in his book *Generos de Algas Marinhas da Costa Atlantica Latino-Americana.* Etcheverry (17) and Alveal (1), among others, have studied the Pacific coast. Etcheverry is currently preparing a more detailed publication on the marine algal flora of Pacific South America. Brazilian sand dune vegetation has been studied recently by de Andrade (13) and the mangroves by Lamberti (42). These are ecological studies with data that will be of interest in other Latin American countries in which such types of vegetation occur, because the environmental conditions are very much the same in these habitats wherever they exist. For this reason, of course, vegetation is very similar in all of them.

The Deciduous *Caatingas*

In the deciduous *caatingas,* among the most frequent species we find several Cactaceae, some of which, such as *Pilocereus gounellei, Cereus squamosus,* and *C. jamacaru,* are very large. Smaller species are *Opuntia bahiensis, O. palmadora, O. inamoena,* and *Melocactus bahiensis.* Bromeliaceae such as *Bromelia laciniosa,* such Euphorbiaceae as *Cnidoscolus phyllacanthus,* and several species of *Jathropha* are important components of this vegetation. Some of these Euphorbiaceae are succulent plants. *Spondias tuberosa, Bumelia sartorun, Zizyphus joazeiro, Caesalpinia pyramidalis, Bursera leptophloeus, Amburana cearensis,* and *Maytenus rigida* are also common species.

This vegetation is restricted to an area with approximately 500 mm of yearly rainfall. Such an area is by no means small, being calculated as 700,000 km^2.

The rainy season lasts some 4 months, from April to July. Sporadic heavy rains of short duration may occur in November. High temperatures are common. In Paulo Afonso (state of Bahia), minimal temperatures average 18°C and maximal 30°C. Temperatures of 40°C are not unusual, and, since relative humidity is in general low, high saturation deficits are frequent. Under such conditions, potential evaporation is high (3000 mm per year in Paulo Afonso).

Most of the rivers, some of which may have a large volume of water during a few weeks in the rainy season, dry out completely in a short time and have no water at all the rest of the year. Sometimes water may be preserved longer in depressions of the river bed, but this water is generally very salty.

The soil is often covered by stones, large and small. It may be very dry except for the short rainy season. In Paulo Afonso, the original rocks are mainly granites, but in several spots gneisses and sienits are also found.

One important morphological characteristic frequently found in this vegetation is succulence. Not only the Cactaceae and some Euphorbiaceae, such as *Jatropha urens* and *J. pohliana,* but also plants of other families may display succulence in the stems. It is doubtful that succulence really plays an important role in protecting plants against drought, but the fact that it is a frequent occurrence in dry habitats is at least suggestive. In some species, such as *Jatropha urens* and *J. pohliana,* plants so young that they still have one or both primary leaves already show a distinct swelling of the stems. Succulent leaves also occur in some Portulacaceae (20).

Tubercular roots, which are common in many herbaceous plants, are found in trees in the *caatinga. Spondias tuberosa* and *Manihot glaziovii* are perhaps the most striking examples. In the case of *Spondias,* some of these tubers weigh 2–3 kg or even more (19,20,27).

It is surprising to find that all those elements of xeromorphy which are frequent in the *cerrado* and which are connected with dry conditions are not common in the anatomy of leaves of the *caatinga,* though this vegetation grows in much drier habitats than that of the *cerrados.* While thick cuticle and cuticular layers (*Maytenus rigida*), stone cells (*Aspidosperma pyrifolium*), and hairs (*Bumelia sartorum* and *Aspidosperma pyrifolium*) are found, the vegetation as a whole is not rich in such characteristics.

On the other hand, we find in many plants (*Aspidosperma pyrifolium, Zizyphus joazeiro, Spondias tuberosa,* etc.) that the stomata are not sunken but that, on the contrary, they are projected above the epidermal level. Many species (*Spondias tuberosa, Zizyphus joazeiro, Jatropha phyllacantha,* etc.) completely lack all the morphological characteristics of adaptation to dry conditions (20).

The Evergreen *Caatinga*

An evergreen *caatinga* in Taraqua in the Upper Rio Negro (0°4'N, 68° 14'W Gr.) (21) is typical of this type as found in the Amazonian region. Among the most frequent species are *Sphaeradenia amazonica, Bactris cuspidata, Clusia spathulaefolia, Compsoneura debilis, Cunuria crassipes, Hevea rigidifolia, Lyssocarpa benthami, Pagamea coriacea, Retiniphyllum truncatum,* and *Zamia lecointei.* Many Orchidaceae and Bromeliaceae are present. The soil is partially covered, in spots, by tufts of *Rapatea longipes,* Hymenophyllaceae, etc.

The average yearly rainfall in Taraqua is approximately 3000 mm, but in some years the rainfall may surpass 4000 mm. There is hardly a month with less than 100 mm. The average minimal temperature is over 20°C, average maximal over 30°C, and average relative humidity 88%. There is not a dry season, and the soil is in general very wet. The soil is very poor, almost pure sand with a thin superficial layer of organic matter in some spots.

Notwithstanding all this, here again, as in the case of the *cerrados,* a large number of plants are xeromorphic. For example, sunken stomata are found in *Pagamea coriacea,* and thick cuticle and cuticular layers in *Retiniphyllum truncatum* and *Sphaeradenia amazonica* (21).

PHYSIOLOGICAL ADAPTATION IN DIFFERENT VEGETATION TYPES

The study of the stomatic openings with Molisch's infiltration method (46) showed that with only a few exceptions the *cerrado* plants keep their stomata widely open all through the day, even during the driest periods, and sometimes through the night. Almost all plants transpire freely all the time (as was determined by rapid weighings with a torsion balance). Thus the daily transpiration curves of these plants closely follow the pattern of the curves of free evaporation. Stomatic reactions to changes of light or of water supply are very slow. Cuticular transpiration is high even when the cuticle is thick; saturation deficits of leaves seldom reach a value greater than 5% of the maximum water content.

In the northeastern dedicuous *caatingas,* on the contrary, most of the plants do not keep the stomata open all day even in the rainy season (27). In the beginning of the dry season, stomata are open only for a short time every day in the early morning (19,20), and as conditions become drier they close their stomata for longer periods. Eventually, the plants keep the stomata closed for days and transpire only through the cuticle. Even this transpiration may endanger the plant, which may have to shed its leaves to reduce the transpiring surface and survive a drought (20).

The cuticular transpiration in the *caatinga* plants is in general low even when the cuticle is thin. Stomatic reactions to changes of light and of water supply are very rapid. For example, *Spondias tuberosa* can reduce its transpiration to about 50% of the initial value in only 2 min and can close its stomata completely in about 5 min (27). In the evergreen *caatinga* of the Amazon, the situation resembles that of the *cerrado.* Stomata are as a rule open all day, there is no restriction of transpiration, stomatic reactions are slow, cuticular transpiration is high, and saturation deficits of the leaves are generally small (21).

Since the situation in these *caatingas* is very similar to that in the *cerrados,* comparison will be confined to *cerrados* and deciduous *caatingas.* In Table I, information on surrounding conditions and morphological and physiological characteristics of *cerrado* and *caatinga* vegetation is compared. Only the permanent vegetation is considered.

**Table I. Comparison of Conditions and Vegetation Characteristics in *Cerrados*
and in Deciduous *Caatingas***

Characteristics	*Cerrados*	Deciduous *caatingas*
Yearly rainfall	1300 mm (Emas, state of São Paulo)	600 mm (Paulo Afonso, state of Bahia)
Yearly evaporation	1100 mm (Emas)	3000 mm (Paulo Afonso)
Soil water reserves	Equivalent to 3 years' rainfall (Emas)	Very small, if any
Floristic		
Bromeliaceae	Not frequent	Frequent
Cactaceae	Not frequent	Frequent
Succulent Euphorbiaceae	Not frequent	Frequent
Morphological		
Root systems	Very deep, sometimes down to the water table (17–18 m in Emas)	Not sufficiently studied
Tubers with water reserves in trees	Not found	Found in several species
Succulent stems	Not found	Found in many species
Microphyllous or aphyllous plants	Not frequent	Frequent
Large leaves	Frequent	Not frequent
Hairy, waxy, or leathery leaves	Frequent	Not frequent
Thick bark	Frequent	Not frequent
Thick cuticle and cuticular layers	Frequent	Not frequent
Stomata sunken	Frequent	Not frequent
Mechanical tissues in the leaves	Frequent	Not frequent
Physiological		
Stomatic reactions	Very slow	Very rapid
Period with stomata open	As a rule, very long even in dry season	As a rule, very short even in rainy season
Restriction of transpiration	Rare, even in dry season	Frequent, even in rainy season
Cuticular transpiration	High, as a rule	Low, as a rule
General fall of leaves	Not frequent	Frequent

INTERPRETATION OF DATA

From the data presented in Table I, we can see that the deciduous *caatinga* vegetation, in a much drier habitat than the *cerrado,* is not as xeromorphic as *cerrado* vegetation, but it is physiologically much better adapted to live in dry habitats. We may conclude, then, that physiological adaptation is the most efficient.

We have now, however, a very important problem to solve: if the *cerrado* vegetation does not live, as a rule, under the stress of water shortage, why is it xeromorphic? Xeromorphic structures may sometimes have nothing to do with dry conditions, but may be related to nutritional problems. Levitt (44) says that xeromorphy has been ascribed to nitrogen deficiency in cold soils but also that Greb was able to show that xeromorphy is primarily due to water deficit. The reader should consult Grieve (34) and Killian and Lemee (41). Arens (4) also reviewed the information on this subject.

Arens (5) attempted in Brazil to interpret the behavior of the *cerrado* and deciduous *caatinga* vegetation based on differences in plant nutrition. He pointed out that *cerrado* plants may have an excess of carbohydrates because, in view of the ample water supply, the stomata are kept open all the time, thus allowing photosynthesis to be performed during a long period. On the other hand, these carbohydrates or their derivatives cannot be used extensively for protein synthesis necessary for growth, because the *cerrado* soils may be deficient in many important elements such as nitrogen, phosphorus, and sulfur (e.g., ref. 45). In this way, the excess carbohydrates might be employed in the building up of dead structures such as thick bark, cuticle, and cuticular layers, stone cells, sclerenchyma, and hairs, which, on the whole, are elements of xeromorphy. The same reasoning would apply to the evergreen *caatinga* in the Amazon. The soil in which this vegetation grows is known to be very poor.

In the deciduous *caatinga,* a plant has little chance of creating excess carbohydrates because photosynthesis may be limited by water shortage. Arens *et al.* (6) tested this hypothesis by giving some of the *cerrado* plants mineral nutrients known to be in limited amounts in the soil and by testing for later morphological or physiological changes or both. Such structures, of course, may be genetically controlled, and therefore there may be only a narrow range within which they can be influenced by external conditions. On the other hand, physiological changes may be detected more easily in many cases. Nitrogen, phosphorus, potassium, and calcium, to name some, were applied in very low concentrations (the highest concentration used was 0.02 M) to two *cerrado* plants, *Ouratea spectabilis* and *Styrax camporum.* Within a few hours, all treatments enhanced protoplasmic activity, bringing about greater stomatic mobility in both species. Thus we have experimental evidence that it is possible to influence some physiological reactions of *cerrado* plants through modifications of their mineral nutrition.

Another way of interpreting the presence of xeromorphic structures in vegetation not found in dry habitats would be to consider that vegetation as a relict (37) of a time when conditions were different. A similar explanation would serve for places in which such vegetation was not primary but was the result of a later invasion, for instance, when the natural vegetation was removed by human activity. In this case, however, we would still have to solve the problem of why xeromorphy is not more frequent in the deciduous *caatinga* in drier habitats. We try to answer this question in the following way. Xeromorphic structures do not protect plants against drought as efficiently as many physiological mechanisms do. They suffice for eventual and mild droughts that may occur in the *cerrado,* in the evergreen *caatinga,* and even in the rainforests where we find many plants with such structures. Thus in these cases, the vegetation was not under a selection stress strong enough to determine the evolutionary development of physiological protection mechanisms. In the drier habitats where the *caatinga* vegetation evolved, however, such selection acted (*cf.* ref. 60).

Why, however, did a greater number of species in which both morphological and physiological mechanisms of drought protection appeared together not survive in the deciduous *caatinga?* Consider that xeromorphy may be in some way deleterious to the plants which live in drier habitats (20,23,24). Because of the water shortage, photosynthesis can be performed for a short period only. As soon as there is danger of drought, the stomata close quickly, but as soon as the danger is over they reopen rapidly and nothing should hinder the penetration of both light and carbon dioxide. The stomata should thus be neither sunken nor covered by hairs; on the contrary, they should be well exposed as is really the general case. Similar reasoning might apply to some other structures.

It may be more helpful to think of the adaptive values of combined characters in relation to combined processes and not of an adaptive value of one character in connection with one single process (59). In the deciduous *caatinga,* xeromorphy combined with physiological mechanisms of protection against drought might have a lower adaptive value than physiological protection alone, since the additional protection against water loss given by xeromorphy might not compensate for the harm done by it to photosynthesis. While these thoughts are highly speculative, they are very stimulating and could lead to much experimental work.

As shown here, water and soil are complex factors which interact with each other. Real understanding of many ecological problems can only be made when such factors are considered together. In fact, they should be considered together with many other environmental factors. Coutinho and Hashimoto (11) have discussed the effect of growth inhibitors produced by some plants of the *cerrados,* a consideration which may also have some bearing on other vegetation types. Vareschi and Huber (62) have already introduced the study of the effect of solar radiation in the Venezuelan *llanos*.

GOODLAND'S THEORY ON THE ROLE OF ALUMINUM

In his thesis which resulted from the work in *cerrados* of the Triangulo Mineiro (state of Minas Gerais), Goodland (31) took as a primary object "to examine and quantify Eiten's physiognomic classes from a physiological point of view." He studied the gradient *campo sujo, campo cerrado, cerrado,* and *cerradao* an arbitrary division based especially on plant vegetation density, which increases from *campo sujo* to *cerradao*. The first is an open grassland type, the last is a type of forest. " 'It rarely burns, but it is very sensitive to fire.' *Campo sujo* frequently burns . . . . The three types of vegetation may be fire degraded forms of *cerrado* . . . ." Fire is thought to be important in this ecosystem and possibly increases in frequency from *cerradao* through *campo sujo*.

Goodland studied 110 *cerrado* stands in the Triangulo Mineiro, representing about 25% *campo sujo,* 22% *campo cerrado,* 27% *cerrado,* and 25% *cerradao*. In all these stands, he collected data on biomass, density, frequency, height, girth, and other characteristics of the species he collected. Goodland analyzed his data very accurately and drew several conclusions of importance for the phytosocio-logical understanding of the four types of vegetation he was studying.

Since the methods he used for analyzing the data produced similar results, he concluded "that the whole range of the vegetation" might be "reacting to a strong, influential, ecological factor." Thus he decided to study the environment, collecting data mainly on several soil factors (pH, C, N, organic matter, Ca + Mg, K, Al, PO_4), since soil "is the medium in which the plants grow. . . ."

Other authors seem to have excluded the possibility of moisture acting as a limiting factor for the vegetation under consideration. These authors "gradually proposed soil as being important." Goodland found that all soil factors he studied increased from *campo sujo* to *cerradao,* with the exception of aluminum. Thus *campo sujo* occurs on more acid soils, which are lower in organic matter and nutrients. The two intermediate types of vegetation, *campo cerrado* and *cerrado,* are intermediate in soil fertility.

At this point, Goodland referred to Arens (4,5) and Arens *et al.* (6), who synthesized and developed observations correlating scleromorphism with nutri-ent deficiencies in the soil. From his own experience and his studies using a quite different approach to the problem, Goodland felt that the theory of "oligotrophic scleromorphism" (pseudoxeromorphism) is strongly supported: "this theory can now be extended to explain also the *cerradao - campo sujo* gradient."

After a detailed study of the aluminum in connection with the four steps of this gradient, Goodland concluded: "The gradient from *cerradao* (forest) to

Vegetation Map of Latin America. Based on maps from papers and books in the Literature, and personal experience: (1) "Savanna" (*latu sensu*); (2) High mountain tropical and subtropical forests; (3) Deciduous tropical forest and semi-arid vegetation; (4) Rain forest; (5) Palm forest ("cocais," in Brazil); (6) Clear forest (with *Araucaria*, in Brazil); (7) Pampa; (8) Merditerranean (transition) vegetation; (9) Desert (several types); (10) Temperate forest (with *Nothofagus*, in Chile); (11) Clear forest (in Chaco).

campo sujo (almost grassland) is one of increasing xeromorphy in a physiognomic sense. This reduction in density and stature of trees may be related to increasing aluminum saturation of the soil which varies from 35 percent in *cerradao* to 58 percent in *campo sujo.*"

Goodland made a detailed study of the Al ion, which, according to Foy and Brown (29,30), "may decrease permeability by coagulating protein" and "inhibit cell division." Aluminum has a "fundamental influence in the soils of the *cerrado.* The main effect of aluminum is to increase the acidity which in turn causes nutrient deficiency. But aluminum also decreases the availability of the critical nutrients phosphate and potassium directly. Aluminum also binds the most abundant cation, calcium, thereby further increasing acidity."

Goodland also emphasized that many plants which are frequent in the *cerrado* belong to families that are aluminum tolerant or are even aluminum accumulators: Vochysiaceae (*Qualea, Vochysia, Salvertia*), Melastomaceae, Rubiaceae, etc. "Important *cerrado* species known to be strong accumulators include *Neea, Strychnos, Miconia, Psychotria, Antonia, Rapanea, Roupala, Rudgia* and *Palicourea.*"

Woody stems, coriaceous leaves with conspicuous venation, leaves which become yellow-green when dry, and bright blue fruits are some characteristics of accumulator plants. They are also characteristic of the *cerrado* vegetation as a whole, particularly in *campo cerrado – campo sujo* gradient. These facts suggest an important role for aluminum in the vegetation under consideration.

To conclude, Goodland (33) thinks that "part of scleromorphism due to oligotrophism is caused by aluminum toxicity." He calls attention to the fact that other elements such as Mn and Fe may complement the action of Al.

REFERENCES

1. Alveal, K. V. (1970). Estudios ficoecológicos en la region costera de Valparaiso. *Rev. Biol. Mar.* **14:**7-88.
2. Alvim, P. T., and de Araujo, W. (1952). El Suelo como factor ecológico en el desarollo de la vegetación en el centro-oeste del Brasil. *Turrialba* **2(4):**153-160.
3. Andrade-Lima, D. (1966). Vegetação (descrição dos tipos e mapa da vegetação do Brasil). In *Atlas Nacional do Brasil,* IBGE, Cons. Nac. Geog., Rio de Janeiro.
4. Arens, K. (1958). Consideracoes sobre as causas do xeromorfismo foliar. *Bol. Fac. Fil. Ciênc. Letr. USP 244 Botânica* **15:**25-26.
5. Arens, K. (1958). O cerrado commo vegetação oligotrofica. *Bol. Fac. Fil. Ciênc. Letr. USP 224 Botânica* **15:**59-77.
6. Arens, K., Ferri, M. G., and Coutinho, L. M. (1958). Papel do factor nutricional na economia d'agua de plantas do cerrado. *Rev. de Biol. (Lisboa)* **1(3-4):**313-324.
7. Bouillenne, R., *et al.* (1930). *Une Mission Biologique Belge au Brésil,* Vol. 2, Brussels.
8. Burkart, A. (1947). Parque mesopotamico. In *Geografia de la Republica Argentina,* Vol. 8, Coni, Buenos Aires.
9. Cabrera, A. L. (1947). La Estepa Patagonica. In *Geografia de la Republica Argentina,* Vol. 8, Coni, Buenos Aires.

10. Coutinho, L. M. (1962). Contribuição ao conhecimento da ecologia da mata pluvial tropical. *Bol. Fac. Fil. Ciênc. Letr. USP 257 Botânica* **18**:11-219.

11. Coutinho, L. M., and Hashimoto, F. (1971). Sobre o efeito inibitorio da germinação de sementes produzido por folhas de *Calea cuneifolia* DC. *Ciência e Cultura* **23(6)**: 759-764.

12. Cuatrecasas, J. (1958). Aspectos de la vegetación natural de Colombia. *Rev. Acad. Ciênc. Exactas, Fisicas y Naturales, Colombiana (Bogota)*.

13. de Andrade, M. A. B. (1968). Contribuição ao conhecimento da ecologia das plantas das dunas do litoral do Estado de São Paulo. *Bol. Fac. Fil. Ciênc. Letr. USP 305 Botânica* **22**:3-170.

14. de Lemps, A. H. (1970). *La Végétation de la Terre,* Masson et Cie, Paris.

15. Ducke, A., and Black, G. A. (1953). Phytogeographical notes on the Brazilian Amazon. *An. Acad. Brasil. Ciênc.* **25(1)**:1-46.

16. Eiten, G. (1968). Vegetation forms. *Bol. Inst. Bot. São Paulo* **4**:3-69.

17. Etcheverry, H. (1960). Algas marinas de las islas oceanicas chilenas (Juan Fernandez, San Felix San Ambrosio, Pascua). *Rev. Biol. Mar.* **10**:83-132.

18. Ferri, M. G. (1944). Transpiração de plantas permanentes dos "cerrados." *Bol. Fac. Fil. Ciênc. Letr. USP 41 Botânica* **4**:159-224.

19. Ferri, M. G. (1953). Water balance of plants from the *caatinga.* II. Further information on transpiration and stomatal behavior. *Rev. Brasil. Biol.* **13(3)**:237-244.

20. Ferri, M. G. (1955). Contribuição ao conhecimento da ecologia do cerrado e da caatinga. Estudo comparativo da economia d'agua de sua vegetação. *Bol. Fac. Fil. Ciênc. Letr. USP 195 Botânica* **15**:103-148.

21. Ferri, M. G. (1960). Contribution to the knowledge of the "Rio Negro Caatinga" [Amazon]. *Bull. Res. Counc. Israel Sec. D Bot.* **8D(3-4)**:195-208.

22. Ferri, M. G. (1961). Aspects of the soil-water-plant relationships in connexion with some Brazilian types of vegetation. In *Tropical Soils and Vegetation,* UNESCO Symposium, Abidjan, 1959, United Nations, Rome, pp. 103-109.

23. Ferri, M. G. (1961). Problems of water relations of some Brazilian vegetation types, with special consideration of the concepts of xeromorphy and xerophytism. In *Plant-Water Relationships in Arid and Semi-arid Regions,* UNESCO Symposium, Madrid, 1959, United Nations, Rome, pp. 191-197.

24. Ferri, M. G. (1962). Evolução do conceito de xerofitismo. *Bol. Fac. Fil. Ciênc. Letr. USP 267 Botânica* **19**:102-113.

25. Ferri, M. G. (1969). Plantas do Brasil. Especies do Cerrado, ed. Edgard Blucher e ed. USP, p. 239.

26. Ferri, M. G., and Coutinho, L. M. (1958). Contribuição ao conhecimento da ecologia do cerrado. Estudo comparativo da economia d'agua de sua vegetação em Emas (Est. de São Paulo), Campo Grande (Est. Mato Grosso) e Goiania (Est. de Goias). *Bol. Fac. Fil. Ciênc. Letr. USP 224 Botânica* **15**:103-150.

27. Ferri, M. G., and Labouriau, L. G. (1952). Water balance of plants from the *caatinga.* I. Transpiration of the most frequent species of the *caatinga* of Paulo Afonso (Bahia) in the rainy season. *Rev. Brasil. Biol.* **12(3)**:301-312.

28. Ferri, M. G., and Lamberti, A. (1960). Informacoes sobre a economia d'agua de plantas de um tabuleiro no municipio de Goiana (Pernambuco). *Bol. Fac. Fil. Ciênc. Letr. USP 247 Botânica* **17**:133-145.

29. Foy, C. D., and Brown, J. C. (1963). Toxic factors in acid soils. I. *Soil Sci. Soc. Am. Proc.* **27**:403-407.

30. Foy, C. D., and Brown, J. C. (1964). Toxic factors in acid soils. II. *Soil Sci. Soc. Am. Proc.* **28**:27-32.

31. Goodland, R. (1969). An ecological study of the cerrado vegetation of south-central Brasil. Thesis, McGill University, Montreal.
32. Goodland, R. (1970). The Savanna Controversy: Background Information on the Brasilian Cerrado Vegetation, Savanna Research Series, No. 15, McGill University, Montreal.
33. Goodland, R. (1971). Oligotrofismo e aluminio no cerrado. In *III Simposio Sobre o Cerrado* (M. G. Ferri, Coordenador), ed. São Paulo; USP, ed. Edgard Blucher.
34. Grieve, B. J. (1955). The physiology of sclerophyll plants. *J. Soc. W. Austral.* **39**:31-45.
35. Hauman, L. (1947). La vegetación de la Argentina, pp. 5-14; La selva misionera, pp. 14-41; Selva Tucumano-Oranense, pp. 41-68; Parque Chaqueno, pp. 69-90; Provincia del "Monte" (O del Espiral), pp. 208-249; Los Bosques Subantarticos, pp. 273-305; El Dominio Andino, pp. 305-338. In *Geografia de la Republica Argentina*, Vol. 8, Coni, Buenos Aires.
36. Huber, O. (1971). Ricerche ecologiche sui problemi della savanna Venezuelana ("llanos"). Thesis, University of Rome.
37. Hueck, K. (1957). Die Ursprunglichkeit der brasilianischen "Campos Cerrados" und neue Beobachtungen an ihrer Sudgrenze. *Erdkunde Arch. Wiss. Geog.* **11**:193-203.
38. Hueck, K. (1972). *As Florestas da America do Sul,* Un. Brasilia and Poligono, São Paulo.
39. Joly, A. B. (1967). *Generos de Algas Marinhas da Costa Atlantica Latino-Americana,* USP, São Paulo.
40. Joly, A. B. (1970). *Conheca a Vegetação Brasileira,* USP and Poligono, São Paulo.
41. Killian, C., and Lemee, G. (1956). Les xérophytes: leur économie d'eau. In *Handbuch der Pflanzenphysiologie,* Vol. 3: *Pflanze und Wasser,* Springer-Verlag, Berlin.
42. Lamberti, A. (1969). Contribuição ao conhecimento da ecologia das plantas do manguezal de Itanhaen. *Bol. Fac. Fil. Ciênc. Letr. USP 317 Botânica* **23**:1-221.
43. Lanjouw, J. (1936). Studies of the vegetation of Surinam savannas and swamps. *Med. Bot. Mus. (Utrecht)* **33.**
44. Levitt, J. (1958). Frost, drought and heat resistance. In *Protoplasmatologia,* Vol. 8(6), *Physiologie des Protoplasmas,* Springer Verlag, Vienna, pp. 1-87.
45. McClung, A. C., Martins de Freitas, L. M., Romano Gallo, J., Quinn, L. R., and Mott, G. O. (1958). Alguns estudos preliminares sobre possiveis problemas de fertilidade em solos de diferentes campos cerrados de São Paulo, e Goias. *Bragantia* **17(3)**:29-44.
46. Molisch, H. (1912). Das Offen und Geschlossensein der Spaltoffnungen, veranschaulicht durch eine neue Methode (Infiltrations-methode). *Z. Bot.,* p. 106. Cited in Nigro, G., *La Fisiologia Vegetale,* Torino, 1925.
47. Morello, J. (1951). El bosque de algarrobo y la estepa de jarilla en el Valle de Santa Maria (Prov. de Tucuman). *Darwiniana* **9.**
48. Morretes, B. L., and Ferri, M. G. (1959). Contribuição ao estudo da anatomia das folhas de plantas do Cerrado. *Bol. Fac. Fil. Ciênc. Letr. USP 243 Botânica* **16**:1-70.
49. Parodi, L. R. (1947). La estepa pampeana. In *Geografia de la Republica Argentina*, Vol. 8, Coni, Buenos Aires.
50. Rachid, M. (1947). Transpiração e sistemas subterraneos de vegetação de verao dos campos cerrados de Emas. *Bol. Fac. Fil. cienc. Letr. USP 80 Botânica* **5**:1-135.
51. Rawitscher, F. (1948). The water economy of the vegetation of the "campos cerrados" in Southern Brazil. *J. Ecol.* **36(2)**:237-267.
52. Rawitscher, F., Ferri, M. G., and Rachid, M. (1943). Profundidade dos solos e vegetação em campos cerrados do Brasil Meridional. *An. Ac. Brasil. Ciênc.* **15(4)**:267-294.
53. Rizzini, C. de T., and Heringer, E. P. (1962). Preliminares Acerca das Formações Vegetais e do Reflorestamento no Brasil Central, Min. Agr. Serv. Inf. Agr., Rio de Janeiro, p. 79.

54. Roseveare, G. M. (1948). The Grasslands of Latin America, Imp. Bur. Pastures and Field Crops, Aberystwyth, p. 356.
55. Schnell, R. (1971). *Introduction à la Phytogéographie des Pays Tropicaux,* Vol. 2: *Les Milieux—Les Groupementes Végétaux,* Gauthier-Villars, Paris, pp. 500-951.
56. Schubart, O. (1959). Segunda contribuição sobre o movimento de água subterrânea de Emas—Pirassununga. *Bol. Fac. Fil. Ciênc. Letr. USP 243 Botânica* 16:71-84.
57. Schubart, O., and Rawitscher, F. (1950). Movimento de água subterrânea em Emas—Pirassununga. *Bol. Fac. Fil. Ciênc. Letr. USP 109 Botânica* 8:69-73.
58. Smith, A. C., and Johnston, I. M. (1945). A phytogeographical sketch of Latin America. In Verdoorn, F. (ed.), *Plants and Plant Science in Latin America,* Vol. 16, Chronica Botanica Co., Waltham, Mass., pp.11-18.
59. Stebbins, G. L., Jr. (1951). Natural selection and the differentiation of angiosperm families. *Evolution* 5(4):299-324.
60. Stebbins, G. L., Jr. (1952). Aridity as a stimulus to plant evolution. *Am. Naturalist* 86(826):33-44.
61. Vareschi, V. (1966). Sobre las formas biológicas de la vegetación tropical. *Bol. Soc. Ven. Cienc. Nat.* 26(110):504-508.
62. Vareschi, V., and Huber, O. (1971). La radiación solar y las estaciones anuales de los llanos de Venezuela. *Bol. Soc. Ven. Cienc. Nat.* 29(119-120):50-135.
63. Warming, E. (1892). *Lagoa Santa. Et Bidrag til den biologiske Plantegeografi,* Copenhagen.
64. Warming, E. (1909). *Lagoa Santa* (Contribuição para a Geographia Phytobiologica) (trans. A. Loefgren), Imprensa Oficial de Minas Gerais, Belo Horizonte.
65. Weberbauer, A. (1945). *El Mundo Vegetal de los Andes Peruanos. Estudio Fitogeografico,* 2nd ed., Min. Agr., Lima, 776 pp.

Basic Molecular Genetic Mechanisms

3

Recent Studies on the Origins of Cellular Organelles

Seymour S. Cohen*

Department of Microbiology
University of Colorado School of Medicine
Denver, Colorado, U.S.A.

A major aspect of the problem of the evolutionary development of eukaryotic cells is that of the origins of mitochondria and chloroplasts. The discovery in these organelles of DNA and of biochemical systems for the synthesis of DNA, RNA, and protein has raised not only the problem of the extent of organelle autonomy within cells but also the possibility that these organelles arose as invasive prokaryotic symbionts. This chapter summarizes the present data on this subject and indicates some experimental approaches for the test of possible distant relationships of the organelles and modern prokaryotic organisms. Examples of the practical importance of this theoretical problem are given.

BIOLOGICAL AND BIOCHEMICAL DISCONTINUITIES

The 25-year period since World War II has produced an enormous acceleration of the pace of discovery in cytology and biochemistry, derived in very large part from fundamental contributions of genetics, microbial physiology, and virology. These disciplines not only enlarged our approaches to eukaryotic cells in multicellular organisms, but also through the characterization of numerous microorganisms introduced numerous biochemical "oddities" into our previously oversimplified systems of cellular structure and function. For instance, the discovery of pantothenate and lipoate led to the detailed demonstration of a

---

* American Cancer Society Professor of Microbiology.

more complete and satisfying Krebs cycle in *Escherichia coli* as well as in pigeon liver, but the discovery of diaminopimelic acid and even of various types of RNA polymerase in prokaryotes introduced biochemical variability as a serious practical and theoretical problem.

Until recent decades, the study of biochemical evolution was largely a summertime seashore activity giving support to the phylogenetic trees accepted by all but a few specialists. The existence of ATP, cytochromes, NAD, and nucleic acids seemed to assure us of the chemical uniformity of the biological world at the cellular level. The advent of battalions of biologists and chemists trained to explore the almost infinite variety of microbes, as well as of virologists schooled in studying the interactions of viruses and cells and of a multiplicity of parasitic and endosymbiotic relations, has inevitably revealed subtle biochemical and biological novelties present in such organisms, i.e., phenomena, mechanisms, and compounds intimately tied to their biological survival and development.

In recent times, we have come to accept the concept of the fundamental diversity of at least two types of cells (123), prokaryotic and eukaryotic. The former are comprised of bacteria and blue-green algae, which lack many elements of structure and organization found in eukaryotic cells. These include a true nucleus, many phenomena of mitosis, specialized organelles such as mitochondria and chloroplasts bounded by doubly layered membranes, and the 11-unit fibrillar system employed in the motile apparatus of eukaryotic cells. Prokaryotic cells possess chemically distinctive cell wall components, such as diaminopimelic acid and muramic acid, and the specific arrest of their synthesis and organization by specific antibiotics provides the basis of a practical antibacterial chemotherapy. Thus an apparent biological discontinuity, defined in terms of cellular organization and chemical structure, has not only clearly emerged in the evolution of our disciplines but has also become a significant consideration in the application of biological science to certain medical problems.

It was recognized almost immediately that many of the numerous major constituents found almost uniquely in eukaryotic cells, such as sterols, characteristic polyunsaturated fatty acids, and ascorbate, which have facilitated the organization of various structures of these cells, require molecular oxygen for their synthesis. These compounds appear to have originated following the evolution of photosynthesis and the production of a new potential metabolite, O_2. As our knowledge of intermediary metabolism developed, it was found that many important compounds, which are made in eukaryotes with the use of molecular O_2, are constructed in bacteria exclusively by different anaerobic paths. The origin of nicotinamide, an essential component of ubiquitous NAD and NADP, is an example of such an anaerobic synthesis in bacteria and an acquisition of biosynthetic capability using molecular oxygen in eukaryotes. There are also some substances synthesized uniquely in eukaryotes in systems which do not require O_2; spermine is an example of this type of eukaryotic acquisition.

The existence of this apparent discontinuity does not disprove the concept of a single line of descent from prokaryote cell to eukaryote cell. Nevertheless, our relatively new knowledge leaves many important problems to be resolved. Can we find prokaryotic microorganisms that have evolved aerobic mechanisms characteristic of eukaryotic cells? How similar will these mechanisms be when defined in terms of enzyme structure and polypeptide homology, as well as in terms of genetic information stored as polynucleotide sequences?

The remarkable parallelism of mechanisms of protein synthesis in prokaryotic and eukaryotic cells, e.g., the universality of the code, the similarities of structure of tRNA and ribosomal RNA, initiation,etc.,seems to indicate a single line of descent rather than the possibilities of convergence from polyphyletic origins. On the other hand, these very similar systems respond totally differently to various inhibitors and antibiotics, often permitting a sharp discrimination between prokaryotic and eukaryotic systems, between protein synthesis by cytoplasmic or organelle ribosomes. How trivial indeed will be these evidences of difference? Can we in fact trace a clear line of monophyletic evolution, biological as well as biochemical, from prokaryote to eukaryote?

About a decade ago, the eukaryotic organelles, mitochondria, and chloroplasts were shown to contain DNA, and in the intervening years an enormous proliferation of data has also revealed the existence of extensive supporting systems of macromolecular biosynthesis in these organelles. These discoveries have led to the serious formulation of still another type of complicating (29, 81) hypothesis.

It has been suggested that present-day mitochondria and chloroplasts may be descendants of ancestral aerobic bacteria and blue-green algae, respectively, which had invaded primitive eukaryotes and established viable symbiotic relationships which have persisted and evolved further. In other words, modern eukaryotes may not be products of direct evolutionary descent from a single ancestral prokaryotic cell but may have shared the genetic equipment and cooperative metabolic systems of several evolutionary paths. This hypothesis need not even raise the question of single or multiple biopoietic lines of descent.[1]

---

[1] In 1969, I explored the biochemical data relating to this problem in some detail, a summary of which was published in 1970 (29). This chapter represents an effort to bring that earlier essay up to date. It must be appreciated that the relevant literature which has appeared in the last 2 years alone and continues to appear as this is being written amounts to well over a thousand papers. For purposes of the present survey, I have culled only a few percent of the significant contributions.

THE VIROLOGIST LOOKS AT MULTIGENOMIC CELLS

I would note that to a modern biochemical virologist the perspective of multiple functional genomes in a single cell merely reflects the activity of his normal working day, dissecting the relative metabolic contributions of host and virus in virus multiplication. Whereas the cytologist interested in RNA metabolism, for example, might think his problems are confined to DNA-dependent RNA polymerase transcribing RNA from a single strand of a double-stranded DNA template, virus-infected cells have the choice of this mechanism and, depending on the virus, at least four additional systems of synthesis, as exemplified in Fig. 1.

Despite the difficulties raised by the problem of the origins of all of these systems of RNA synthesis, we know today that we can approach these problems experimentally by study of the structure, metabolic origin, and immunochemistry of these molecules, by the determination and matching of primary amino acid sequences, and by hybridization of the nucleic acids which encode the information for their synthesis. We can hope that these same techniques may reveal gross elements of relation or independence as applied to molecular aspects of the origins of organelle components.

Invoking further the less rigid preconceptions of the virologists, we note that the possible existence of various latent viral genomes in virtually all cells is accepted as the framework within which every hypothesis must be formulated. Genetic approaches have burgeoned and developed to reveal the existence and location of all kinds of inheritable information. Biology and chemistry are no longer the staid patterned and specialized disciplines of the 1950s and earlier; everything related to the cell and its dissection has in recent years become grist for our mill.

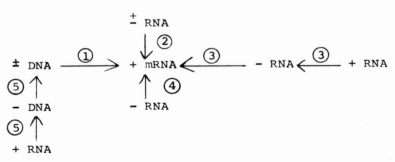

Fig. 1. Viral mechanisms of synthesis of mRNA. (1) Vaccinia, (2) reo, (3) polio, (4) VSV, (5) RNA tumor virus.

THEORETICAL AND PRACTICAL ASPECTS OF THE DIVISION OF LABOR IN CELLS

Although many technical strategies are known to approach the problems of biochemical and genetic origin, we note also that to speak of a component as mitochondrial or chloroplastic can introduce a potential threefold confusion. Are we speaking of the presence of the bulk of the substance in the organelle, are we speaking of the site of its synthesis, or are we defining the site of the genetic information determining its synthesis? Having formulated our questions this precisely, we find that the emerging answers have nevertheless been surprising, even confusing. We shall see that the organelles have proved to possess quite limited stores of genetic information and that many organelle proteins are coded for in the cell nucleus and constructed in the cytoplasm outside of the organelle itself. This is the case for cytochrome c, which is central to the respiratory activity of mitochondria or for photosynthetic components which define a major special role of chloroplasts. Our apparently simple inquiry has come to a qualitatively new question concerning the possibility of invasion and endosymbiosis: What selective advantages have been gained in placing the genes and synthetic apparatus for certain organellar proteins so distant from the organelles?[2] The problem of the division of labor within the cell has assumed new dimensions.

The limitations of autonomy stated briefly above demand the existence of a most active traffic between organelles and the rest of the cell. Such a traffic between mitochondria and cytoplasm is known for low molecular weight components such as glutamate, glutamine, and citrulline or even for adenine nucleotides. Indeed, the cross-feeding of deficient mitochondria, leading in one experimental example to complementation for the synthesis of valine (69), has been discussed as a possible explanation of the mechanism of the hybrid vigor observed in heterosis in maize and wheat. It has been suggested also (69) that structural components and membrane-bound enzymes might participate as well in intramitochondrial complementation in these plants.

Protein transfer from cytoplasm to organelle can be expected to occur at

---

[2] It may be remarked in passing that we may eventually obtain some insights into this question from the developing knowledge of the evolution of cellular and biochemical efficiency. This includes the development of numerous control mechanisms for transcription and translation, the formation of enzymatic aggregates containing one or many enzymatic activities, or the separation and compartmentation of similar activities involved in potentially competing functions. For example, carbamyl phosphate is required for both arginine and pyrimidine synthesis, and two discrete pools of this substance are maintained in *Neurospora crassa*. It has been reported recently (14) that in this organism the mitochondrion contains a complex of a characteristic carbamyl phosphate synthetase and ornithine transcarbamylase, whereas the nucleus contains a complex of a different carbamyl phosphate synthetase and aspartate transcarbamylase. Thus both aggregation and compartmentation have been evolved in this organism to solve its metabolic needs.

specific stages of development and to be aberrant in distinctive pathologies. For example, the liver of a ureotelic or a uricotelic animal develops a characteristic mitochondrial enzyme essential to the detoxification of ammonia at a specific stage of its development (139). Such organ-specific enzymes are probably determined by nuclear genes. Will the transfer of such enzymes to the mature organelle be aborted in tumors of hepatic origin; i.e., will the mitochondria appear to retain fetal rather than differentiated characters? Can such aberrations of normal development be made diagnostic of developing pathology?

A more sharply focused interest in the degrees of organelle autonomy must lead to new types of experiment, many of wnich will be of practical interest in agriculture and medicine. From a long familiarity with infectious disease, we attempt to infect man with immunizing avirulent viral strains, to control mosquitoes with rickettsia used as lethal intracellular parasites (147), and to explore the possibilities of establishing new symbioses in order to extend nitrogen fixation to new crops such as grasses or cereal grains (97). Thinking of organelles as invasive symbionts, we can ask if we can seed new organelles in deficient tissues in which they can be maintained. Chloroplasts from ingested algae appear to be functional naturally in some cells of marine slugs (133) and survive for some weeks intracytoplasmically when these isolated organelles are fed to mouse fibroblasts (89). Although we would not expect to be able to exploit such laboratory tricks, is it possible that there might be occasions when it would be desirable to be able to restock an animal (or human) liver with mitochondria after long treatments with drugs known to poison mitochondrial activity and biogenesis?

MITOCHONDRIAL COMPOSITION AND SYNTHESES OF NUCLEIC ACIDS

Following the rigorous demonstrations of DNA in chloroplasts (113) and mitochondria (91), these nucleic acids were isolated and characterized with respect to size, shape, density, and base composition. In some recent studies, evidence has been obtained for the existence of multiple populations of each organelle in the same organism (19, 47). These results do not appear to stem from sedimentation artifacts (92, 100); as always, the investigator is compelled to choose and to examine his experimental material with great care.

Multiple, apparently homogeneous, copies (two to six) of double-stranded circular DNA are found in compartments of animal mitochondria. These molecules are small (about 10×10^6 mol wt) and hence unable to code for all but a small fraction of the proteins and enzymatic activities found in these organelles. They differ from nuclear DNA in base composition and do not hybridize with it. The DNAs of plant, fungal, and protozoan mitochondria are frequently linear and hence pose the problem of whether the observed linear molecules are intact or merely fragments of the original circles. In addition, they are significantly larger (3.5 to 5 × 10^7 mol wt) than those of animal mitochondria. Nevertheless, it appears that most of the proteins of even yeast mitochondria, which may contain the largest size of DNA, must also be coded by nuclear genes, despite the fact that organelle DNA may comprise up to 18% of the total cell DNA.

Although the analysis of yeast DNA has presented some technical problems, e.g., the presence of a novel circular DNA possibly derived from nonmitochondrial particles (28), the ease of manipulation of yeast mitochondrial form and function by genetic and physiological techniques has led to many studies exploring mitochondrial DNA in this organism. It has been found, for example, that the fluorescent dye ethidium bromide induces an inheritable respiratory deficiency (petite mutation) characterized initially by the inability to utilize non-fermentable substrates and to incorporate cytochromes into the mitochondria. This mutation has been shown recently to be accompanied by a total loss or reduced size and altered composition of mitochondrial DNA (88). Indeed, a deoxyribonuclease stimulated by ethidium has recently been detected in yeast mitochondria (95). Such dye-induced cytoplasmic mutants, as well as mutants whose mitochondria are resistant to selected antibiotics, have provided the biological tools for the recent discovery of mitochondrial recombination (18).

The total and irreversible loss of organelle DNA as a result of treatment by dyes not only shows that the organelle is dispensable under selected physiological conditions, e.g., anaerobic growth in the presence of sterols, but also suggests that organelle DNA is at least essential for the duplication of that DNA. The notion that a master DNA copy residing in the nucleus is, of all parts of the nuclear genome, selectively inhibited by ethidium is not considered likely. By this criterion, the DNA of a trypanosome mitochondrion or of *Euglena* and *Chlamydomonas* chloroplasts is also unique within those organelles and essential for its own maintenance.

Protozoa of the order Kinetoplastidae, which are known as hemoflagellates or trypanosomatids, possess a very large mitochondrion, a portion of which contains a high concentration of DNA (20–30% of the total cell DNA) organized in the kinetoplast, an elongated chromosome-like structure. Treatment of the log phase flagellates with basic dyes, such as acriflavines, can cause the selective and inheritable loss of this DNA-containing structure, as has been studied by many workers. Most recently, the entire DNA complement of individual kinetoplasts has been isolated as compact particles of homogeneous size (66), comprised largely of interlocking catenanes of DNA minicircles which appear also to be threaded by linear DNA (108). It may be mentioned that the minicircles (about 0.4 μ) can code for no more than two proteins of 20,000 mol wt, suggesting that the individual circles may consist of individual cistrons or operons. The mechanism of the division of kinetoplast and duplication of its DNA presents an obviously difficult problem. The trypanocide Berenil, on treatment of *Trypanosoma cruzi,* has been shown to produce an accumulation of double-branched circular molecules of the kinetoplast DNA blocked at specific sites in their replication (24).

Interlocking catenanes and their dimers, trimers, etc., have been observed as relative rarities in mitochondria of many species. Increases in the proportions of such "aberrant" mitochondrial forms have been observed on treatment of fibroblasts with some but not all inhibitors of protein synthesis (90). Cells transformed by DNA tumor viruses, i.e., polyoma, SV40, or adenoviruses, or even infected by herpes simplex virus I (103) also show this effect (90,112); the data on infection by RNA tumor viruses are somewhat less clear.

Animal mitochondria have been shown to contain a DNA polymerase. This enzyme has been purified several thousandfold and has been reported to be associated with DNA at the mitochondrial membrane (85). The polymerase can be induced very considerably (35-fold) in *Tetrahymena,* by a period of thymine starvation; enzyme production requires RNA and protein synthesis (142). Similar enzymes have also been obtained from the mitochondria of both normal and a "petite" yeast; the mitochondria of the latter strain still contained DNA, albeit altered in composition (143).

The mitochondrial and nuclear polymerases of yeast are similarly inhibited by basic dyes, although in intact cells the dyes inhibit the organelle relatively specifically (143). In yeast, then, we imagine that the organization of the replication mechanism in the organelle may be significantly different from that in the nucleus. On the other hand, the mitochondrial polymerase of rat liver is reported to be far more sensitive to dyes than is the nuclear enzyme (84).

Isolated mitochondria will incorporate deoxynucleoside triphosphates into DNA (129); the study of this system led to the detection of a noncovalently linked single-stranded DNA intermediate within double-stranded circular DNA (130). These surprising biochemical observations have been confirmed by direct electron microscopy and centrifugal analysis (57, 114) and extended to point to a new mechanism of DNA replication (Fig. 2). This asymmetrical mechanism of DNA synthesis exists in addition to three other patterns of DNA synthesis detected in replication of various bacterial viruses, i.e., the symmetrical replication found for λ circles, the rolling circle detected in φX-174 multiplication, and the Y-shaped replicating rod of T7 (145). It is of great interest that this extensive biochemical variability is found even in so fundamental a process as DNA replication.

In the study of organelle RNA, it has been frequently necessary to remove contaminating microsomal materials. Although intact mitochondria from ovaries of *Xenopus laevis* can incorporate exogenous polynucleotides and translate these on mitochondrial ribosomes (127), transcription of mitochondrial DNA appears to produce most of the RNA species seen in the organelle (63). Indeed, it is

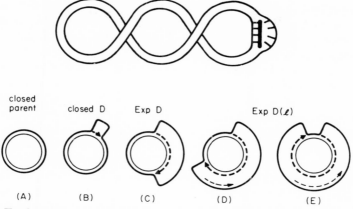

Fig. 2. A new mechanism of DNA replication in mitochondria. A displacement loop, D, is formed, within which is contained a newly synthesized heavy strand hydrogen-bonded to the circular light strand. When the D loop has expanded, Exp D, to about 0.55 of the genome, synthesis of the complementary light strand, Exp D(e), begins in the opposite direction.

reported that both strands of mitochondrial DNA are transcribed but that only the product of the heavy strand is conserved within the mitochondrion (1).

The ribosomes of animal mitochondria have been characterized as among the smallest ribosomes, e.g., 55S. The subunits contain correspondingly small species of rRNA which have very low degrees of methylation (36) and a significant turnover (35, 148). However, lower eukaryotes contain fairly large mitochondrial ribosomes (73–81S) and larger species of rRNA (63). Some of these may be isolated in polysomes (94) which are still functional in *in vitro* systems (6). Mitochondria also contain unique species of tRNA. Nevertheless, the mitochondrial ribosomes of *Neurospora* (73) are reported to lack the species of 5S RNA common to prokaryotic and eukaryotic ribosomes.

Isolated rat liver mitochondria will synthesize characteristic mitochondrial ribosomal RNA and other nucleic acids from ribonucleoside triphosphates, suggesting further the role of the organelle DNA in this transcription (40,41). Since mitochondrial rRNA from *Neurospora* is complementary to but 2.5% of the organelle DNA, it appears that there is only a single cistron for each rRNA species in the genome (117). In this respect, then, i.e., the absence of redundancy of these cistrons, these genomes are more like that of a bacterium than that of a eukaryotic nucleus. Nevertheless, during the development of embryos of *Xenopus laevis* the synthesis of mitochondrial rRNA is not coordinated to that of mitochondrial tRNA. Further, since the synthesis of the former can occur in an anucleolate embryo it is not necessarily tied to the synthesis of other ribosomal RNA (27). However, the synthesis of mitochondrial RNA *in vivo* is often synchronized in the cell cycle; in HeLa cells, marked increases of the rate occur mainly in the S and G2 phases, even as is observed for maximal replication of mitochondrial DNA (98).

Hybridization studies of mitochondrial 4S RNA from *Saccharomyces* with mitochondrial DNA have shown that the latter contains 20–26 genes for mitochondrial tRNA (107). This is a larger value than found for animal mitochondrial DNA. The authors interpreted these results to mean that the yeast organelle DNA, in contrast to that of animal mitochondria, contains genes for a set of tRNAs for each of 20 amino acids and does not contain genes for several tRNAs per amino acid as in nuclear DNA.

As we might expect, then, mitochondria (liver, yeast, *Neurospora*) contain a DNA-dependent RNA polymerase which is found to be somewhat different from the nuclear enzyme. After solubilization from the organelle membrane, the enzyme is found to be somewhat smaller than the bacterial polymerase (106). *In vitro* synthesis by both nuclear and mitochondrial enzymes is inhibited by actinomycin D and ethidium, but, unlike the former, synthesis by the latter enzyme is insensitive to α-amanitin and camptothecin. Although early reports had indicated that rifamycin inhibited both bacterial and mitochondrial polymerases, it appears that the effect of this inhibitor of prokaryotic RNA polymerase may be significantly less on the mitochondrial polymerase.

THE SYNTHESIS OF MITOCHONDRIAL PROTEINS

Isolated mitochondria incorporate amino acids into structural proteins definable by gel electrophoresis. Such incorporation is inhibited by chloramphenicol, a well-known inhibitor of prokaryotic protein synthesis. Under conditions in which protein synthesis is blocked in liver cells outside of the organelle by emetine, the labeled organelle proteins are the same whether made in the intact inhibited cell or by isolated mitochondria (32). These are mainly insoluble materials which can be solubilized by detergents to reveal at least ten distinct proteins of 14,000–50,000 mol wt apparently coded by the mitochondrial genome (32).

When the inner and outer membranes of *Neurospora crassa* mitochondria are separated, it is found that the outer membranes are essentially unlabeled as a result of amino acid incorporation by the isolated organelle. This result is also found in intact *Neurospora* inhibited by cycloheximide, which also blocks protein synthesis outside of the organelle. The inner membrane may then be resolved into about 20 proteins (93), many of which are heavily labeled. However, it has been estimated by various workers that only 7–15% of the total mitochondrial protein is made in the organelle and coded by the mitochondrial genome (32,48,76,126,132). It must be cautioned that these estimates have usually derived from the use of inhibitors whose specificity as inhibitors of protein synthesis by cytoplasmic ribosomes has occasionally been questioned.

Not a single such protein coded by the mitochondrial genome has yet been identified rigorously. Possible membrane-associated candidates have been suggested (126) to be a cytochrome oxidase subunit, cytochrome b, succinate dehydrogenase subunit, nonheme iron protein, adenosine triphosphatase subunit, and an oligomycin-sensitivity-conferring protein. However, in studies of liver mitochondria which differentiated the inner membranes into parts of varying biosynthetic origins (141) few of the activities suggested above were found associated with the labeled proteins made during amino acid incorporation by the isolated organelles. Studies with mitochondrial inhibitors such as chloramphenicol and ethidium in yeast have indicated that among enzymes of the respiratory chain neither cytoplasmic nor mitochondrial ribosomes alone are responsible for total translation of the essential messengers (75). Other studies in yeast of the synthesis of mitochondrial adenosine triphosphatase have led to similar conclusions (134,135).

In *Neurospora crassa*, cycloheximide blocked incorporation into cytochrome oxidase,[3] leading to the view that cytoplasmic ribosomes contributed to synthesis of this enzyme (15). A similar conclusion was reported recently for the origin of some protein subunits of the cytochrome oxidase of yeast (118). It is reported that in rat liver only 15–20% of the protein associated with purified cytochrome oxidase[3] is synthesized by the cycloheximide-insensitive system of the mitochondria (10). The results may suggest even as in the composite genetic origins of some phage-induced enzymes, e.g., the Qβ RNA polymerase (31), that some organelle enzymes, i.e., their subunits, may be derived from several genetic systems (135).

Indeed, such a multigenomic origin is considered to be proven for mitochondrial ribosomes whose proteins do differ from those of cytoplasmic ribosomes (20,64). Although the rRNA is clearly derived from mitochondrial DNA, with which it hybridizes, most of the proteins of mitochondrial ribosomes are reported to be formed on the cytoplasmic ribosomes (64). This conclusion is based mainly on the observation that the synthesis of the proteins of mitochondrial ribosomes is blocked by cycloheximide but not by chloramphenicol, in contrast to the inner membrane proteins alluded to above. It should be men-

---

[3] Cytochrome oxidase is a component of the mitochondrial inner membrane, expresses the quintessence of mitochondrial function, i.e., aerobic respiration, and exists tightly associated (7) with a lipid, cardiolipin. Cardiolipin is found otherwise only in prokaryotic membranes and can be synthesized in isolated mitochondria (52). These facts have probably led many workers to hope that this enzyme will provide a mitochondrial marker with respect to its distribution, site of synthesis, and site of genetic control. However, the copper of the mitochondrial enzyme, which has not been found as yet in any bacterial enzyme, such as *Pseudomonas* cytochrome oxidase, suggests that the mitochondrion may have acquired a new function rather than inherited an old one. Furthermore, cytochromes $a + a_3$ and cardiolipin have recently been found in bovine liver nuclear membranes in rather high concentrations (13,59), indicating that this enzyme and phospholipid are not as exclusively mitochondrial as had been thought.

tioned that certain inhibitors, e.g., erythromycin, do not affect rat liver mitochondria *in vivo,* although their ribosomes are as sensitive to the antibiotics as
are bacterial ribosomes. In these instances, permeability barriers at the mitochondrial level appear to explain such resistance.

A cytoplasmic mutation ("poky") in *Neurospora crassa* affecting mitochondrial function has been found to cause a deficiency in small mitochondrial
ribosomal subunits (111). It has been hypothesized that this effect on synthesis
or assembly is controlled by the supply of mitochondrial rRNA rather than of a
mitochondrially determined ribosomal protein. On the other hand, some studies
of inherited resistance to mitochondrial inhibitors in *Paramecium* have appeared
to be examples of cytoplasmic determination and to be expressed in altered
proteins of the mitochondrial ribosomes (9), even as reported for some instances
of drug resistance for *Chlamydomonas* chloroplasts (115).

In the face of the startling complexity of the distribution of genetic information and sites of synthesis controlling mitochondrial proteins in various eukaryotes, a view derived from the use of inhibitors, these data to date seem to
suggest that the mechanisms of protein synthesis themselves in the respective
compartments are quite distinct. Nevertheless, as noted earlier, the analyses of
the mechanisms of protein synthesis in prokaryotes and eukaryotes have stressed
similarities rather than differences (65). For example, mitochondrial initiation
involves formylmethioninyl tRNA, even as does prokaryotic translation, and
such a tRNA is found only in mitochondria. Nevertheless, it has been argued
that this is but a minor difference from eukaryotic cytoplasmic initiation, which
requires another unique methioninyl tRNA that, while unformylated in the
cytoplasm, can be formylated by a prokaryote transformylase (74). Despite this
result, we are astonished not only that mitochondrial and chloroplast tRNA
hybridize uniquely with their homologous organelle DNA but also that they lack
such structures as the Y base found in the cytoplasmic tRNAs of eukaryotes
(39). Thus evolutionary divergence in tRNA is rigorously maintained for reasons
which must relate to selection of mechanisms of protein synthesis. Nevertheless,
it is reported that the elongation factors essential for mitochondrial protein
synthesis are formed in cytoplasm (109), although specific for prokaryotic and
mitochondrial ribosomes (74). These factors are made in "petite" mutants of
yeast totally lacking in mitochondrial DNA (109).

As remarked earlier, it is inconceivable that this interplay of synthetic
mechanisms detailed above should not be closely controlled, that distortions of
the patterns of protein traffic should not be fairly easily detectable. Thus when
cycloheximide is used to block synthesis of cytoplasmic proteins in yeast, the
synthesis of nuclear DNA is arrested while the synthesis of mitochondrial DNA
continues for some hours (46). In mammalian cells (70), inhibition of transcription of mitochondrial DNA by ethidium and of translation on mitochondrial
ribosomes by chloramphenicol permits a continuing growth of the cells with

dilution of some mitochondrial enzymes. Nevertheless, while the outer membrane remains intact, a gradual disappearance of the inner membrane is observed. In *Neurospora crassa*, chloramphenicol permits a significant increase in mitochondrial protein, a doubling of mitochondrial RNA, and almost a tripling of mitochondrial ribosomes (8). Enzymes such as RNA polymerase, ribosomal translocase, and methionyl transformylase are also made under these conditions (8), affirming the nuclear control of the organelle. The fact that organelle division in this organism normally is synchronized with the cell cycle suggests that the organelle may normally elaborate controls on nuclear transcription of mitochondrial-related function which are derepressed under conditions of inhibition of mitochondrial syntheses. We may ask if the stimulation of mitochondrial syntheses by polyoma virus (137), in oncocytomas (128), does not reflect such loss of controls, whereas the formation of dimers and higher catenanes may reflect the availability of proteins from one system rather than from both closely cooperating genetic systems.

CONCLUSIONS CONCERNING MITOCHONDRIA AND A FRESH START WITH CHLOROPLASTS

Current data on the origins of chloroplasts have developed in a manner much like that of studies on mitochondrial origin. Both organelles have been found to possess the requirements for potential autonomy: (a) a DNA characteristic of the organelle, (b) a distinctive DNA polymerase, (c) an RNA polymerase which synthesizes mRNA, rRNA, and tRNA in the isolated organelle, and (d) ribosomes for the translation of mRNA. Nevertheless, as in the case of mitochondria, whose structure is very largely determined by nuclear genes, it has been found that chloroplast structures crucial to the performance of plastid function are also determined by nuclear genes. In yeast, at least 63 nuclear genes affect mitochondrial function, structure, and biogenesis (11); in barley, 86 nuclear genes controlling chloroplast development have been identified (138). For this class of reasons, therefore, it has been generally concluded that these organelles do not in fact possess genetic autonomy.

Indeed, Raff and Mahler (104) have concluded that mitochondria are probably not of symbiotic origin. They believe, among other arguments, that such a hypothesis demands, even as I had suggested earlier (29), the existence of an aerobic but grossly inefficient protoeukaryotic host whose survival was unlikely before infection. In my turn, I do not find their arguments compelling and have concluded only that it will take a great deal more evidence to permit conclusions to be reached with respect to mitochondria. In support of a theory of symbiotic origins, it would be particularly important to obtain data on the degree of molecular hybridization between mitochondrial DNA and that of some microbe. Although studies of relatedness determined by hybridization are moving rapidly for bacteria, a sufficiently broad analysis to seek cross-reactions with mitochondria has not yet been reported. In this area, it is difficult to see how a convincing positive answer to the postulate of symbiotic origin can be obtained in the absence of the detection of a descendant of the presumed primitive infecting organism. It is possible that no cross-reaction will ever be found in mitochondrial studies, suggesting either the lack of a symbiotic origin for the organelle or the disappearance of the primitive infecting organism. In this case, the lack of evidence will prevent any conclusion from being reached.

Nevertheless, despite the apparent similarities in the summation of data concerning mitochondria and chloroplasts, the data on the latter possess some distinguishing features which suggest that it will be more fruitful at this time to pursue the possible relations between chloroplasts and blue-green algae; i.e. there are reasons to hope that some primitive precursor of the latter may eventually be proven to be the progenitor of the organelle.

CHLOROPLAST COMPOSITION AND SYNTHESIS

A number of useful relevant reviews have recently appeared on this rapidly burgeoning field (22,44,62,115,131). Direct observations of several modes of chloroplast division (fission) within leaves and in *in vitro* systems (33,110) have also been reported recently, as well as correlations of such divisions with the stage of cell elongation (56). In detached leaves of the moss *Funaria,* replication of nuclear DNA is followed by chloroplast DNA replication and the formation of dumbbell-shaped chloroplasts. These initial steps of division were not blocked by rifampicin or by chloramphenicol, which block lipid synthesis as well as transcription and translation, respectively, in these organelles (42). On the other hand, as might be expected from earlier remarks on the absence of complete genetic autonomy, continued growth and division of chloroplasts *in vitro* or of surviving organelles in animal cells have not been detected. Nevertheless, the inference of genetic recombination and linkage (116) of the organelles in zygotes of the alga *Chlamydomonas* has been supported by observations of chloroplast fusion (26), not as yet detected for mitochondria.

Circular DNA has been isolated from chloroplasts of *Euglena* (78) and of spinach (77), the former of about 9×10^7 mol wt while the latter is about 10% larger. Although the total DNA complements of chloroplasts have ranged from 2 to 6×10^9 daltons, nonredundant DNA in the range of $1-2 \times 10^8$ daltons has been detected in several estimates of "kinetic complexity" based on the rates of DNA renaturation (22). It would appear that these apparent units have in fact been isolated as the circular molecules noted earlier. The replication and turnover of chloroplast DNA of *Euglena gracilis* have been shown to be more rapid than those of nuclear DNA (79). Another novel DNA enriched in cistrons for plastid rRNA has also been isolated from this organism.

Analysis of the variability of quantity of DNA in plastids of *Acetabularia* revealed that as many as 65–80% of these bodies did not contain any DNA (146). Rejecting the notion that the DNA of the plastids was inaccessible to their detection methods, the reporters suggest that division of plastids is unequal and that plastids without DNA may gain DNA by fusion with plastids containing multiple genomes.

In any case, the chloroplast genome appears to contain 10–20 times more DNA than that of animal mitochondria and perhaps a fifth to a tenth that of some bacteria. It is theoretically capable, then, of coding for several hundred proteins. As in bacteria or mitochondria, the DNA is attached to the chloroplast membrane (16). The organelle contains a DNA polymerase (122) and tolueneized *Chlamydomonas* incorporates deoxynucleoside triphosphates mainly into chloroplast DNA (53), while synthesis of nuclear DNA is severely inhibited. Despite the apparent autonomy of DNA replication in the organelle, cycloheximide, an inhibitor of synthesis by cytoplasmic ribosomes, blocks synthesis of chloroplast DNA (34). These results have been interpreted to suggest a nuclear control of DNA replication in the chloroplast.

DNA ligase has been detected in both nuclei and chloroplasts (61). The enzyme can produce circular conformations in various DNA preparations only in the presence of some hormones, such as gibberellin A (60).

Isolated chloroplasts incorporate ribonucleoside triphosphates into RNA and contain a DNA-dependent RNA polymerase. A comparison of solubilized nuclear and chloroplast RNA polymerases from wheat leaf has revealed similar requirements and reactivities of these enzymes (102). It has been suggested that the various enzymes may have identical catalytic cores but different subunits determining template specificities. Although rifamycin bleaches some algae, no selective effect of this antibiotic has been obtained on isolated nuclei or chloroplasts (21) or on the derived enzymes (101). It should be noted that although the antibiotic is somewhat inhibitory to the RNA polymerase of a blue-green alga, this inhibition is more difficult to demonstrate than that with bacteria (49).

The organelles contain several thousand ribosomes per plastid; such ribosomes contain RNA resembling that in prokaryotic organisms (22). Ribosomes of broad bean and *Chlamydomonas* also contain 5S RNA (23,96), which is reported to be lacking in mitochondrial ribosomes. The genes for synthesis of chloroplast ribosomal RNA (16 and 23S) reside in the organelle and appear to exist in several pairs of tandem genes, each of which seems to be preceded by spacer polynucleotides (125).

It is of great interest that studies of the hybridization of the rRNA of widely divergent organisms with DNA have revealed significant degrees of homology between the rRNA of such organisms as *E. coli* and pea (12). This result is interpreted to indicate that polynucleotide sequences in these molecules have been highly conserved during evolution and are strong evidence of a single line of evolution from prokaryote to eukaryote. Although it will be important to have a comparison of the degree of hybridization between rRNA of an appropriate eukaryote with nuclear mitochondrial and plastid DNA, the conservation of polynucleotide sequences alluded to above may conceivably confuse interpretations of such data. Nevertheless, a comparison of the rRNA of *Euglena* plastids with that of the cytoplasm has revealed almost complete specificity in reaction with plastic DNA (99). In extending such tests, the rRNAs of several blue-green algae were found to be highly reactive with the DNA of *Euglena* plastids, while the rRNAs of bacteria were much less so (99).

Whereas the ribosomal proteins of mitochondria are controlled almost, if not entirely, by nuclear genes, it has been reported that a *Chlamydomonas* plastid gene controls the synthesis of a specific component of the plastid 50S ribosomal subunit determining resistance to the antibiotic carbomycin (119). A non-Mendelian gene is also known for the control of resistance to erythromycin, i.e., controlling binding to the ribosome (83). In the first instance, these phenomena are considered to relate primarily to alteration of a ribosomal protein; however, Mets and Bogorad (83) ask if the change can be in RNA or protein. The belief that it is the latter is strengthened by the observation that in the alga *Ochromonas* chloramphenicol blocks synthesis of chloroplast ribosomes without an effect on synthesis of mitochondrial ribosomes (121).

The similarities of protein synthesis by ribosomes of prokaryotes and plastids have been elaborated in now familiar tests of antibiotic sensitivity, requirements for initiation and cofactors (22), etc. These results have been underlined by a recent demonstration of the formation and activity of hybrid ribosomes produced from the 30S subunit of *Euglena* plastid ribosomes and the 50S subunit of *E. coli* (68). Such a hybrid has not been obtained by mixture of subunits of prokaryote 70S and eukaryote 80S ribosomes (82).

Chloroplasts contain apparently unique tRNAs and aminoacyl tRNA synthetases (22), some of which in *Euglena* are light inducible (105). However, bleached *Euglena* mutants lacking chloroplast DNA and structure do contain some of these enzymes, suggesting their determination by nuclear genes (105).

Many nuclear genes have been identified which control the synthesis of at least seven components of the photosynthetic apparatus (72), although it is not known that these are structural genes. Nevertheless, it has been shown that the control of numerous protein components of chloroplast membranes does reside in both nuclear genes and organelle genes (4, 37, 38, 50, 121), and indeed significant interactions of the two genomes have been detected by many of these in production of the membranes of the organelle. On the other hand, the synthesis of the galactolipids specifically associated with chloroplast membranes is specifically inhibited by chloramphenicol and not by cycloheximide, suggesting a greater organelle control over production of these lipids (17).

Even as in the study of the control of biosynthesis of cytochrome oxidase in mitochondria, many studies (22) with various mutants and antibiotics have attempted similar analyses of numerous specific proteins essential to photosynthetic activity. From studies of components of the photosystems, it has been concluded that both chloroplast DNA and nuclear DNA control the synthesis of some chloroplast cytochromes (5,71). Nevertheless, components such as ferredoxin, ferredoxin-NADP reductase, and chlorophyll are determined by synthetic events on cytoplasmic ribosomes (5). It has been reported that the ferredoxin of the blue-green alga *Nostoc* is far more similar to the ferredoxins of the chloroplast type than to the two classes of bacterial ferredoxins (87). It will obviously be important to determine if a polynucleotide sequence specifying a photosynthetic protein possibly derived from blue-green algae has truly found its way to nuclear DNA.

Components involved in CO_2 fixation, some of which are easily available, have received very considerable attention. For example, a dozen studies examine the origin of ribulose-1,5-diphosphate carboxylase, which has proven to be the fraction 1 protein, the protein present in largest amount in some plant leaves (58). The enzyme derived from higher plants is quite large (about 5×10^5 mol wt) and is comprised of two subunits. Enzymes of similar function but markedly lower molecular weight (down to 8×10^4) are known in photosynthetic and other autotrophic bacteria. Several reports have appeared indicating that the eukaryote enzyme is synthesized on both plastid and cytoplasmic ribosomes (5,80). However, in *Chlamydomonas* the synthesis of both subunits is blocked by chloramphenicol (51), and the kinetics of production of the two subunits are so similar as to suggest that the synthesis occurs at the same site or in a very closely coordinated manner (43). Furthermore, it is reported that isolated chloroplasts of pea will incorporate amino acids exclusively into the large subunit of the enzyme (22).

The apparently chloroplast determination of a large part, at least, of this important enzyme does not exhaust our interest in this protein. Since this carboxylase is known in autotrophic bacteria and blue-green algae (58), it is obvious that it will be important to see if there is a primary sequence homology between the prokaryotic and eukaryotic enzymes. Further, it has been reported that the spinach enzyme contains tightly bound copper (144). We can ask, if this metal is associated with a particular subunit, do any of the prokaryotic carboxylases contain copper?

If I may pursue the copper matter briefly, we know that blue-green algae contain a component functional as plastocyanin, but it has not been shown that this particular protein contains copper. Superoxide dismutase seems to be present in all oxygen-metabolizing organisms; it contains copper when isolated from eukaryotes, but the bacterial enzyme contains $Mn_2{}^+$ (86). Which metal is found in the enzyme of blue-green algae?[4] Will the pursuit of copper enzymes

---

[4] It appears that both enzymes are present in liver, the Cu^{2+} enzyme in cytosol and the Mn^{2+} enzyme in mitochondria (Fridovich personal communication). However, it will now be necessary to determine the sites of synthesis and genetic determination of the Mn^{2+} enzyme in the eukaryotic cell.

reveal a chemical similarity of blue-green algae and chloroplasts not readily interpretable in terms of the possible evolutionary origin of the latter from the former, or will we reveal a serious biochemical difference in this respect between microorganism and organelle?

In contrast to bacteria and blue-green algae, which contain an aldolase for a fructose-1,6-diphosphate that requires a metal for its activity (class II aldolase), higher plants contain an aldolase lacking a metal (class I aldolase) (67). In the pea, this chloroplast enzyme which differs only slightly from the cytoplasmic enzyme (3) appears determined by a nuclear gene (2). Since enzymes of both classes are found in both *Euglena* and *Chlamydomonas,* it would obviously be of interest to determine if their class II enzyme is determined by a chloroplast gene. In *Euglena,* the synthesis of aldolase is in fact reported to be inhibited by chloramphenicol (22), suggesting a potential relation of chloroplast and prokaryote warranting further study.

The above examples of nuclear determination indicate that as in mitochondria numerous components essential to chloroplast function will not be determined by chloroplast DNA. Nevertheless, it will be important to know if some instances of prokaryotic biochemistry are possibly determined by the chloroplasts. Among many other examples of such metabolic capability, isolated plastids can synthesize methionine from homocysteine (120) and chlorophyll from δ-aminolevulinate (140). Where in fact are the numerous enzymes determined?

We may also search for as yet unsought chloroplast functions. For example, higher plants synthesize lysine via diaminopimelic acid and pyridine nucleotides from glycerol and aspartate, i.e., by prokaryotic mechanisms. Will these be found in the chloroplasts and will the enzymes be determined by chloroplast DNA?

SOME CONCLUSIONS AND PERSPECTIVES

This brief summary of the existing data on the chloroplast indicates that this organelle has a very significant DNA component potentially coding for several hundred chloroplast components, capable of hybridizing with some genes of blue-green algae (rRNA) and coding for specific components for which homologous protein and other polynucleotide sequences may exist in the algae. The metabolic potentialities of the organelle, e.g., synthesis of methionine and porphyrins, are promising, and the organelle may actually contain specifically prokaryotic metabolic remnants, such as pathways of lysine and NAD synthesis, which for these reasons warrant closer study. For all of these reasons, then, the study of chloroplasts and their possible relation to blue-green algae appears more promising from the point of view of seeking organelle origins and evolution than does the current explosion in the exploration of mitochondrial origins.

It should be noted that biological (124), genetic (55), and biochemical data on blue-green algae are in an exceedingly primitive state, despite the obvious theoretical and practical importance of these organisms. It can be expected that the search for chloroplast origins will help to phrase quite penetrating questions about these prokaryotes.

Although a study of the apparent acquisition of copper enzymes may tell us more about the evolution of blue-green algae than of chloroplasts, we at least have the opportunity of exploring more comprehensively the nature and extent of the biochemical discontinuity between prokaryotes and eukaryotes.

The startling finding that the individual phycobilins of blue-green algae (Cyanophyta) are strongly cross-reactive immunologically with the corresponding proteins of the eukaryotic red algae (Rhodophyta) (45) demands detailed studies of the red algae and their chloroplasts. The considerable similarities (54) of chloroplast rRNA of red algae and the rRNA of blue-green algae also extend the possibilities of direct homologies between these relatively neglected eukaryotes and the prokaryotes.

From the point of view of a virologist, I have been struck by the recent evidence suggesting that some plant viruses, e.g., turnip yellow mosaic virus, multiply in chloroplasts within infected plants (25, 65, 136). I wonder, then, if these viruses will multiply in the chloroplasts isolated from infected plants or if they can be used to infect unicellular blue-green algae.[5] As is well known, the difficulties of initiating simultaneous plant virus infection in many cells have enormously hindered the development of plant virology.

In conclusion, then, it should be clear that the apparently academic and theoretical search for organelle origins really holds many possibilities of enriching both theoretical and practical biology. At the moment, work on plants, chloroplasts, and algae appears potentially more promising, but I do not doubt that such a shift in emphasis will also rapidly rebound to enrich work on the animal organelles.

REFERENCES

1. Aloni, Y., and Attardi, G. (1971). Symmetrical *in vivo* transcription of mitochondrial DNA in HeLa cells. *Proc. Natl. Acad. Sci. (USA)* 68:1757-1761.
2. Anderson, L. E., and Levin, D. A. (1970). Chloroplast aldolase is controlled by a nuclear gene. *Plant Physiol.* 46:819-820.

[5] We have reported that blue-green algae, like other prokaryotes, contain spermidine alone, in contrast to eukaryotes, which contain spermidine and spermine (30). It may be relevant that the RNA of turnip yellow mosaic virus contains far more spermidine than spermine (30), despite the greater affinity of the latter for RNA. Thus chloroplasts may only make the former. Since the enzymes of spermidine synthesis in prokaryotes differ significantly from those in eukaryotes (30), it will be of great interest to see if chloroplasts synthesize polyamines and to determine the nature and origin of these chloroplast enzymes, if they do in fact exist.

3. Anderson, L. E., and Pacold, I. (1972). Chloroplast and cytoplasmic enzymes. IV. Pea leaf fructose 1,6-diphosphate aldolases. *Plant Physiol.* 49:393-397.
4. Apel, K., and Schweiger, H. (1972). Nuclear dependency of chloroplast proteins in *Acetabularia. Europ. J. Biochem.* 25:229-238.
5. Armstrong, J. J., Surzycki, S. J., Moll, B., and Levine, R. P. (1971). Genetic transcription and translation specifying chloroplast components in *Chlamydomonas reinhardi. Biochemistry* 10:692-701.
6. Avadhani, N. G., and Buetow, D. E. (1972). Isolation of active polyribosomes from the cytoplasm, mitochondria and chloroplasts of *Euglena gracilis. Biochem. J.* 128:353-365.
7. Awasthi, Y. C., Chuang, T. F., Keenan, T. W., and Crane, F. L. (1971). Tightly bound cardiolipin in cytochrome oxidase. *Biochim. Biophys. Acta* 226:42-52.
8. Barath, Z., and Küntzel, H. (1972). Cooperation of mitochondrial and nuclear genes specifying the mitochondrial genetic apparatus in *Neurospora crassa. Proc. Natl. Acad. Sci. (USA)* 69:1371-1374.
9. Beale, G. H., Knowles, J. K. C., and Tait, A. (1972). Mitochondrial genetics in *Paramecium. Nature* 235:396-397.
10. Beattie, D. S. (1970). Cycloheximide-resistant amino acid incorporation into rat liver mitochondrial proteins *in vivo. FEBS Letters* 9:232-234.
11. Beck, J. C., Parker, J. H., Balcavage, W. X., and Matoon, J. R. (1971). Mendelian genes affecting development and function of yeast mitochondria. In *Autonomy and Biogenesis of Mitochondria and Chloroplasts,* North-Holland, Amsterdam, pp. 194-204.
12. Bendich, A. J., and McCarthy, B. J. (1970). Ribosomal RNA homologies among distantly related organisms. *Proc. Natl. Acad. Sci. (USA)* 65:349-356.
13. Berezney, R., and Crane, F. L. (1971). Cytochromes in bovine liver nuclear membranes. *Biochem. Biophys. Res. Commun.* 43:107-1023.
14. Bernhardt, S. A., and Davis, R. H. (1972). Carbamoyl phosphate compartmentation in *Neurospora:* Histochemical localization of aspartate and ornithine transcarbamoylases. *Proc. Natl. Acad. Sci. (USA)* 69:1868-1872.
15. Birkmayer, G. D. (1971). The site of cytochrome oxidase biosynthesis in *Neurospora crassa. Europ. J. Biochem.* 21:258-263.
16. Bisalputra, T., and Burton, H. (1970). On the chloroplast DNA-membrane complex in *Sphacelaria SP. J. Microscop.* 9:661-666.
17. Bishop, D. G., and Smillie, R. M. (1970). The effect of chloramphenicol and cycloheximide on lipid synthesis during chloroplast development in *Euglena gracilis. Arch. Biochem. Biophys.* 137:179-189.
18. Bolotin, M., Coen, D., Deutsch, J., Dujon, B., Netter, P., Petrochilo, E., and Slonimski, P. P. (1971). La recombinaison des mitochondries chez *Saccharomyces cerevisiae. Bull. Inst. Pasteur* 69:215-239.
19. Bondi, E. E., Devlin, T. M., and Ch'ih, J. J. (1972). Distribution of two mitochondrial populations in rabbit kidney cortex and medulla. *Biochem. Biophys. Res. Commun.* 47:574-580.
20. Borst, P., and Grivell, L. A. (1971). Mitochondrial ribosomes. *FEBS Letters* 13:73-88.
21. Bottomley, W., Spencer, D., Wheeler, A. M., and Whitfeld, P. R. (1971). The effect of a range of RNA polymerase inhibitors on RNA synthesis in higher plant chloroplasts and nuclei. *Arch. Biochem. Biophys.* 143:269-275.
22. Boulter, D., Ellis, R. J., and Yarwood, A. (1972). Biochemistry of protein synthesis in plants. *Biol. Rev.* 47:113-175.
23. Bourque, D. P., Boynton, J. E., and Gillham, N. W. (1971). Studies on the structure

and cellular location of various ribosome and ribosomal RNA species in the green alga *Chlamydomonas reinhardii. J. Cell Sci.* **8**:153-183.

24. Brack, C. H., Delain, E., and Riou, G. (1972). Replicating, covalently closed, circular DNA from kinetoplasts of *Trypanosoma cruzi. Proc. Natl. Acad. Sci. (USA)* **69**: 1642-1646.
25. Carroll, T. W. (1970). Relation of barley stripe mosaic virus to plastids. *Virology* **42**:1015-1022.
26. Cavalier-Smith, T. (1970). Electron microscopic evidence for chloroplast fusion in zygotes of *Chlamydomonas reinhardii. Nature* **228**:333-335.
27. Chase, J. W., and Dawid, I. B. (1972). Biogenesis of mitochondria during *Xenopus laevis* development. *Develop. Biol.* **27**:504-518.
28. Clark-Walker, G. D. (1972). Isolation of circular DNA from a mitochondrial fraction from yeast. *Proc. Natl. Acad. Sci. (USA)* **69**:388-392.
29. Cohen, S. S. (1970). Are/were mitochondria and chloroplasts microorganisms? *Am. Scientist* **58**:281-289.
30. Cohen, S. S. (1971). *Introduction to the Polyamines,* Prentice-Hall, Englewood Cliffs, N.J.
31. Cohen, S. S. (1971). Some enzymes specified by DNA phages. *Ciba Foundation Symposium on Strategy of the Viral Genome,* Churchill Livingstone, London, pp. 5-24.
32. Coote, J. L., and Work, T. S. (1971). Proteins coded by mitochondrial DNA of animal cells. *Europ. J. Biochem.* **23**:564-574.
33. Cran, D. G., and Possingham, J. V. (1972). Two forms of division profile in spinach chloroplasts. *Nature New Biol.* **235**:142.
34. Drlica, K. A., and Knight, C. A. (1971). Inhibition of chloroplast DNA synthesis by cycloheximide. *J. Mol. Biol.* **61**:629-641.
35. Dubin, D. T. (1972). Mitochondrial ribonucleic acid from cultured animal cells. Comparison of pulse-labeled with steady state-labeled ribonucleic acid. *J. Biol. Chem.* **247**:2662-2666.
36. Dubin, D. T., and Friend, D. A. (1971). Degree of methylation of mitochondrial ribosomal RNA. *FEBS Letters* **18**:287-289.
37. Eytan, G., and Ohad, I. (1970). Biogenesis of chloroplast membranes. VI. Cooperation between cytoplasmic and chloroplast ribosomes in the synthesis of photosynthetic lamellar proteins during the greening process in a mutant of *Chlamydomonas reinhardi* y-1. *J. Biol. Chem.* **245**:4297-4307.
38. Eytan, G., and Ohad, I. (1972). Biogenesis of chloroplast membranes. VIII. Modulation of chloroplast lamellae composition and function induced by discontinuous illumination and inhibition of ribonucleic acid and protein synthesis during greening of *Chlamydomonas reinhardi* y-1 mutant cells. *J. Biol. Chem.* **247**:122-129.
39. Fairfield, S. A., and Barnett, W. E. (1971). On the similarity between the tRNAs of organelles and prokaryotes. *Proc. Natl. Acad. Sci. (USA)* **68**:2972-2976.
40. Fukamachi, S., Bartoov, B., and Freeman, K. B. (1972). Synthesis of ribonucleic acid by isolated rat liver mitochondria. *Biochem. J.* **128**:299-309.
41. Fukamachi, S., Bartoov, B., Mitra, R. S., and Freeman, K. B. (1970). The synthesis of ribosomal-type RNA by isolated rat liver mitochondria. *Biochem. Biophys. Res. Commun.* **40**:852-857.
42. Giles, K. L., and Taylor, A. O. (1971). The control of chloroplast division in *Funaria hygrometrica.* I. Patterns of nucleic acid, protein and lipid synthesis. *Plant Cell Physiol.* **12**:437-445.
43. Givan, A., and Criddle, R. S. (1972). Ribulose-diphosphate carboxylase from *Chlam-*

ydomonas reinhardi: Purification, properties and its mode of synthesis in the cell. *Arch. Biochem. Biophys.* **149**:153-163.

44. Givan, C. V., and Leech, R. M. (1971). Biochemical autonomy of higher plant chloroplasts and their synthesis of small molecules. *Biol. Rev.* **46**:409-428.

45. Glazer, A. N., Cohen-Bazire, G., and Stanier, R. Y. (1971). Comparative immunology of algal biliproteins. *Proc. Natl. Acad. Sci. (USA)* **68**:3005-3008.

46. Grossman, L. I., Goldring, E. S., and Marmur, J. (1969). Preferential synthesis of yeast mitochondrial DNA in the absence of protein synthesis. *J. Mol. Biol.* **46**:367-376.

47. Hatch, M. D., and Slack, C. R. (1970). Photosynthetic CO_2-fixation pathways. *Ann. Rev. Plant Physiol.* **21**:141-162.

48. Hawley, E. S., and Greenwalt, J. W. (1970). An assessment of *in vivo* mitochondrial protein synthesis in *Neurospora crassa. J. Biol. Chem.* **245**:3574-3583.

49. Herzfeld, F., and Zillig, W. (1971). Subunit composition of DNA-dependent RNA polymerase of *Anacystis nidulans. Europ. J. Biochem.* **24**:242-248.

50. Hoober, J. K. (1970). Sites of synthesis of chloroplast membrane in polypeptides in *Chlamydomonas reinhardi* y-1. *J. Biol. Chem.* **245**:4327-4334.

51. Hoober, J. K. (1972). A major polypeptide of chloroplast membranes of *Chlamydomonas reinhardi. J. Cell Biol.* **52**:84-96.

52. Hostetler, K. Y., Van Den Bosch, H., and Van Deenen, L. L. M. (1971). Biosynthesis of cardiolipin in liver mitochondria. *Biochim. Biophys. Acta* **239**:113-119.

53. Howell, S. H., and Walker, L. L. (1972). Synthesis of DNA in toluene-treated *Chlamydomonas reinhardi. Proc. Natl. Acad. Sci. (USA)* **69**:490-494.

54. Howland, G. P., and Ramus, J. (1971). Analysis of blue-green and red algal ribosomal-RNAs by gel electrophoresis. *Arch. Mikrobiol.* **76**:292-298.

55. Ingram, L. O., Pierson, D., Kane, J. F., Van Baalen, C., and Jensen, R. A. (1972). Documentation of auxotrophic mutation in blue-green bacteria: Characterization of a tryptophan auxotroph in *Agmenellum quadruplicatrum. J. Bacteriol.* **111**:112-118.

56. Kameya, T. (1972). Cell elongation and division of chloroplasts. *J. Exptl. Bot.* **23**:62-64.

57. Kasamatsu, H., Robberson, D. L., and Vinograd, J. (1971). A novel closed-circular mitochondrial DNA with properties of a replicating intermediate. *Proc. Natl. Acad. Sci. (USA)* **68**:2252-2257.

58. Kawashima, N., and Wildman, S. G. (1970). Fraction I protein. *Ann. Rev. Plant Physiol.* **21**:325-358.

59. Keenan, T. W., Berezney, R., and Crane, F. L. (1972). Lipid composition of further purified bovine liver nuclear membranes. *Lipids* **7**:212-215.

60. Kessler, B. (1971). Interactions *in vitro* between hormones and DNA. III. Effects of plant and animal hormones on the action of DNA ligase and its relationship to age. *Biochim. Biophys. Acta* **240**:330-342.

61. Kessler, B. (1971). Isolation, characterization and distribution of a DNA ligase from higher plants. *Biochim. Biophys. Acta* **240**:496-505.

62. Kirk, J. T. O. (1971). Chloroplast structure and biogenesis. *Ann. Rev. Biochem.* **40**:161-196.

63. Kroon, A. M. (1971). Structure and function of mitochondrial nucleic acids. *Chimia* **25**:114-124.

64. Küntzel, H. (1969). Proteins of mitochondrial and cytoplasmic ribosomes from *Neurospora crassa. Nature* **222**:142-146.

65. Laflèche, D., and Bové, J. M. (1971). Virus de la mosaïque jaune de Navet: Site cellulaire de la réplication du RNA viral. *Physiol. Veg.* **9**:487-503.

66. Laurent, M., Van Assel, S., and Steinert, M. (1971). Kinetoplast DNA. A unique macromolecular structure of considerable size and mechanical resistance. *Biochem. Biophys. Res. Commun.* **43**:278-284.

67. Lebherz, H. G., and Rutter, W. J. (1969). Distribution of fructose diphosphate aldolase variants in biological systems. *Biochemistry* **8**:109-121.

68. Lee, S. G., and Evans, W. R. (1971). Hybrid ribosome formation from *Escherichia coli* and chloroplast ribosome subunits. *Science* **173**:241-242.

69. Leiter, E. H., LaBrie, D. A., Berquist, A., and Wagner, R. P. (1971). *In vitro* mitochondrial complementation in *Neurospora crassa. Biochem. Genet.* **5**:549-561.

70. Lenk, R., and Penman, S. (1971). Morphological studies of cells grown in the absence of mitochondrial-specific protein synthesis. *J. Cell Biol.* **49**:541-546.

71. Levine, R. P., and Armstrong, J. (1972). The site of synthesis of two chloroplast cytochromes in *Chlamydomonas reinhardi. Plant Physiol.* **49**:661-662.

72. Levine, R. P., and Goodenough, U. W. (1970). The genetics of photosynthesis and of the chloroplast in *Chlamydomonas reinhardi. Ann. Rev. Genet.* **4**:397-408.

73. Lizardi, P. M., and Luck, D. J. L. (1971). Absence of a 5S RNA component in the mitochondrial ribosomes of *Neurospora crassa. Nature New Biol.* **229**:140-142.

74. Lucas-Lenard, J., and Lipmann, F. (1971). Protein synthesis. *Ann. Rev. Biochem.* **40**:409-448.

75. Mahler, H. R., and Perlman, P. S. (1971). Mitochondrio-genesis analyzed by blocks on mitochondrial translation and transcription. *Biochemistry* **10**:2979-2990.

76. Mahler, H. R., Jones, L. R., and Moore, W. J. (1971). Mitochondrial contribution to protein synthesis in cerebral cortex. *Biochem. Biophys. Res. Commun.* **42**:384-389.

77. Manning, J. E., Wolstenholme, D. R., and Richards, O. C. (1972). Circular DNA molecules associated with chloroplasts of spinach, *Spinacia oleracea. J. Cell Biol.* **53**:594-601.

78. Manning, J. E., and Richards, O. C. (1972). Isolation and molecular weight of circular chloroplast DNA from *Euglena gracilis. Biochim. Biophys. Acta.* **259**:285-296.

79. Manning, J. E., and Richards, O. C. (1972). Synthesis and turnover of *Euglena gracilis* nuclear and chloroplast deoxyribonucleic acid. *Biochemistry* **11**:2036-2049.

80. Margulies, M. M. (1971). Concerning the sites of synthesis of proteins of chloroplast ribosomes and of fraction I protein (ribulose-1,5-diphosphate carboxylase). *Biochem. Biophys. Res. Commun.* **44**:539-545.

81. Margulis, L. (1970). *Origin of Eucaryotic Cells,* Yale University Press, New Haven.

82. Martin, T. E., Becknell, J. N., and Kumar, A. (1970). Hybrid 80S monomers formed from subunits of ribosomes from protozoa, fungi, plants and mammals. *Biochem. Genet.* **4**:603-615.

83. Mets, L. J., and Bogorad, L. (1971). Mendelian and uniparental alterations in erythromycin binding by plastid ribosomes. *Science* **174**:707-709.

84. Meyer, R. R., and Simpson, M. V. (1969). DNA synthesis in mitochondria: Differential inhibition of mitochondrial and nuclear DNA polymerases by the mutagenic dyes ethidium bromide and acriflavin. *Biochem. Biophys. Res. Commun.* **34**:238-244.

85. Meyer, R. R., and Simpson, M. V. (1970). Deoxyribonucleic acid biosynthesis in mitochondria. Purification and general properties of rat liver mitochondrial deoxyribonucleic acid polymerase. *J. Biol. Chem.* **245**:3426-3435.

86. Misra, H. P., and Fridovich, I. (1972). The purification and properties of superoxide dismutase from *Neurospora crassa. J. Biol. Chem.* **247**:3410-3414.

87. Mitsui, A., and Arnon, D. I. (1971). Crystalline ferredoxin from a blue-green alga, *Nostoc* sp. *Physiol. Plant.* **25**:135-140.

88. Nagley, P., and Linnane, A. W. (1972). Biogenesis of mitochondria. XXI. Studies on

the nature of the mitochondrial genome in yeast: The degenerative effects of ethidium bromide on mitochondrial genetic information in a respiratory competent strain. *J. Mol. Biol.* **66**:181-193.

89. Nass, M. M. K. (1969). Uptake of isolated chloroplasts by mammalian cells. *Science* **165**:1128-1131.

90. Nass, M. M. K. (1970). Abnormal DNA patterns in animal mitochondria: Ethidium bromide-induced breakdown of closed circular DNA and conditions leading to oligomer accumulation. *Proc. Natl. Acad. Sci. (USA)* **67**:1926-1933.

91. Nass, M. M. K., and Nass, S. (1963). Intramitochondrial fibers with DNA characteristics. I. Fixation and electron staining reactions. *J. Cell Biol.* **19**:593-611.

92. Neal, W. K., Hoffmann, H. P., and Price, C. A. (1971). Sedimentation behavior and ultrastructure of mitochondria from repressed and derepressed yeast, *Saccharomyces cerevisiae*. *Plant Cell Physiol.* **12**:181-192.

93. Neupert, W., and Ludwig, G. D. (1971). Sites of biosynthesis of outer and inner membrane proteins of *Neurospora crassa* mitochondria. *Europ. J. Biochem.* **19**:523-532.

94. Ojala, D., and Attardi, G. (1972). Expression of the mitochondrial genome in HeLa cells. X. Properties of mitochondrial polysomes. *J. Mol. Biol.* **65**:273-289.

95. Paoletti, C., Couder, H., and Guerineau, M. (1972). A yeast mitochondrial deoxyribonuclease stimulated by ethidium bromide. *Biochem. Biophys. Res. Commun.* **48**:950-958.

96. Payne, P. I., and Dyer, T. A. (1971). Characterization of cytoplasmic and chloroplast 5 S ribosomal ribonucleic acid from broad-bean leaves. *Biochem. J.* **124**:83-89.

97. Phillips, D. A., Torrey, J. G., and Burris, R. H. (1971). Extending symbiotic nitrogen fixation to increase man's food supply. *Science* **174**:169-171.

98. Pica-Mattoccia, L., and Attardi, G. (1971). Expression of the mitochondrial genome in HeLa cells. V. Transcription of mitochondrial DNA in relationship to the cell cycle. *J. Mol. Biol.* **57**:615-621.

99. Pigott, G. H., and Carr, N. G. (1972). Homology between nucleic acids of blue-green algae and chloroplasts of *Euglena gracilis*. *Science* **175**:1259-1261.

100. Pollack, J. K., and Woog, M. (1971). Changes in the proportions of two mitochondrial populations during the development of embryonic chick liver. *Biochem. J.* **123**:347-353.

101. Polya, G. M., and Jagendorf, A. T. (1971). Wheat leaf RNA polymerases. I. Partial purification and characterization of nuclear, chloroplast and soluble DNA-dependent enzymes. *Arch. Biochem. Biophys.* **146**:635-648.

102. Polya, G. M., and Jagendorf, A. T. (1971). Wheat leaf RNA polymerases. II. Kinetic characterization and template specificities of nuclear, chloroplast and soluble enzymes. *Arch. Biochem. Biophys.* **146**:649-657.

103. Radsak, K. D., and Freise, H. W. (1972). Stimulation of mitochondrial DNA synthesis in HeLa cells by herpes simplex virus (1). *Life Sci.* **11**:717-724.

104. Raff, R. A., and Mahler, H. R. (1972). The non-symbiotic origin of mitochondria. *Science* **177**:575-582.

105. Reger, B. J., Fairfield, S. A., Epler, J. L., and Barnett, W. E. (1970). Identification and origin of some chloroplast aminoacyl-tRNA synthetases and tRNAs. *Proc. Natl. Acad. Sci. (USA)* **67**:1207-1213.

106. Reid, B. D., and Parsons, P. (1971). Partial purification of mitochondrial RNA polymerase from rat liver. *Proc. Natl. Acad. Sci. (USA)* **68**:2830-2834.

107. Reijnders, L., and Borst, P. (1972). The number of 4-S RNA genes on yeast mitochondrial DNA. *Biochem. Biophys. Res. Commun.* **47**:126-133.

108. Renger, H. C., and Wolstenholme, D. R. (1971). Kinetoplast and other satellite DNAs of kinetoplastic and dyskinetoplastic strains of *Trypanosoma. J. Cell Biol.* **50**:533-540.

109. Richter, D. (1971). Production of mitochondrial peptide-chain elongation factors in yeast deficient in mitochondrial deoxyribonucleic acid. *Biochemistry* **10**:4422-4425.

110. Ridley, S. M., and Leech, R. M. (1970). Division of chloroplasts in an artificial environment. *Nature* **227**:463-465.

111. Rifkin, M. R., and Luck, D. J. L. (1971). Defective production of mitochondrial ribosomes in the *poky* mutant of *Neurospora crassa. Proc. Natl. Acad. Sci. (USA)* **68**:287-290.

112. Riou, G., and Delain, E. (1971). Mitochondrial DNA from cells transformed by adenoviruses and SV 40. *Biochimie* **53**:831-836.

113. Ris, H., and Plaut, W. (1962). Ultrastructure of DNA-containing areas in the cloroplast of *Chlamydomonas. J. Cell. Biol.* **13**:383-391.

114. Robberson, D. L., Kasamatsu, H., and Vinograd, J. (1972). Replication of mitochondrial DNA. Circular replicative intermediates in mouse L cells. *Proc. Natl. Acad. Sci. (USA)* **69**:737-741.

115. Sager, R. (1972). *Cytoplasmic Genes and Organelles,* Academic Press, New York.

116. Sager, R., and Ramanis, Z. (1970). A genetic map of non-Mendelian genes in *Chlamydomonas. Proc. Natl. Acad. Sci. (USA)* **65**:593-600.

117. Schäfer, K. P., and Küntzel, H. (1972). Mitochondrial genes in *Neurospora:* A single cistron for ribosomal RNA. *Biochem. Biophys. Res. Commun.* **46**:1312-1319.

118. Schatz, G., Groot, G. S. P., Mason, T., Rouslin, W., Wharton, D. C., and Saltzgaber, J. (1972). Biogenesis of mitochondrial inner membranes in bakers' yeast. *Fed. Proc.* **31**:21-29.

119. Schlanger, G., Sager, R., and Ramanis, Z. (1972). Mutation of a cytoplasmic gene alters chloroplast ribosome function. *Proc. Natl. Acad. Sci. (USA)* **69**:3551-3555.

120. Shah, S. P. J., and Cossins, E. A. (1970). Pteroylglutamates and methionine biosynthesis in isolated chloroplasts. *FEBS Letters* **7**:267-270.

121. Smith-Johannsen, H., and Gibbs, S. P. (1972). Effects of chloramphenicol on chloroplast and mitochondrial ultrastructure in *Ochromonas danica. J. Cell Biol.* **52**:598-614.

122. Spencer, D., and Whitfeld, P. R. (1969). The characteristics of spinach chloroplast DNA polymerase. *Arch. Biochem. Biophys.* **132**:477-488.

123. Stanier, R. Y., and van Niel, C. B. (1962). The concept of a bacterium. *Arch. Mikrobiol.* **42**:17-35.

124. Stanier, R. Y., Kunisawa, R., Mandel, M., and Cohen-Bazire, G. (1971). Purification and properties of unicellular blue-green algae (Order Chroococcales). *Bacteriol. Rev.* **35**:171-205.

125. Surzycki, S. J., and Rochaix, J. D. (1971). Transcriptional mapping of ribosomal RNA genes of the chloroplast and nucleus of *Chlamydomonas reinhardi. J. Mol. Biol.* **62**:89-109.

126. Swank, R. T., Sheir, G. I., and Munkres, K. D. (1971). *In vivo* synthesis, molecular weights, and proportions of mitochondrial proteins in *Neurospora crassa. Biochemistry* **10**:3924-3931.

127. Swanson, R. F. (1971). Incorporation of high molecular weight polynucleotides by isolated mitochondria. *Nature* **231**:31-34.

128. Tandler, B., Hutter, R. V. P., and Erlandson, R. A. (1970). Ultrastructure of oncocytoma of the parotid gland. *Lab. Invest.* **23**:567-580.

129. Ter Schegget, J., and Borst, P. (1971). DNA synthesis by isolated mitochondria. I.

Effect of inhibitors and characterization of the product. *Biochim. Biophys. Acta* **246**:239-248.

130. Ter Schegget, J., and Borst, P. (1971). DNA synthesis by isolated mitochondria. II. Detection of product DNA hydrogen-bonded to closed duplex circles. *Biochim. Biophys. Acta* **246**:249-257.

131. Tewari, K. K. (1971). Genetic autonomy of extranuclear organelles. *Ann. Rev. Plant Physiol.* **22**:141-168.

132. Thomas, D. Y., and Williamson, D. H. (1971). Products of mitochondrial protein synthesis in yeast. *Nature New Biol.* **233**:196-199.

133. Trench, R. K., Trench, M. E., and Muscatine, L. (1972). Symbiotic chloroplasts: Their photosynthetic products and contribution to mucus synthesis in two marine slugs. *Biol. Bull.* **142**:335-349.

134. Tzagoloff, A. (1971). Assembly of the mitochondrial membrane system. IV. Role of mitochondrial and cytoplasmic protein synthesis in the biosynthesis of the rutamy-cin-sensitive adenosine triphosphatase. *J. Biol. Chem.* **246**:3050-3056.

135. Tzagoloff, A., and Meagher, P. (1972). Assembly of the mitochondrial membrane system. VI. Mitochondrial synthesis of subunit proteins of the rutamycin-sensitive adenosine triphosphatase. *J. Biol. Chem.* **247**:594-603.

136. Ushiyama, R., and Matthews, R. E. F. (1970). The significance of chloroplast abnormalities associated with infection by turnip yellow mosaic virus. *Virology* **42**:293-303.

137. Vesco, C., and Basilico, C. (1971). Induction of mitochondrial DNA synthesis by polyoma virus. *Nature* **229**:336-338.

138. von Wettstein, D., Henningsen, K. W., Boynton, J. E., Kannangara, G. C., and Nielsen, O. F. (1971). The genic control of chloroplast development in barley. In *Autonomy and Biogenesis of Mitochondria and Chloroplasts,* North-Holland, Amsterdam, pp. 205-223.

139. Vorhaben, J. E., and Campbell, J. W. (1972). Glutamine synthetase: A mitochondrial enzyme in uricotelic species. *J. Biol. Chem.* **247**:2763-2767.

140. Wellburn, F. A. M., and Wellburn, A. R. (1971). Chlorophyll synthesis by isolated intact etioplasts. *Biochem. Biophys. Res. Commun.* **45**:747-750.

141. Werner, S., and Neupert, W. (1972). Functional and biogenetical heterogeneity of the inner membrane of rat-liver mitochondria. *Europ. J. Biochem.* **25**:379-396.

142. Westergaard, O., Marcker, K. A., and Keiding, J. (1970). Induction of a mitochondrial DNA polymerase in *Tetrahymena. Nature* **227**:708-710.

143. Wintersberger, U., and Wintersberger, E. (1970). Studies on deoxyribonucleic acid polymerases from yeast. 2. Partial purification and characterization of mitochondrial DNA polymerase from wild type and respiration-deficient yeast cells. *Europ. J. Biochem.* **13**:20-27.

144. Wishnick, M., Lane, M. D., Scrutton, M. C., and Mildvan, A. S. (1969). The presence of tightly bound copper in ribulose diphosphate carboxylase from spinach. *J. Biol. Chem.* **244**:5761-5763.

145. Wolfson, J., Dressler, D., and Magazin, M. (1971). Bacteriophage T7 DNA replication: A linear replicating intermediate. *Proc. Natl. Acad. Sci. (USA)* **69**:499-504.

146. Woodcock, C. L. F., and Bogorad, L. (1970). Evidence for variation in the quantity of DNA among plastids of *Acetabularia. J. Cell Biol.* **44**:361-375.

147. Yen, J. H., and Barr, A. R. (1971). New hypothesis of the cause of cytoplasmic incompatibility in *Culex pipiens L. Nature* **232**:657-658.

148. Zylber, E. A., Perlman, S., and Penman, S. (1971). Mitochondrial RNA turnover in the presence of cordycepin. *Biochim. Biophys. Acta* **240**:588-593.

4

Some Molecular Aspects of Mitochondrial Complementation and Heterosis

Igor V. Sarkissian and H. K. Srivastava*

Department of Biology
Texas A & M University
College Station, Texas, U.S.A.

Studies of heterosis in plants and animals generally emphasize one of four aspects of the phenomenon: yield of final product, the genetic basis of heterosis, the gene product and its function, or the biochemical systems involved in the accomplishment of heterotic phenotype. The latter two, together with information on the rate of formation of the final product, should be a guide for more meaningful studies of heterosis. The ultimate aim of such studies is to remove the mystique of heterosis. This aim can be achieved through operational devices whereby an experimentally induced biochemical event resembling heterosis in inbred individuals can be manipulated at will in the laboratory. It is a great honor to have been asked by the Organizing Committee of this Symposium to discuss some of the work and reasoning that my students and I have done over the past few years that may contribute to the eventual attainment of the ultimate aim.

The first category of study as designated above has been carried on for a very long time and by many workers. It focuses on instances where F_1 hybrids exceed their parents in a given measurable attribute. The second category has also received a great deal of attention, but the genetic aspects of heterosis have not been clearly defined. The other two categories, namely, studies of gene products and biochemical systems, are very closely related, and it is through studies of these aspects that we may gain a glimmer of how heterotic phenotype is achieved (8).

Chloroplasts and mitochondria are obvious but often neglected targets for

* Present address: Merrut University, Merrut, India.

such investigations because they are directly related to growth in general, the most commonly measured attribute of heterotic hybrids, and because they can be easily isolated for *in vitro* studies. Comparing efficiency of these organelles among a hybrid and its parents may yield some knowledge about the means by which the heterotic hybrid surpasses its parents (10). Such studies have already been made, especially on the respiratory system using mitochondria (5, 6, 12-14).

It was observed that plant hybrids which are heterotic in early growth rate had higher respiration rates at early stages of germination as well as higher efficiency of energy conservation in their mitochondria (13). From measurements of mitochondrial activities (ADP:O ratio and cytochrome *c* oxidase activity), two interesting observations have been reported. First, heterotic hybrids showed "mitochondrial heterosis"; i.e., mitochondrial activity was higher than the expected midparent value. Second, *in vitro* mixtures of parental mitochondria showed enhanced oxidative phosphorylation over the midparent, approaching that of the hybrid. This phenomenon has been called "mitochondrial complementation" (5). Complementation is of interest because (a) it may provide an operational means for the study of heterosis, and (b) it may be a useful tool in predicting the potential combining ability of parents (4).

Although mitochondrial heterosis appears to be the result of complementation between parent mitochondria which may be present in the hybrid (11), little is known about the mechanism by which complementation is accomplished. It was recently suggested that particle-to-particle contact between mitochondria of maize is a physical basis for complementation (7). The present investigations were undertaken to shed light on molecular mechanisms of complementation between mitochondria of wheat with the hope that the findings would contribute to the elucidation of biochemical aspects of heterosis.

MATERIALS AND METHODS

The genotypes of wheat used were 28, 31MS, and 31MS × 28. The culturing of seedlings and isolation of mitochondria have been described earlier (13). For each experiment, 1 g of shoot tip served as the source of mitochondria. Complementation was studied in mixtures of mitochondria of parents made 1:1 with respect to mitochondrial protein in all experiments. In the final comparison of activities, mitochondria of the mixture were compared with equivalent mitochondria (based on protein) of shoots of each parent and the hybrid.

Oxygen uptake and phosphorylation were measured by polarographic techniques using a Clark-type oxygen electrode (Yellow Springs Instrument Company). Respiratory rates were calculated from a recorder trace on the basis of 240 μM oxygen in aerated medium (1). Respiratory control indices (RCI) were calculated as given by Chance and Williams (1). ADP:O ratios were determined from the amount of oxygen utilized (μatoms of oxygen) during state 3 of respiration responding to a known amount of added ADP (μmoles).

For measurement of adenosine triphosphatase (ATPase) activity, mitochondria were isolated and assayed as described earlier (13). Mitochondrial nitrogen was estimated following determination of mitochondrial protein with bovine serum albumin as a standard (3).

RESULTS AND DISCUSSION

Both the RCI and ADP:O ratio of the hybrid and the parental mixture utilizing a-ketoglutarate were significantly greater than those of parental mitochondria. Activities of mitochondria of the hybrid and the mixture were not significantly different (Table I). Complementation in the mixture of mitochondria appears to be some type of interaction between organelles. It is evident that complementation occurs in all the mixtures, but maximum complementation was achieved in a mixture of 2 parts of mitochondria 31MS to 1 part of mitochondria of 28 (unpublished). Similar results were obtained by McDaniel and Sarkissian (7) for a 2:1 mixture of mitochondria of maize lines Wf 9 and Ohio 45. It was shown that a mixture of mitochondria of *Triticum timopheevi* Zhuk. and *Triticum aestivum* L. reflects the activity of mitochondria of 31MS (16), which is a product of hybridization between the two species (17). These findings suggested that a cooperative interaction between species-specific mitochondria is involved during complementation. Complementation in maize resulted from interaction between intact mitochondria from the parents, no detectable soluble factors being responsible for the enhancement of oxidative phosphorylation in the mixture of mitochondria (7). In other words, a physical contact (particle-to-particle) between mitochondria of the parents was required for complementation. When mitochondria of wheat parents were mixed, a rapid onset of enhancement of respiratory activity was noted (Table II). But when mitochondria of separate preparations of each parent were mixed, no marked change in oxygen uptake, RCI, or ADP:O ratio was observed.

Table I. Oxidative Phosphorylation by Mitochondria of Wheat[a]

	Mitochondrial source			
	28	31MS	31MS × 28	31MS + 28
Mean RCI (8 expt.)	3.7	4.6	5.3	5.5
Mean ADP:O ratio (8 expt.)	3.2	3.8	5.4	5.8

[a] Basal reaction mixture (3 ml) was composed of 0.3 M mannitol, 10 mM KCl, 5 mM MgCl$_2$, 10 mM each of KH$_2$PO$_4$ and tris-Cl (pH 7.4), 0.75 mg bovine serum albumin/ml, and 4–6 mg mitochondrial protein. Substrate was a-ketoglutarate (a-KG) (10 mM). State 3 of respiration was initiated by 100 μM ADP. Experiments were at $27°$C. Polarographic data were analyzed by Duncan's multiple range test. Treatment means were ranked and compared by using a set of significant ranges, each range dependent on the number of means in the particular comparison. Means not underlined by the same line are significantly different at 5% level of significance.

Table II. Kinetics of Mitochondrial Complementation (α-KG Substrate)[a]

Mixing: 45 sec (between columns II and III)

Mitochondria		I 3	I 4	II 3	II 4	III 3	III 4	IV 3	IV 4
28 and 31 MS	RCI	32[b]	8[b]	35[b]	8.3[b]	43[b]	7.2[b]	42[b]	7[b]
	ADP:O	4.0	3.4	4.2	3.5	5.9	5.6	6.0	5.4
28 and 28	RCI	37[b]	10.5[b]	36[b]	9.7[b]	38[b]	10.5[b]	35[b]	10.3[b]
	ADP:O	3.5	1.1	3.7	3.2	3.6	3.2	3.4	3.1
31 MS and 31 MS	RCI	47[b]	12.4[b]	46[b]	12.1[b]	46.5[b]	12.2[b]	47[b]	12.5[b]
	ADP:O	3.8	3.8	3.9	3.8	3.8	3.7	3.7	3.8

[a] Specific activity of mitochondria as given in Table I. Mitochondria separated by a dialysis membrane were mixed after 2 cycles of respiration. Data are averages of 5 separate experiments.
[b] $\mu M\ O_2$/mg N/min.

Table III shows the effect of diethylstilbestrol (DES) on respiratory activity of mitochondria from the hybrid, its parents, and the parental mixture. The RCI and ADP:O ratios were inhibited in the mixture but less in the hybrid and the individual parents. Table IV demonstrates the effect of DES on the mitochondrial ATPase system. Percent decrease of ATPase activity in the mixture was greater than in the hybrid and the parents, but percent decrease of ATPase

Table III. Effect of Diethylstilbestrol on Mitochondria of Wheat[a]

Mitochondria	Treatment	RCI	ADP:O ratio	Percent decrease in ADP:O ratio
28	Control	3.3	3.0	
	DES ($2 \times 10^{-5}\ M$)	1.9	1.8	40.0
31MS	Control	4.5	3.8	
	DES	1.9	2.6	31.0
31MS × 28	Control	5.4	5.4	
	DES	3.3	3.4	37.0
31MS + 28	Control	5.1	5.6	
	DES	3.2	2.0	64.0

[a] Reaction mixture was as in Table I. Diethylstilbestrol was dissolved in ethanol, and 50 μl of stock solution was added to give the desired concentration. Data are averages of five experiments.

Table IV. Effect of Diethylstilbestrol on Mitochondrial ATPase System[a]

Source of activity	ATPase activity[b]	Percent decrease
28	97.5	—
+ DES	73.4	25
31MS	130.8	—
+ DES	103.4	21
31MS × 28	150.7	—
+ DES	114.6	24
31MS + 28	142.5	—
+ DES	93.0	35

[a] The concentration of DES was $2 \times 10^{-5}\ M$. The procedure for the enzymatic assay is given elsewhere (13). Data are averages of six separate experiments.

[b] μmoles Pi released/mg protein/hr.

activity due to DES in the hybrid was similar to that of parents. These results suggest that complementation by membrane-bound ATPase may depend on the proper conformation of mitochondrial membrane when mitochondria come in close proximity to one another. When the conformation of the membrane was altered by DES as a result of solubilization of protein or enzyme (15), complementation was reduced.

Mitochondrial complementation did not occur when the mixture was treated with the sulfhydryl reagent p-chloromercuribenzoate (PCMB). Both RCI and ADP:O ratio were diminished, each by about 38% (Table V). The effects of PCMB on ATPase of mitochondria are shown in Table VI. These data are similar

Table V. Effect of p-Chloro-mercuribenzoate on Mitochondrial Activity of Wheat[a]

Source of mitochondria	RCI	ADP:O ratio
28	3.4	3.2
10^{-5} PCMB	3.3	3.2
31MS	4.5	3.8
10^{-5} PCMB	4.5	3.7
31MS × 28	5.4	5.7
10^{-5} PCMB	3.5	3.6
31MS + 28	5.2	5.6
10^{-5} PCMB	3.2	3.4

[a] Reaction mixture was as given in Table I. Data are averages of four separate experiments.

Table VI. Effect of PCMB on ATPase Activity[a]

Source of ATPase activity	ATPase activity[b]
28	98.0 ± 7.8
10^{-5} M PCMB (20 min)	96.0 ± 6.8
31MS	115.5 ± 16.2
10^{-5} M PCMB (20 min)	114.2 ± 15.0
31MS × 28	147.5 ± 10.2
10^{-5} M PCMB (20 min)	143.2 ± 12.4
31MS + 28	142.8 ± 7.2
10^{-5} M PCMB (20 min)	96.6 ± 5.2

[a] Data are averages of five separate experiments ± SE.
[b] μmoles Pi released/mg protein/hr.

to those in Table V with respect to degree of inhibition by PCMB. A reasonable explanation could be that sulfhydryl binding of PCMB under the present conditions prevents complementation by ATPase. It is of interest that modification of SH groups by PCMB has been demonstrated to be closely related to a major alteration in the conformation of the enzyme cytochrome oxidase (2). At this point, it can be postulated that SH groups of the membrane-bound ATPase are involved in internal hydrogen bonding to maintain the proper conformation of the active site(s) of the enzyme in the interacting mixture of mitochondria.

While it inhibited the mixture of mitochondria, PCMB did not seem to have any marked effect on state 3 oxidation, RCI, and ADP:O ratio, and ATPase of mitochondria of the parents (Tables V and VI). Such observations give some indication that sulfhydryl groups of the protein available to PCMB binding probably do not participate in the enzymatic reaction. However, the possible role of SH groups in conferring a significant conformational arrangement of the enzyme in interacting mixture of mitochondria cannot be excluded.

The present evidence indicates that the modification of sulfhydryl groups when PCMB reacts with mitochondria results in a complete loss of the kinetic expression of cooperative interaction of the enzymes in the mixture of parental mitochondria. Since sulfhydryl groups are intrinsic to almost all mitochondrial functions (9), it is a reasonable inference that SH groups of these enzymes (a-ketoglutarate dehydrogenase, ATPase, and other respiratory enzymes) may be involved in internal hydrogen bonding to maintain a proper conformation of the active site(s) of the enzyme in the complementing mixture of mitochondria. Mitochondrial complementation and heterosis described here appear to be regulated through the conformation of membrane-bound enzymes. It is suggested that mitochondrial heterosis on the molecular level depends on the proper conformation of the enzymes. Complementation can be viewed as an event between dissimilar mitochondria causing a rapid conformational change in the enzymes permitting efficient energy conservation.

ACKNOWLEDGMENTS

This work was supported in part by a grant from DeKalb AgResearch, Inc.

REFERENCES

1. Chance, B., and Williams, G. R. (1956). The respiratory chain and oxidative phosphorylation. *Advan. Enzymol.* **17**:65-132.
2. Knight, V. A., Settlemire, C. T., and Brierley, G. D. (1968). Differential effects of mercurial reagents upon mitochondrial thiol groups and mitochondrial permeability. *Biochem. Biophys. Res. Commun.* **33**:287-293.
3. Lowry, O. H., Rosebrough, N. J., Farr, A. J., and Randall, R. J. (1951). Protein measurement with the Folin phenol reagent. *J. Biol. Chem.* **193**:265-275.

4. McDaniel, R. G. (1972). Mitochondrial heterosis and complementation as biochemical measure of yield. *Nature New Biol.* **236:**190-191.
5. McDaniel, R. G., and Sarkissian, I. V. (1966). Heterosis: Complementation by mitochondria. *Science* **152:**1640-1642.
6. McDaniel, R. F., and Sarkissian, I. V. (1968). Mitochondrial heterosis in maize. *Genetics* **59:**465-475.
7. McDaniel, R. F., and Sarkissian, I. V. (1970). Kinetics of mitochondrial complementation. *Physiol. Plant.* **23:**335-342.
8. Robbins, W. J. (1962). Hybrid nutritional requirements. In Gowen, J. W. (ed.), *Heterosis,* Iowa State College Press, Iowa City, pp. 14-48.
9. Sanadi, D. R., Lam, K. W., and Kurup, C. K. R. (1968). The role of factor B in the energy transfer reactions of oxidative phosphorylation. *Proc. Natl. Acad. Sci. (USA)* **61:**277-283.
10. Sarkissian, I. V. (1967). Some answers and questions on heterosis. *Agr. Sci. Rev.* **5:**21-25.
11. Sarkissian, I. V., and McDaniel, R. G. (1967). Mitochondrial polymorphism in maize. I. Putative evidence for *de novo* origin of hybrid-specific mitochondria. *Proc. Natl. Acad. Sci. (USA)* **57:**1262-1266.
12. Sarkissian, I. V., and Srivastava, H. K. (1967). Mitochondrial polymorphism in maize. II. Further evidence of correlation of mitochondria complementation and heterosis. *Genetics* **57:**843-850.
13. Sarkissian, I. V., and Srivastava, H. K. (1969). High efficiency, heterosis, and homeostasis in mitochondria of wheat. *Proc. Natl. Acad. Sci. (USA)* **63:**302-309.
14. Sarkissian, I. V., and Srivastava, H. K. (1971). Mitochondrial polymorphism. III. Heterosis complementation, and spectral properties of purified cytochrome oxidase of wheat. *Biochem. Genet.* **5:**57-63.
15. Smoly, J. M., Byington, K. H., Tan, W. C., and Green, D. E. (1968). On the fragmentation of mitochondria by diethylstilbesterol. II. On the relation of the releases of proteins to the mitochondrial membrane. *Arch. Biochem. Biophys.* **128:**774-789.
16. Srivastava, H. K., Sarkissian, I. V., and Shands, H. L. (1969). Mitochondrial complementation and cytoplasmic male sterility in wheat. *Genetics* **63:**611-618.
17. Wilson, J. A., and Ross, W. M. (1962). Male sterility interactions of *Triticum aestivum* L. nucleus and *Triticum timopheevi* cytoplasm. *Wheat Inform. Serv.* **14:**29-30.

5

Studies on Protein Synthesis Elongation Factor 1 from Plant Seeds

Simon Litvak, Adela Tarrago, Beatriz Levy, Lucia Manzocchi, Marta Gatica, and Jorge E. Allende

Departamento de Química
Facultad de Medicina and Departamento de Biología
Facultad de Ciencias
Universidad de Chile, Santiago, Chile

The study of the process of protein synthesis in seed plant embryos is interesting for two reasons. First, the mechanism operative in eukaryotic protein synthesis has not been worked out in the detail achieved with bacterial systems. Obviously, it is important to explore possible differences in the mechanisms and to establish how the whole machinery fits in the context of the cells of these organisms. The second reason is more relevant to the specific system reported on here. The involvement of protein synthesis in the trigger mechanism of germination that changes dormant seed embryos into highly active seedlings offers an opportunity to study protein synthesis in relation to dramatic and fundamental developmental events.

In this chapter, we present some of our studies on protein synthesis elongation factor 1 (EF1) found in wheat and pea seeds. The results obtained suggest that the activity of this factor, which has a key function in the binding of aminoacyl-tRNA to ribosomes, can be modulated and that changes of activity of the factor accompany the germination process.

METHODS AND MATERIALS

The methods for the preparation of ribosomes, tRNA, and partially purified EF1 from wheat embryos have been reported previously (1, 2).

Sucrose gradients were placed in a SW39 rotor using 5-20% sucrose solutions in a buffer containing 10 mM MgCl$_2$, 50 mM NH$_4$Cl, and 10 mM tris-HCl, pH 7.5. The gradients were centrifuged at 37,000 rpm for 18 hr. Fractions of 6 drops were collected. The assays for ^{3}H-GTP binding to EF1 and for ternary complex formation were as described previously (2, 3).

The germination of a genetically pure strain of peas (*Pisum sativum* var. Alaska) was carried out in the dark under sterile conditions. At the various times, the embryos and the cotyledons were separated by hand and homogenized in a medium containing 0.5 M sucrose, 25 mM KCl, 10 mM MgCl$_2$, 10 mM tris-HCl, pH 7.5, and 1 mM 2-mercaptoethanol. The homogenate was spun at 30,000 $\times$ g for 20 min, and the supernatant fraction was used for the determination of GTP-binding activity.

^{3}H-GTP and ^{14}C-amino acids were purchased from New England Nuclear, GMP-PCP was purchased from Miles Laboratories, and ppGpp was a generous gift from Dr. M. Cashel.

RESULTS AND DISCUSSION

Previous results from this laboratory have shown that a partially purified GTP-binding protein obtained from the supernatant fraction of wheat embryo extracts has all the properties of eukaryote EF1 (2). A summary of the evidence is as follows:

a. This protein not only interacts specifically with GTP but also interacts with aminoacyl-tRNA, forming a ternary complex of EF1 · GTP · aminoacyl-tRNA. The formation of this complex can be detected by a nitrocellulose filter assay (3) or by Sephadex G100 chromatography (4).

b. The partially purified factor stimulates considerably the binding of aminoacyl-tRNA to ribosomes at low Mg^{2+} concentrations (2). In the absence of the factor, codon-dependent aminoacyl-tRNA binding to ribosomes requires Mg^{2+} concentrations of 20 mM, while in the presence of the factor and GTP, this requirement is shifted down to 5-7 mM of the cation.

c. The protein factor complements wheat EF2 in permitting polypeptide synthesis (2,5). This has been shown by assaying polyphenylalanine synthesis from phenylalanyl-tRNA in the presence of partially purified wheat translocase (EF2).

Multiple Forms of Wheat EF1

Recently, we have been studying the distribution of the GTP-binding activity of this factor on sucrose gradients.

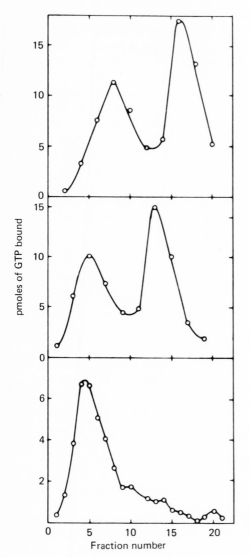

Fig. 1. Sucrose gradient analysis of different stages of purification of wheat EF1. The gradients were run as described in *Methods and Materials.* Top: Approximately 1.5 mg of protein obtained by precipitation between 40 and 80% saturation with $(NH_4)_2SO_4$ of a crude supernatant fraction was added to the gradient. Fractions of 6 drops were collected, and aliquots of 75 μl were used to assay for ^{3}H-GTP-binding activity. Middle: 0.4 mg of protein of the EF1 preparation obtained after DEAE-cellulose chromatography was used in a similar gradient. Bottom: 50 μg of EF1 preparation obtained after phosphocellulose chromatography was analyzed in a similar fashion.

Figure 1 shows gradient analysis of the EF1 preparations at different stages of purification. It is evident that the $(NH_4)_2SO_4$ fraction and DEAE-cellulose fraction present two distinct peaks of GTP-binding activity, while the phosphocellulose fraction contains only the lighter peak. Molecular weight estimation with marker proteins indicates that the light peak (L) is 40,000-50,000 mol wt, while the heavy material (H) is approximately 200,000 mol wt.

Addition of 5×10^{-5} *M* GTP or GDP to the EFl and gradient solutions has a dramatic effect on the patterns obtained with sucrose gradients of the DEAE-cellulose preparation of wheat EF1 (Fig. 2). The disappearance of the heavy fraction is not unspecific, since other nucleotides such as GMP or ATP at similar concentrations do not have this effect.

Figure 3 (top) shows that the H species isolated by pooling the appropriate

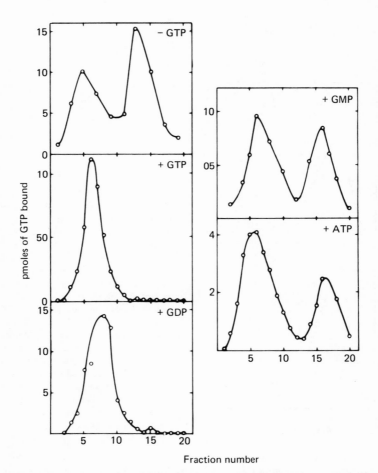

Fraction number

Fig. 2. The effect of different nucleotides on the sucrose gradient profiles of GTP-binding activity of a DEAE-cellulose preparation of wheat EF1. Where indicated, the different nucleotides at a concentration of 5×10^{-4} *M* were incubated with the factor for 10 min at $0°$C. Subsequently, the incubation mixture was added to a gradient that contained throughout 5×10^{-5} *M* of the same nucleotide. The analysis was carried out as in Fig. 1.

fractions from a preparative gradient and recentrifuged in the absence of nucleotide gives essentially only heavy material. Thus if there is an equilibrium between
the two species, it must be greatly in favor of the larger form. Figure 3 (bottom)
shows that the same preparation of H recentrifuged in the presence of 5×10^{-5}
M GTP gives rise to a considerable amount of L species. This finding indicates
that the H species is not inactivated by GTP but rather that it is converted into
the L material. It is interesting to note that in this case there is a large amount of
H material left in the presence of the nucleotide, while in the previous cases this
material disappeared completely. This result, which is reproducible, may indicate
that the conversion from H to L may require some component not present in the
isolated H material.

The two species of GTP-binding protein have EF1 activity when assayed in
the presence of EF2 in polyphenylalanine synthesis. However, they do show an
important difference in their reactivity with aminoacyl-tRNA. As demonstrated
in Table I, ternary complex formation with peak L is very efficient and is

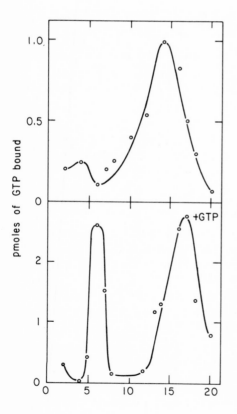

*Fig. 3. Centrifugation of isolated H
peak in the presence and absence of
GTP.* The H-peak fractions from
three gradient tubes were pooled and
precipitated with 80% saturation of
$(NH_4)_2SO_4$. Approximately 0.1 mg
of this preparation was recentrifuged
in a gradient without nucleotide
(top), and 0.2 mg of the same preparation was analyzed in a gradient
with GTP as in Fig. 2 (bottom).

Table I. Formation of EF1·GTP·Aminoacyl-tRNA with the Two Species of Wheat EF1[a]

	pmoles of Phe-tRNA added	pmoles of ^{3}H-GTP retained on filter	pmoles of ternary complex formed
A. With peak L of EF1	–	3.2	–
	0.6	2.52	0.68
	0.9	2.08	1.12
	1.5	1.74	1.46
	3.0	1.37	1.83
	15.0	0.74	2.46
B. With peak H of EF1	–	2.90	–
	0.6	2.62	0.28
	0.9	2.54	0.36
	1.5	2.51	0.39
	3.0	2.60	0.30
	15.0	1.54	1.36

[a] The two species were obtained by sucrose gradient centrifugation of a DEAE-cellulose fraction of EF1 as described in Fig. 1. The two peak fractions were pooled and concentrated by precipitation with 80% saturation of $(NH_4)_2SO_4$. The assay for ternary complex formation with nitrocellulose filters was as previously described (3). The amount of ternary complex is calculated by subtracting the amount of ^{3}H-GTP retained in the presence of Phe-tRNA from the amount sticking to the filter in its absence.

stoichiometric at the lower concentrations of aminoacyl-tRNA. Peak H, on the other hand, is very unreactive with aminoacyl-tRNA and requires large excess of the compound to make significant amounts of ternary complex.

The two species of EF1 also differ markedly in their heat stability. At similar protein concentrations, the H species is much more resistant to inactivation at 37°C than the very labile L species.

Although we are far from knowing the possible significance of the existence of multiple forms of EF1, the specific effect of nucleotides and the different activity observed suggest that interconversion between these forms may play a regulatory role on the activity of this factor.

Moon *et al.* (6) have reported finding multiple forms of calf-brain EF1 and nucleotide effects similar to those reported here. It would seem, therefore, that this may be a general phenomenon of eukaryotic EF1.

Interaction of Wheat EF1 with Aminoacylated Viral RNAs

The RNA of several plant viruses apparently has a tRNA-like structure in the 3'-OH end of the molecule. Thus turnip yellow mosaic virus (TYMV) RNA has

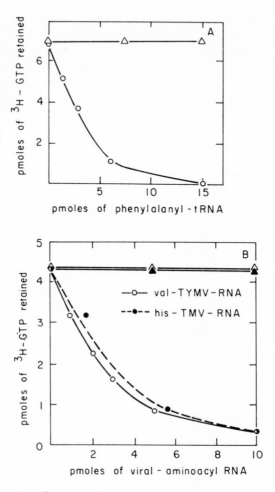

Fig. 4. The interaction of aminoacylated viral RNAs with wheat EF1. The formation of a ternary complex of wheat EF1, ^{3}H-GTP, and aminoacyl viral RNA was measured as described previously (3). Phosphocellulose fractions of wheat EF1, ^{3}H-GTP (specific activity 1 mc/μmole), and the amounts indicated of aminoacylated viral RNAs were used. ○, TYMV RNA acylated with valine; ●, TMV acylated with histidine; △, ▲, the same preparations of viral RNAs. The amount of unacylated viral RNAs was calculated by their acceptor capacity for their respective amino acid.

been found to accept enzymatic esterification with valine by bacterial and eukaryotic valyl-tRNA synthetase (7). In a similar manner, tobacco mosaic virus (TMV) RNA can be esterified with histidine (8, 9) and bromegrass mosaic virus RNA with tyrosine (10).

The physiological significance of this finding is unknown. However, the recent discovery of the participation of elongation factor T_U, the bacterial counterpart of EF1, in the replicase of the RNA phage Qβ (11) induced us to look at a possible relation between plant EF1 and the RNA from plant viruses.

Figure 4, taken from Litvak *et al.* (9), shows that valyl-TYMV RNA and histidyl-TMV RNA are capable of forming a ternary complex with wheat EF1 and GTP, while the unacylated viral RNAs are unable to react. The formation of the ternary complex is measured by its property of going through nitrocellulose filters while the unreacted EF1 · ^{3}H-GTP complex is retained on the membranes.

The interaction of EF1 · GTP with the acylated viral RNAs strengthens the idea that the 3′-OH of these RNAs possesses a "tRNA-like" structure which can be recognized by tRNA enzymes and factors. In addition, it suggests that the aminoacylation of the viral RNAs regulates the capacity of EF1 to interact with the polynucleotide. Whether this interaction is important for viral RNA replication as in the case of Qβ or whether it may be important in the translation of the viral RNA cannot be answered presently.

Variations of a GTP-Binding Activity During Germination of Peas (*Pisum sativum*)

Homogenates of pea embryos and pea cotyledons contain a factor which binds radioactive GTP to nitrocellulose membranes under conditions similar to

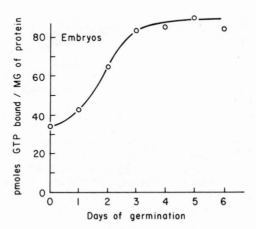

Fig. 5. The variation of GTP-binding activity in extracts of germinating pea embryos. The germination and extraction were carried out as described in *Methods and Materials.* Protein was determined by the method of Lowry; each time, 25 embryos were processed.

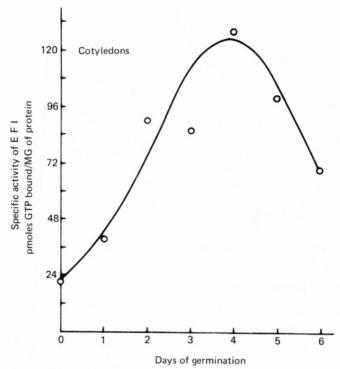

Fig. 6. The GTP-binding activity of pea cotyledons during germination.
The germination and extraction of cotyledons were carried out as
described in *Methods and Materials* and in the caption of Fig. 5.

those for wheat EF1. This activity is largely EF1 since more than 60% can be
made to go through the filter by aminoacyl-tRNA, and partial purification of the
GTP-binding factor results in a preparation that is active in binding aminoacyl-
tRNA to ribosomes and in complementing EF2 in amino acid polymerization.

Experiments were set up to determine whether EF1, as measured by its
GTP-binding capacity in crude preparations, was regulated during the process of
pea germination.

The GTP-binding activity of the 30,000 X g supernatant of three sets of ten
seedlings (embryos and cotyledons) was measured at different times of germination as described in *Methods and Materials*. In addition to GTP binding, the
protein and DNA concentration of these extracts was determined in order to
obtain the specific activity of EF1.

Figure 5 shows the average of the results obtained in three separate experiments. It is clear that the specific activity of EF1 in the seed embryos increases
approximately 2.5-fold in the first 3 days of germination. Subsequently, the high

level of the factor is maintained. In the cotyledons, however, the results are different (Fig. 6). There is a fivefold increase again in the first 3-4 days, but thereafter the levels drop sharply as the cotyledons become senescent. It is interesting that these results are in very close agreement with those obtained for the aminoacyl-tRNA synthetases in pea cotyledons by Goodwin and his associates (12) demonstrating some coordination among the proteins that participate in protein synthesis. We have not shown the results obtained by expressing EF1 activity per DNA concentration instead of protein concentration because the patterns are essentially identical. In addition, the advantage in presenting the data in this fashion is lost due to the polyploidy known to occur in germinating pea seeds.

These very preliminary results would seem to indicate that the activity of EF1 is regulated and increases considerably during the period when great demands are made on the protein synthesis machinery by the triggering of germination. Obviously, there are many questions to be asked about the regulatory mechanisms that are operative and about the effect that this modulation may have physiologically.

ACKNOWLEDGMENT

This study was supported by CIC, the University of Chile, and CONICYT, Chile.

REFERENCES

1. Allende, J. E. (1969). In P. N. Campbell and J. R. Sargent (eds.), *Techniques in Protein Biosynthesis,* Vol. 2, Academic Press, London and New York.
2. Allende, J. E., Tarragó, A., Monasterio, O., Gatica, M., and Ojeda, J. M. (1973). Studies on the binding of aminoacyl-tRNA to wheat ribosomes. In Kenney, F. T., Hamkalo, B. A., Favelukes, G., and August, J. T. (eds.), *Gene Expression and Its Regulation,* Plenum Press, New York, p. 411.
3. Jerez, C., Sandoval, A., Allende, J. E., Henes, C., and Ofengaud, J. (1969). *Biochemistry* 8:3006.
4. Tarragó, A., Monasterio, O., and Allende, J. E. (1970). *Biochem. Biophys. Res. Commun.* 41:765.
5. Legocki, A., and Marcus, A. (1970). *J. Biol. Chem.* 245:2841.
6. Moon, H. M., Redfield, B., and Weissbach, H. (1972). *Proc. Natl. Acad. Sci. (USA)* 69:1249.
7. Yot, P., Pinck, M., Haenni, A. L., Duvanton, H. M., and Chapeville, F. (1970). *Proc. Natl. Acad. Sci. (USA)* 67:1345.
8. Oberg, B., and Philipson, L. (1972). *Biochem. Biophys. Res. Commun.* 48:927.
9. Litvak, S., Tarragó, A., Tarragó-Litvak, L., and Allende, J. E. (1973). *Nature New Biology* 241:88.
10. Hall, T. C., Shih, D. S., and Kaesberg, P. (1973). *J. Virol.* (in press).
11. Blumenthal, T., Landers, T. A., and Weber, K. (1972). *Proc. Natl. Acad. Sci. (USA)* 69:1313.
12. Henshall, J. D., and Goodwin, T. W. (1964). *Phytochemistry* 3:677.

6

Genetic Regulatory Mechanisms in the Fungi

J. Polacco

Departamento de Ciencias Fisiológicas
Sección de Bioquimica, Universidad del Valle
Cali, Colombia

and

S. R. Gross

Division of Genetics
Department of Biochemistry, Duke University
Durham, North Carolina

There are at least two interdependent signals controlling the production, by three unlinked structural genes, of the three leucine biosynthetic enzymes of *Neurospora* (1). Leucine represses the first enzyme, a-isopropylmalate synthetase (the synthetase), the product of the *leu-4* cistron. The synthetase catalyzes the production of a-isopropylmalate (a-IPM), which is the second signal—an obligate inducer for the synthesis of a-IPM isomerase (the isomerase) and β-IPM dehydrogenase (the dehydrogenase), specified, respectively, by the *leu-2* and *leu-1* cistrons. Endogenous a-IPM concentrations respond inversely to endogenous leucine concentration, not only because leucine represses synthetase formation but more importantly because leucine feedback inhibits the catalytic activity of the synthetase (1, 2).

Another leucine auxotrophic class, *leu-3,* is pleiotropic, being deficient in synthesis of both the isomerase and dehydrogenase and exhibiting only one-fourth to one-third maximum synthetase derepression under conditions of leucine limitation (1). The aim of this work is to assign definitively a structural or regulatory role to the *leu-3*[+] gene product.

Table I. Leucine Biosynthetic Enzyme Levels of Derivatives of *leu-3^{cc}* and *leu-3$^+$*

Strain	Genotype	Minimal medium[a]			300 mg leucine/liter		
		Synthetase	Isomerase	Dehydrogenase	Synthetase	Isomerase	Dehydrogenase
R203,r219-1-6A	*leu-3^{cc} inos*	19	45	10	4	55	15
R229,r21-6-201a	*leu-3^{cc} pan-1*	7	53	13	4	56	14
R229,r21-1-11a	*leu-3^{cc} inos*	7	51		4	59	12
R229,r11-1-219a	*leu-3^{cc} pan-1*				8	60	12
R229-1-2a	*leu-3*	32	Trace		3	2	5[b]
R203-1-5a	*leu-3*		2	7	3	Trace	5[b]
STD8A	*leu-3$^+$* (wild type)	14	111	22	20	9	5[b]
STD7a	*leu-3$^+$* (wild type)	5	129	27	13	6	6

[a] Where required, supplemented with either 25 mg/liter inositol, 50 mg/liter calcium pantothenate, or 20 mg/liter L-leucine.

[b] A specific activity of 5 is near the limit of detection of dehydrogenase activity according to the assay procedure employed, and values below 10 are subject to considerable error.

RESULTS

The expressed goal would have been greatly facilitated by temperature-sensitive *leu-3* auxotrophs or *leu-3* revertants. However, none of 1500 leucine-fed survivors of inositol-less death selection (3) at 39°C after MNG or UV mutagenesis was a temperature-sensitive *leu-3* mutant, nor did any of 905 revertants of the three *leu-3* auxotrophs R156, R203, and R229 exhibit temperature-sensitive leucine prototrophy. One class of revertants, however, after a considerable growth lag, grew at wild-type (*leu-3⁺*) rate and produced intermediate levels of isomerase and dehydrogenase (Table I). Production of the isomerase and dehydrogenase by this class (for reasons stated below termed *leu-3^cc*) is not reduced by growth in excess leucine even though the synthetase produced is feedback inhibited and partially repressed by leucine, suggesting that the synthesis of the isomerase and dehydrogenase is insensitive to changes in inducer (*a*-IPM) concentration.

The mutation responsible for this phenotypic class appears to be a secondary mutation within the *leu-3* cistron, since in crosses to *leu-3⁺* strains no *leu-3⁻* segregants were obtained from among nearly 1000 random ascospores. One *leu-3^cc* strain, R229, r21, was crossed to the tight *leu-3* mutant, R156, and only 19 *leu-3⁺* recombinants were obtained among 152,000 viable ascospores.

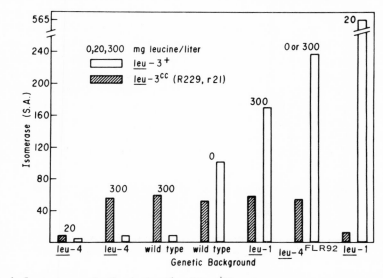

Fig. 1. Isomerase production by leu-3⁺ and leu-3^cc strains. Isomerase specific activity was measured in extracts of *leu-3⁺* (open bars) and *leu-3^cc* (crosshatched bars) grown with 0, 20, or 300 mg leucine/liter. Both *leu-3⁺* and *leu-3^cc* strains had wild-type backgrounds or contained either *leu-4* (synthetaseless), *leu-1* (dehydrogenaseless), or *leu-4^FLR92* (feedback-insensitive synthetase) mutations.

To characterize further the phenotype of the $leu-3^{cc}$ mutants, we sought to vary the endogenous a-IPM concentration. Although mycelia are impermeable to a-IPM, the endogenous inducer level can be varied by proper choice of mutants and by varying available leucine. Thus there may be zero production in synthetaseless ($leu-4$) mutants, low steady-state in wild type, intermediate levels in feedback-insensitive synthetase $leu-4^{FLR92}$ strains, or very high accumulation in strains ($leu-1$ or $leu-2$) blocked in a-IPM utilization. As indicated in Fig. 1, so manipulating a-IPM levels in $leu-3^{cc}$ strains has no effect on isomerase production. But when available leucine is growth limiting, isomerase production is drastically reduced whether a-IPM production is maximal (as in leucine-limited $leu-1$ strains) or zero ($leu-4$ strains). Parallel results have been obtained for the pattern of dehydrogenase production.

The amino acid effect is specific, inasmuch as limiting a $lys-1$, $leu-3^{cc}$ double mutant for lysine does not affect isomerase and dehydrogenase production. To study a possible dependence on the related branched-chain amino acids, isoleucine and valine, the triple mutant $iv-2$, $leu-1$, $leu-3^{cc}$ was synthesized. In addition to a block in isoleucine-valine biosynthesis, it was necessary to introduce one in the leucine pathway to avoid the conversion of valine to leucine (via a-ketoisovalerate).

The data indicate (Table II) that isomerase production in $leu-3^{cc}$ is lowered only when isoleucine, valine, and leucine are all limiting. Because the synthesis of the isomerase and dehydrogenase in $leu-3^{cc}$ is not dependent on a-IPM as an inducer, but exhibits a heretofore undetected dependence on leucine or isoleucine and valine, these revertants are called "conditionally constitutive" ($leu-3^{cc}$).

It is concluded that mutation at the $leu-3$ locus seems to alter specifically the regulation of the isomerase and dehydrogenase. Assigning a regulatory role to the product of the $leu-3$ cistron is reinforced by experiments (4, 7) that show that several *in vitro* properties (k_m, thermolability, cysteine inhibition) of the isomerase are not altered in the $leu-3^{cc}$ strain, nor is there altered thermolability of the isomerase production in low levels by a leaky $leu-3$ (R14) auxotroph.

Heterokaryotic Interactions of the Different *leu-3* Alleles

leu-3⁺ vs. *leu-3*⁻

Dominance relationships and complementation in *Neurospora* can be studied by fusing mycelia of different strains so that different haploid nuclei reside in a common cytoplasm, thus forming a heterokaryon. Heterokaryons between auxotrophic $leu-3^-$ and prototrophic $leu-3^+$ strains do not require leucine. Further, $leu-3^+$ is at least codominant to $leu-3^-$ with respect to isomerase synthesis in preformed obligatory heterokaryons where a-IPM is in excess (Table IIIC). These

Table II. Effect of Leucine and Isoleucine-Valine Supplementation on Leucine Biosynthetic Enzyme Levels in *leu-3^{cc}*

Strain	Genotype	Supplements[a] (mg/liter)			Synthetase	Isomerase	Limitation(s)
		Leu	Ileu	Val			
R229,r21-6-2a	*iv-2 leu-1 leu-3^{cc}*	20	20	20	41	17	Ileu-Val, Leu
		50	20	20	7	53	Ileu-Val
		20	50	50	40	45	Leu
		300	300	300	6	76	None
T322-iv-2-52a	*iv-2 leu-1 leu-3^{+}*	20	20	20	56	368	Ileu-Val, Leu
		50	20	20	10	43	Ileu-Val
		20	50	50	168	525	Leu
		300	300	300	11	97	None

[a] Abbreviations: Leu, leucine; Ileu, isoleucine; Val, valine.

results indicate a "positive" regulatory function of the *leu-3⁺* product—that it is necessary to turn on synthesis of the isomerase and dehydrogenase.

leu-3⁺ vs. *leu-3ᶜᶜ*

The two alleles *leu-3⁺* and *leu-3ᶜᶜ* may be distinguished by the metabolites which stimulate enzyme production—α-IPM in the former and leucine in the latter. Various obligatory heterokaryons formed between *leu-3⁺* and *leu-3ᶜᶜ* and grown on excess leucine (where α-IPM production is low) produce the isomerase at a somewhat constant level virtually independent of the *leu-3⁺:leu-3ᶜᶜ* nuclear

Table III. Leucine Biosynthetic Enzyme Levels in *leu-3ᶜᶜ/leu-3⁺* Heterokaryons Grown on Low Leucine[a]

Heterokaryon or strain	Genotype	Synthetase	Isomerase	Percent *leu-3ᶜᶜ* nuclei
A. R229,r21-3-49a + D221-P1-76a	*leu-1 leu-3ᶜᶜ pan-1* + *leu-1 leu-3⁺ inos*	131	399	61
R229,r21-3-49a	*leu-1 leu-3ᶜᶜ pan-1*	52	13	100
D221-P1-76a	*leu-1 leu-3⁺ inos*	158	608	0
B. R229,r21-3-62a + D221-P1-76a	*leu-1 leu-3ᶜᶜ leu-2 pan-1* + *leu-1 leu-3⁺ leu-2⁺ inos*	99	333	32
R229,r21-3-49a + D221-P1-68a	*leu-1 leu-3ᶜᶜ leu-2⁺ pan-1* + *leu-1 leu-3⁺ leu-2 inos*	119	268	79
C. R156-K-190a + D221a	*leu-1 leu-3⁻ pan-1* + *leu-1 leu-3⁺ inos*	118	351	45[b]
R156-8-1A[c]	*leu-1 leu-3*	46	Trace	
R229-1-2a	*leu-3*	32	Trace	

[a] All heterokaryons and *leu-1* strains were grown on 20 mg/liter leucine.
[b] Represents the percentage of *leu-3⁻* nuclei in a *leu-3⁻/leu-3⁺* heterokaryon.
[c] Data from Gross (1).

ratio (three examples are given at the top of Table IV). This result seems to indicate a partial dominance of leu-3⁺ over leu-3^cc under conditions of low a-IPM production. Indeed, if leucine is in excess and a-IPM is absent, as is obtained when both nuclei are leu-4 (synthetaseless), leu-3⁺ is almost completely dominant (Table IV). In the opposite situation, when a-IPM is in excess and leucine very low (as when both component nuclei are leu-1 or dehydro-genaseless), isomerase production is induced to levels intermediate between "turned-off" leu-3^cc and "turned on" leu-3⁺ (Table IIIA). The observations suggest that in the absence of a-IPM and presence of excess leucine, leu-3⁺ is functionally dominant to leu-3^cc, but that in the opposite situation the two alleles function codominantly.

Table IV. Leucine Biosynthetic Enzyme Levels in leu-3^cc/leu-3⁺ Hetero-karyons Grown on High Leucine[a]

Heterokaryon or strain	Genotype	Synthetase	Isomerase	Percent leu-3^cc nuclei
R229,r11-1-11a + Y152-m4⁰-2-5a	leu-3^cc pan-1 + leu-3⁺ ad-5	11	21	65
R229,r21-2-5a + DK52-20-647a	leu-3^cc pan-1 + leu-3⁺ nic-1	17	19	32
R229,r21-1-11a + DK52-20-647a	leu-3^cc inos + leu-3⁺ nic-1	17	16	48
R229,r11-1-219a	leu-3^cc pan-1	8	60	100
R229,r21-1-11a	leu-3^cc inos	4	59	100
R229,r21-4-11A + R59-11-19A	leu-4 leu-3^cc inos + leu-4 leu-3⁺ ad-5	0	7	53
R229,r21-4-11A	leu-4 leu-3^cc inos	0	46	100
R59-11-19A	leu-4 leu-3⁺ ad-5	0	5	0
STD7a	leu-3⁺ (wild type)	13	6	0
STD8A	leu-3⁺ (wild type)	20	9	0

[a] Growth medium was supplemented with 300 mg/liter leucine.

Note that in *leu-3^{cc}/leu-3^{+}* heterokaryons (Table IIIB) that are heterokaryotic as well for *leu-2^{+}* and *leu-2* (isomeraseless), isomerase synthesis is elevated regardless of the nuclear location of the two *leu-3* alleles. Therefore, the effect of the products of the two *leu-3* alleles on isomerase production must be transnuclear.

leu-3^{-} vs. *leu-3^{cc}*

Unexpectedly, preformed obligatory *leu-3^{cc}/leu-3^{-}* heterokaryons do not grow on either liquid or solid minimal medium before the *leu-3^{-}* component itself will grow. As indicated in Fig. 2, however, the addition of isoleucine plus valine, which enhances the growth of *leu-3^{cc}* but not *leu-3^{-}*, stimulates growth of the heterokaryons after a considerable lag period. Isoleucine alone is less effective, and valine hardly stimulates growth of the heterokaryon at all. On the basis of the growth responses, *leu-3^{-}* is dominant to *leu-3^{cc}* in minimal medium, but in the presence of isoleucine plus valine the *leu-3^{cc}* phenotype is expressed.

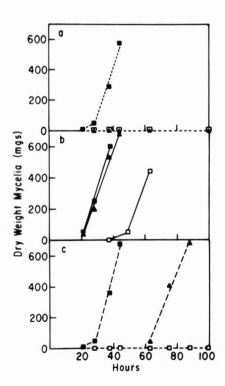

Fig. 2. Growth on liquid medium. (a) *leu-3* (-----), (b) *leu-3^{cc}* (———), and (c) the *leu-3/leu-3^{cc}* obligatory heterokaryon (– – –). Supplements: □, none; ■, 300 mg leucine/liter; ▲, and 300 mg isoleucine-valine/liter.

Isomerase and dehydrogenase levels in *leu-3^{cc}/leu-3$^-$* heterokaryons grown on limiting or excess leucine are higher than those of the *leu-3$^-$* component alone but significantly less than expected for a *leu-3^{cc}* homokaryon (Table V). Surprisingly, however, after growth on isoleucine and valine the levels of the

Table V. Leucine Biosynthetic Enzyme Levels in *leu-3$^-$/leu-3^{cc}* Heterokaryons

Heterokaryon[a] or strain	*leu-3$^-$* allele	Supplement (mg/liter)	Synthe-tase	Isomerase	Dehydro-genase	Percent *leu-3^{cc}* nuclei
			Leucine			
R156a + R229,r21-6-201a	R156	20	9	14	6	
		300	9	20	7	30
R203-1-5a + R229,r21-6-201a	R203	20	11	16	10	
		300	8	19	9	22
R229-1-2a + R229,r21-6-201a	R229	20	14	11	7	
		300	12	16	7	45
R156a	R156	20	37	Trace	Trace	
		300	13	Trace	Trace	
R203-1-5a	R203	20	19	2	7	
		300	4	Trace	5	
R229-1-2a	R229	20	32	2		
		300	3	Trace	5	
			Isoleucine and valine			
R156a + R229,r21-6-201a	R156	300	6	40	19	65
R203-1-5a + R229,r21-6-201a	R203	300	5	67	18	62

a All heterokaryons have the genotype $\dfrac{leu\text{-}3^-\,inos}{leu\text{-}3^{cc}\,(R229,r21)\,pan\text{-}1}^{+}$

two enzymes are near that of the $leu\text{-}3^{cc}$ parent (Table V). Synthetase production by the heterokaryons, whether grown on low leucine or isoleucine and
valine, is low, suggesting that once growth is initiated leucine ceases to be
limiting. Indeed, the mycelial yield in each case was higher than expected on the
basis of growth limitation by leucine. The $leu\text{-}3^{cc}/leu\text{-}3^{-}$ heterokaryons, then,
have the extraordinary property of expressing the $leu\text{-}3^{-}$ auxotrophic phenotype
on unsupplemented medium, but upon amino acid supplementation they express
the $leu\text{-}3^{cc}$ phenotype with respect to growth and enzyme production.

CONCLUSIONS

From the data so far presented, one may derive a rough model for the
regulatory action of the $leu\text{-}3^{+}$ product if it is assumed that regulation is at the
level of transcription and that the effector molecules interact directly with
aporegulator. Accordingly, the $leu\text{-}3^{+}$ product must have (a) a binding site(s) for
stretches of DNA adjacent to or within the unlinked $leu\text{-}1$ and $leu\text{-}2$ cistrons, (b) a
binding site(s) for the inducer a-IPM, and (c) a binding site(s) for the branched-
chain amino acids (prediction of this site on the $leu\text{-}3^{+}$ product seems inescap-
able, since it could hardly have risen *de novo* in the mutational sequence $leu\text{-}3^{+}$
to $leu\text{-}3^{-}$ to $leu\text{-}3^{cc}$).

All of the information reported here indicates that a-IPM must be bound by
a $leu\text{-}3^{+}$ product to switch on isomerase and dehydrogenase synthesis. In view of
the lack of dependency on a-IPM for the "on" function of $leu\text{-}3^{cc}$, it is tempting
to conclude that the mutation of $leu\text{-}3^{+}$ to $leu\text{-}3^{-}$ resulted in the loss of an
effective a-IPM binding site and that the subsequent mutation of $leu\text{-}3^{-}$ to
$leu\text{-}3^{cc}$ altered the defective regulatory molecule so that a "switch-on" function
results when the branched-chain amino acid binding site is occupied.

The behavior of the three $leu\text{-}3$ alleles in heterokaryons suggests first of all
that the $leu\text{-}3^{+}$ product functions transnuclearly. In the presence of a-IPM, it is
capable of switching on isomerase synthesis in $leu\text{-}3^{+}/leu\text{-}3^{cc}$ heterokaryons
nearly equally well, irrespective of its nuclear location relative to a functional
$leu\text{-}2$ cistron. Second, the $leu\text{-}3^{+}$ product, in the absence of a-IPM (i.e., when
both nuclei of a heterokaryon are $leu\text{-}4^{-}$), is nearly completely dominant to
$leu\text{-}3^{cc}$. This implies either preferential binding of the $leu\text{-}3^{+}$ regulator-minus
a-IPM to the DNA regulatory sites or some multimeric interaction with the
$leu\text{-}3^{cc}$ product which renders it inactive. The dominance of the $leu\text{-}3^{-}$ product
to $leu\text{-}3^{cc}$ in the absence of added branched-chain amino acids suggests the same
sorts of interactions. Here the expression of the $leu\text{-}3^{cc}$ phenotype depends on
the presence of the appropriate effectors, the branched-chain amino acids. The
heterokaryon behavior suggests different conformational states of the $leu\text{-}3$

products in the presence or absence of effectors but does not distinguish between differential DNA binding of the *leu-3* products or the formation of mixed multimers with different DNA affinities.

DISCUSSION

The unexpected branched-chain amino acid dependence of *leu-3^{cc}* deserves further consideration. Heretofore, no such signal by the branched-chain amino acids *per se* could be demonstrated in the regulation of isomerase and dehydrogenase synthesis, not only because of the masking signal of the primary effector, a-IPM, but also because as mentioned at the beginning of this chapter endogenous a-IPM levels are related to endogenous leucine levels. It appears, then, that removal of dependence on the primary positive effector for a response revealed the involvement of the branched-chain amino acids.

The branched-chain amino acid dependence explains the anomalous growth lag of *leu-3^{cc}* on minimal medium (Fig. 2b). It can also account for the remarkable change from the exclusive requirement for leucine for growth of *leu-3^{-}* to the enhancement of growth of *leu-3^{cc}* by isoleucine and valine (Fig. 2a,b). Early logarithmically growing mycelia would drain endogenous leucine, isoleucine, and valine levels, which in turn would result in lowered isomerase and dehydrogenase synthesis. We have verified this; isomerase and dehydrogenase levels from young *leu-3^{cc}* mycelia are very low (4). The addition of the branched-chain amino acids raises these levels.

Isoleucine and valine supplementation, although not as effective as leucine in initiating growth of *leu-3^{cc}*, appears more effective than leucine in evoking synthesis of the two enzymes (4). This suggests that their derivatives, rather than isoleucine and valine themselves, are involved in switching on isomerase and dehydrogenase synthesis. Accordingly, conversion to the active effectors would depend on protein synthesis, which, because of the enzyme deficiencies of *leu-3^{cc}*, would be limited by available leucine during germination. Thus leucine, by satisfying a growth requirement, would function only to facilitate the formation of effectors from endogenous isoleucine and valine.

The "new" effector role of isoleucine and valine in *leu-3^{cc}* is indicative of a central regulatory role of the *leu-3* cistron in branched-chain amino acid metabolism. For instance, neither isoleucine nor valine alone is as effective as both compounds in concert in stimulating isomerase and dehydrogenase production. This suggests the possibility that the production of enzymes common to isoleucine and valine biosynthesis (5), as well as those for leucine biosynthesis, may be shut down early in the growth of *leu-3^{cc}*. Actually, Olshan and Gross (6) have shown that the *leu-3^{+}* product and a-IPM are required for maximum production of most of the enzymes of isoleucine and valine biosynthesis. As has been mentioned briefly here, the $leu\text{-}3^+$ product is also involved in leucine regulation of the synthetase, since $leu\text{-}3$ (and $leu\text{-}3^{cc}$) mutants never attain more than one-third maximum synthetase production (1, 6). Further levels of a branched-chain amino acid permease depend, at least in part, on endogenous α-IPM levels and the $leu\text{-}3$ allele present (7).

A comparison of the regulation of the leucine biosynthetic pathways of *Salmonella* (8) on the one hand and *Neurospora* on the other illustrates several of the general differences between fungal and bacterial regulatory mechanisms. The enzyme-catalyzed reactions leading to leucine are identical in both systems. However, the structural genes are dispersed in *Neurospora* (1) and tightly clustered in *Salmonella* (9). As the linkage patterns perhaps indicate, bacterial genetic regulation is generally less complex than that of the fungi (10). The bacterial leucine structural genes are under coordinate repressive control—leucine being the only detectable regulatory signal (8). Existence of a class of mutants exhibiting polarity and another having 0^c properties (11) suggests that the leucine gene cluster is an operon under negative control.

In this and other fungal systems examined, more than one effector is involved in expression of related genes (10). In addition, internal induction by the pathway intermediate, α-IPM, of the subsequent pathway enzymes is a quite sophisticated control mechanism, especially since the production of the inter-mediate is subject to end-product inhibition and repression. Gross (10) has characterized such a situation as the flux of carbon through the pathway controlling the levels of the pathway enzymes. Such sequential induction has also been observed in yeast pyrimidine biosynthesis (12). Also, in contrast to bacterial systems, positive control plays a much more predominant role, as evidenced by the wide occurrence of pleiotropic negative mutants such as $leu\text{-}3$, which have been shown to be at control loci and recessive to the wild-type allele (13-16). Finally, with possibly one exception (16) there have been no reported 0^c mutations in the fungi; such pleiotropic, constitutive, *cis*-dominant mutations have been mapped near one extreme of several bacterial operons. Although "operon-type" gene clusters are not common in the fungi, under certain condi-tions 0^c-type mutations could have been selected for single-gene expression. For instance, a suppressor of $leu\text{-}3$ auxotrophy, unlinked to $leu\text{-}2$ or to $leu\text{-}3$, elevates partially only isomerase activity and has no effect on that of the dehydrogenase (7). It is conceivable, then, that an 0^c-like mutation at the $leu\text{-}2$ locus could be selected among a population of $leu\text{-}3$ "revertants." None has yet been found. It may be argued that genes under positive control should not be expected to yield 0^c-type mutations. However, in the bacterial L-arabinose system of *Escherichia coli*, which is under positive control, *cis*-dominant, low constitutive mutations have been mapped near one extreme of the L-arabinose operon (17, 18).

ACKNOWLEDGMENT

This work was supported by NSF Grant GB-27575. J.P. was a predoctoral trainee supported by USPHS Training Grant GM 02007 from the NIGMS.

REFERENCES

1. Gross, S. R. (1965). *Proc. Natl. Acad. Sci. (USA)* **54**:1538.
2. Webster, R. E., and Gross, S. R. (1965). *Biochemistry* **4**:2309.
3. Lester, H. E., and Gross, S. R. (1959). *Science* **129**:572.
4. Polacco, J., and Gross, S. R. (1973). *Genetics* **74** (in press).
5. Wagner, R. P., *et al.* (1964). *Genetics* **49**:865.
6. Olshan, A., and Gross, S. R. In preparation.
7. Polacco, J. (1971). The *leu-3* cistron as a genetic regulatory element for the leucine biosynthetic enzymes of *Neurospora*. Doctoral thesis, Duke University.
8. Burns, R. O., *et al.* (1966). *J. Bacteriol.* **91**:1570.
9. Margolin, P. (1963). *Genetics* **48**:441.
10. Gross, S. R. (1969). *Ann. Rev. Genet.* **3**:395.
11. Calvo, J. M. (1969). *Genetics* **61**:777.
12. LaCroute, F. (1968). *J. Bacteriol.* **95**:824.
13. Marzluf, G. A., and Metzenberg, R. L. (1968). *J. Mol. Biol.* **33**:423.
14. Valone, J. A., *et al.* (1971). *Proc. Natl. Acad. Sci. (USA)* **68**:1555.
15. Pateman, J. A., and Cove, D. J. (1967). *Nature* **215**:1234.
16. Douglas, H., and Hawthorne, D. C. (1966). *Genetics* **54**:911. Douglas H., and Hawthorne, D. C. (1972). *J. Bacteriol.* **109**:1139.
17. Englesberg, E., *et al.* (1969). *J. Mol. Biol.* **43**:281.
18. Englesberg, E., *et al.* (1969). *Proc. Natl. Acad. Sci. (USA)* **62**:1100.

7

Feedback-Resistant Mutants of Histidine Biosynthesis in Yeast

Francine Rasse-Messenguy and Gerald R. Fink

Department of Genetics, Development, and Physiology
Cornell University
Ithaca, New York

Mutants resistant to the histidine analog 1, 2, 4-triazole-3-alanine have been isolated and characterized. All members of one group, *TRA1*, map in the gene encoding the first enzyme of histidine biosynthesis, have a feedback-resistant first enzyme, and are dominant in diploids. As a consequence of the altered feedback properties, some *TRA1* mutants have an internal histidine pool 12–15 times higher than that of wild type. In addition to their inability to control the size of their histidine pool, these mutants are unable to derepress normally. Some implications of these results for the study of feedback-resistant strains of higher plants are discussed.

INTRODUCTION

One goal of plant breeders is to select varieties of plants which have greater nutritive value than the standard varieties. Recent advances in plant cell genetics suggest that the most efficient approach to this problem may be the selection of the desired strains on a petri plate and not in the field. The remarkable selective schemes designed to obtain regulatory mutants of bacteria may then serve as the paradigm for higher plant work. Using these procedures, it is possible in a matter of days to select bacterial strains which make enormous amounts of a specified amino acid or have levels of a particular enzyme 50–100 times that of the normal (1, 2). The ease and rapidity with which such results can be achieved in *Escherichia coli* are due to this organism's rapid rate of growth as well as to the judicious use of amino acid analogs. These compounds have provided the tools for selection of interesting regulatory mutants out of millions of uninteresting normal strains (3). In prokaryotic systems, mutants resistant to amino acid analogs have been shown to be altered in either of two regulatory controls: (a) feedback inhibition, which involves inhibition of the enzyme catalyzing the first step in a pathway by the end product of the pathway; and (b) repression, which involves control of the rate of synthesis of the enzymes in the pathway. Although a great deal is known about these controls in bacteria, it is only recently that information concerning the effects of regulatory mutations in eukaryotes has become available (4, 5). Of particular importance for plant geneticists working with diploid organisms is whether eukaryotic regulatory mutations are dominant or recessive and whether they lead to higher levels of the desired end products, amino acids and proteins.

In this chapter, we would like to summarize our studies on feedback-resistant mutations affecting the first enzyme of histidine biosynthesis in baker's yeast (*Saccharomyces cerevisiae*). Yeast is a simple eukaryote which can be grown as either a haploid or a diploid, and this feature of its life cycle permits a rapid test of the dominance or recessiveness of any new mutation. Thus, studies with yeast may serve as models for certain kinds of biochemical genetic situations in higher plants.

MUTANT ISOLATION AND PROPERTIES

The haploid yeast strain αS288C (wild type) was spread on a minimal medium plate containing the histidine analog (Fig. 1) 1, 2, 4-triazole-3-alanine (TRA) at a concentration of 0.25 mM. Medium containing citrulline or proline rather than ammonia was used because the wild type is more sensitive to TRA when these amino acids are used as a source of nitrogen. The inhibition of growth by TRA is overcome if 0.1 mM histidine is added to the plate; no other amino acid at a comparable concentration can overcome TRA inhibition. Therefore, TRA *in vivo* is specific for histidine metabolism. Mutant strains resistant to the analog appeared after 6–8 days of incubation. These were purified and

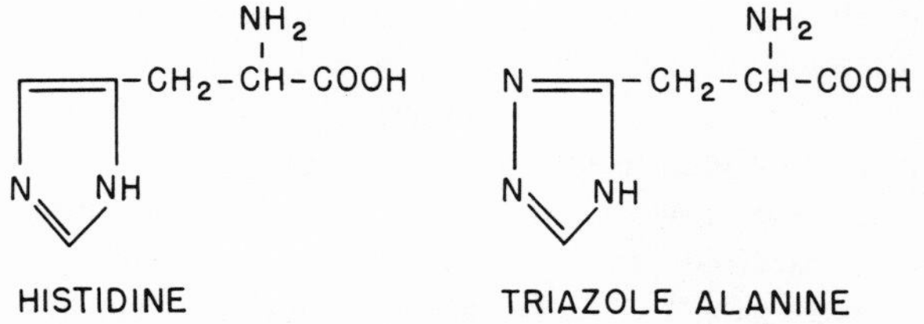

Fig. 1. The structure of histidine and the analog 1,2,4-triazole-3-alanine (TRA).

characterized genetically and biochemically. All of the strains were resistant to TRA upon retesting.

The strains could be divided into two groups on the basis of their growth responses on medium containing a high histidine concentration (30 mM histidine). One group of TRA-resistant mutants grew on high histidine, and the other did not. We have found that yeast strains are inhibited by high concentrations of only two of the 20 amino acids, histidine and methionine. External histidine at a concentration of 6 mM will inhibit the growth of wild-type yeast strains, but mutant strains with an impaired permeation system are resistant. Fifteen of the 40 TRA^R strains, classified as $TRA2$, were resistant to high histidine concentrations. Further analysis indicates that all $TRA2$ mutants are like the strains containing a mutation in the gene called AAP (6, 7) which controls the entry of amino acids into yeast cells. This genetic assignment suggests that the $TRA2$ mutants are resistant to TRA because they are unable to concentrate it. Uptake studies show directly that $TRA2$ mutants have a reduced ability to take up labeled amino acids as compared with isogenic wild-type strains. All of our $TRA2$ mutations are recessive.

Dominance of $TRA1$ Mutations

Of the 25 TRA-resistant mutants which were sensitive to high histidine, 18 appeared to map in or close to the $his1$ gene. This gene codes for the phosphoribosyltransferase, the enzyme catalyzing the first step of histidine biosynthesis (8). The map location is based on crosses in which each of the TRA-resistant mutants was mated with a strain carrying a temperature-sensitive his-1 mutation. In a cross of TRA^R $HIS1^+ \times TRA^S$ $his1^-$, it is difficult to diagnose the TRA resistance or sensitivity of the his^- (histidine-requiring) spores, because histidine supplementation would make all spores resistant. Strains carrying the temperature-conditional his^- mutation have the virtue that they require a histidine supplement at 37°C but not at 23°C. Thus the segregation of TRA resistance can be tested at 23°C and the segregation of $his1$ at 37°C. The 25 histidine-sensitive TRA^R strains were tested in crosses by this $his1$ strain, and 18 failed to recombine with the $his1$ mutation (all asci in these crosses were 2 TRA^R $HIS1^+$: 2 TRA^S $his1^-$). These mutants were all designated $TRA1$.

The $TRA1$ mutants differ among themselves in a number of properties. Some, but not all, of the mutants excrete histidine (Fig. 2). The excretion property segregates together with TRA resistance, and thus both traits are considered a consequence of the same mutation. Among the excreters are those which excrete a great deal of histidine ($TRA1-15$, -17) and those which excrete smaller amounts ($TRA1-1$, -3, -4, -13). All of the strains show normally on minimal medium except $TRA1-8$, which grows slowly on minimal medium but normally on minimal plus histidine. All 18 $TRA1$ mutations are *dominant* in

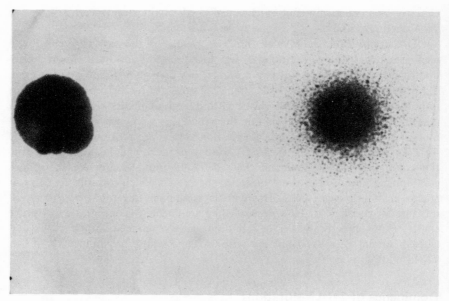

Fig. 2. The excretion of histidine by TRA1-17. The two colonies of yeast are growing on a petri plate covered with a confluent suspension of a histidine-requiring strain. Because the medium has no histidine, the histidine-requiring strain cannot grow. The colony on the left is a standard yeast strain, that on the right is *TRA1-17.* The fuzzy growth of the histidine auxotroph around the excreting colony shows that *TRA1-17* excretes enough histidine to support the growth of a histidine mutant.

diploids for their resistance to TRA. Those mutations which lead to histidine excretion in the haploids also lead to excretion when heterozygous in diploids. To show that the dominance of *TRA1* mutants can be used as a selective screen, we have selected four TRA^R mutations by direct plating of diploids on TRA. Genetic studies indicate that these *TRA1* mutants map in the *his1* gene and have properties similar to other *TRA1* mutations selected in haploid strains.

Regulatory Defects in *TRA1* Mutants

Since the *TRA1* mutations all mapped in the gene coding for the first enzyme in the pathway but did not significantly affect the catalytic activity of this enzyme, it seemed likely that these mutations might affect the regulatory site. The phosphoribosyltransferase extracted from a wild-type strain is specifically inhibited by histidine (apparent $K_i = 6 \times 10^{-4} M$). Extracts of *TRA1-8, -15, -17,* and *-19* were prepared, and in each extract the reaction catalyzed by the first enzyme was tested in the presence and absence of L-histidine. No inhibition of this reaction was detectable in mutant extracts in the range of histidine concentrations where the enzyme from wild type was 90% inhibited. In fact, only at concentrations of histidine a hundredfold higher ($10^{-1} M$) was there any appreciable inhibition of the enzyme from these mutant strains. These results are similar to those of Sheppard (9) for thiazole alanine resistant mutants of *Salmonella typhimurium*. In most *TRA1* strains, the specific activity of the first enzyme in the biosynthetic reaction is normal and the strains show no histidine requirement. Only *TRA1-8* has a lower specific activity than wild type. These results provide strong evidence that the molecular consequence of the *TRA1* mutation is the loss of feedback sensitivity of the first enzyme.

The loss of the feedback control on the histidine pathway in a *TRA1* mutant

Table I. Pool Size of Histidine in Wild-Type and Mutant Strains of Yeast[a]

Strain	Genotype	Histidine excretion	Histidine pool (mM)	Arginine pool (mM)
S288C	Wild type	−	6.3	13.6
his6	his⁻	−	58.5	15.5
TRA1-17	TRA^R FB^R	+++	88.5	15.7
TRA1-8	TRA^R FB^R	−	2.0	56.3
TRA1-19	TRA^R FB^R	−	19.0	14.35

[a] The cells were harvested during the logarithmic phase of growth ($5 \times 10^6 - 10^7$ cells/ml), and the amino acid pools were extracted with boiling water as described by Ramos *et al.* (10). The concentration of histidine and arginine in the extracts was determined in an amino acid analyzer and related to the concentration in the cells. The volume of the cells is taken as four times their dry weight. For each culture, two values were obtained; they do not differ by more than 10% when the cells are taken in log phase. However, if the pools are determined at other stages of growth, the values are slightly lower (see Table II). All strains were grown in standard minimal medium (Difco yeast nitrogen base without amino acids). The *his6* strain carries a mutation in the fourth step of the histidine pathway and was grown on medium containing histidine at a concentration of 0.3 mM. As shown in the table, cells grown with a histidine supplement concentrate the histidine 200-fold. The designation FB^R means that the phosphoribosyltransferase has been extracted from the strain and shown to be resistant to feedback inhibition by histidine.

Table II. Relationship Between the Histidine Pool and the
Extent of Derepression[a]

	Histidine pool (mM)		his4A activity	
Strain	Initial	6 hr starvation	Initial	6 hr starvation
S288C	4.25	1.44	1.42	11.35
his6	38.0	1.50	1.72	8.55
TRA1-8	2.0	N.T.	2.61	6.70

[a] The histidine pools were extracted and measured as described in
Table I. Cells for inoculation were grown in minimal medium
(S288C and TRA1-8) or minimal plus 0.3 mM histidine (his6).
These cells were washed and placed in starvation medium—
minimal plus 20 mM AT (S288C and TRA1-8) or minimal (his-6).
The histidine pool and the activity of the his4A gene product, the
cyclohydrolase, were determined at the time of inoculation into
starvation medium (initial) and after 6 hr of starvation. The
cyclohydrolase activity (his4A) is measured in a Gilford recording
spectrophotometer by following the increase in absorbancy at 290
mμ resulting from the conversion of phosphoribosyl-AMP to phos-
phoribosyl-formimino aminoimidazole carboxamide ribotide
(BBM II). The numbers in the table represent the specific activity
as μmoles of BBM II formed/hr/mg protein.

should destroy the strain's ability to regulate the size of the histidine pool. To
see whether this prediction was correct, the size of histidine pool in wild type
and several TRA1 mutants grown on minimal medium was compared (Table I).
The size of the arginine pool was also measured as a control. The normal pool in
wild type can be increased tenfold by addition of low concentrations of histidine
to the medium. Mutants TRA1-17 and TRA1-19 have histidine pools that are,
respectively, 15 and 3 times larger than that of wild type. The histidine pool of
TRA1-17 is so high that this strain excretes the amino acid into the medium.
The mutant TRA1-8 has a pool of histidine lower than that of wild type. In this
strain, the catalytic site as well as the regulatory site of the first enzyme is
impaired. Since the strain cannot carry out the synthesis of histidine at the
normal level, the pool size is low despite the altered feedback control.

TRA1-8, as is shown in Table II, does not respond normally to the low internal
histidine pool. A low histidine pool is the signal to turn on the genes encoding
the histidine biosynthetic enzymes to a higher level, allowing the cell to make
more histidine. Situations evoking this "derepression" of the histidine enzymes
can be created experimentally in two ways. A histidine-requiring mutant placed
on medium lacking histidine rapidly exhausts its internal supply of histidine. As
shown in Table II, when a his6 mutant is grown in the absence of histidine for 6
hr the internal pool size drops to one-third that of wild type and the strain

derepresses about five- to sixfold. The histidine pool in wild type can also be reduced by creating a physiological block in the pathway with the inhibitor 3-amino-1, 2, 4 triazole (AT). When added to a culture, this compound is taken up by the cells, inhibits the sixth step in the pathway, and leads to a decreased production of histidine. As can be seen in Table II, the histidine pool in wild type is reduced about threefold by growth in AT and the biosynthetic enzymes are correspondingly derepressed about six- to eightfold. The surprising result is that *TRA1-8,* which has a pool as low as *his6* starved for histidine or wild type grown on AT, is not derepressed. Under these conditions, the *his6* mutant and wild type have three to four times the level of histidine enzymes as compared with *TRA1-8.* Even when further deprived of histidine by growth in AT, *TRA1-8* never achieves maximal derepression.

The inability of *TRA1-8* and other *TRA1* mutants to derepress normally was explored by examining the extent of derepression at various times after cultures were exposed to the inhibitor AT. The results are shown in Fig. 3. These curves show that, in addition to *TRA1-8,* mutants *TRA1-17* and *TRA1-19* fail to

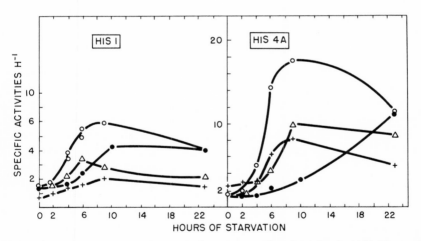

Fig. 3. Derepression of yeast strains in the presence of amino triazole (AT). The strains were pregrown in minimal medium plus 20 m*M* AT. At the times indicated, aliquots were removed, cycloheximide was added, and the cells were chilled and centrifuged. Enzymes were extracted by disruption of the cells in a Braun homogenizer. The resulting homogenate was clarified by centrifugation, and the enzymes were assayed directly. The *his1* activity (phosphoribosyltransferase) (on the left) was measured as described by Kovach *et al.* (13). The *his4A* activity (cyclohydrolase) was measured as described in Table II. Both activities are expressed as μmoles of product/hr/mg protein. ○, Wild type; ●, *TRA1-17;* △, *TRA1-19;* +, *TRA1-8.*

derepress normally. In fact, these strains never achieve the highest level of derepression possible. One objection to these experiments is that in *TRA1-17* the high internal pool of histidine might partially overcome the inhibition by AT, thereby preventing the full effect of the inhibitor and the concatenation of events leading to derepression. To study this possible complication and others of a similar nature, the *TRA1* mutations were combined genetically with a *his6* mutation to make double mutants of the type *TRA1 his6*. The *his6* mutation causes a block in the pathway so that these double mutants cannot produce histidine internally even though they are feedback resistant. The time course of derepression was followed in these strains, along with that of a *his6* mutant as a control, at various times after the strains were placed on medium lacking histidine. The growth rates of the double mutants and the *his6* mutant were identical under starvation conditions. As is shown in Fig. 4, the *TRA1* mutants do not derepress normally under these conditions. The *his6* mutant can derepress ten- to fifteenfold over a 20-hr period, whereas *TRA1-17* derepresses only

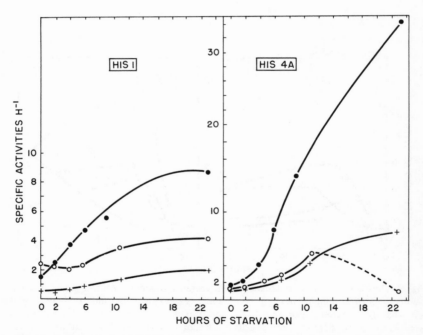

Fig. 4. Derepression of TRA1 his6 double mutants. The strains were grown on minimal medium supplemented with 0.3 mM histidine and then diluted into minimal medium without histidine. Samples were taken at various times after inoculation into minimal and treated as described in Fig. 3. •, *his6*; ○, *his6 TRA1-17*; +, *his6 TRA1-8*. The *his6* mutation in all strains was the same.

twofold and *TRA1-8* derepresses only fivefold. The *his6* mutants cannot accumulate any of the intermediates structurally related to histidine, making it unlikely that any of the intermediates in the pathway of histidine biosynthesis are responsible for the altered derepression. Mutations in the *his1* gene other than the feedback *TRA1* types also appear defective in their ability to derepress. Several histidine-requiring mutants with mutational sites located throughout the *his1* gene were tested for their ability to derepress when starved for histidine. None derepressed to the level of *his6* or of wild type grown on AT.

DISCUSSION

Our studies show that feedback-resistant mutants are a frequent class of regulatory mutants obtained by selection for resistance to the analog triazole alanine. The finding that all feedback mutations are dominant agrees with earlier findings by Bussey (11) for similar mutations in leucine biosynthesis and suggests that feedback-resistant strains should be a frequent class of amino acid analog resistant mutants in diploid plant cells or seeds. The contention that such mutations will be dominant regardless of the biosynthetic pathway or organism affected is supported by the molecular basis of the resistance—production of a feedback-insensitive first enzyme. The high amino acid pools which result from the abolition of feedback control could be of extreme importance to nutritionists seeking to alter the amino acid composition of plant cells. Amino acid analogs are known for virtually every one of the 20 amino acids, allowing the experimentalist to choose the appropriate reagent with which to select his mutant. It is possible to envision some potential problems in the use of feedback-resistant mutants of plants as replacements for presently used crops. High internal pools of certain amino acids might be toxic to the organism and prevent good yields. Our studies on yeast indicate that even though external histidine at very high concentrations is toxic, internal histidine is not. It is likely that excretion of histidine, facilitated by one of the permeation systems, prevents the pool from swelling to a toxic level. This situation suggests that *a priori* judgments about the viability of feedback mutants of plants should not be based on the sensitivity of plants to exogenous amino acids. Once feedback-resistant plant strains have been obtained, it will have to be determined whether the endosperm manifests the high amino acid pool. The *opaque-2* mutant of corn does not have an altered amino acid pool; rather, the content of lysine-rich proteins in the endosperm has been increased (12). Though there may be problems in designing exactly the right strain, the potential benefits of feedback-resistant strains urge a serious effort to obtain and investigate these mutants in plants.

The effect of feedback-resistant mutants on derepression has been reported by other workers. Goldberger and his colleagues have found altered kinetics of repression in feedback-resistant mutants of *Salmonella typhimurium* (13,14).

These workers have suggested the possibility of a direct involvement of the first enzyme in repression control. Repression of the histidine operon in *S. typhimurium* is known to require aminoacylated histidine tRNA (15). Recent experiments (16,17) show that the enzyme catalyzing the first step of histidine biosynthesis binds histidyl-tRNA in preference to other species of aminoacylated tRNA and binds aminoacylated histidine tRNA in preference to deacylated tRNA^{His}. These results are consistent with the possibility that the regulatory role of the first enzyme is carried out as a complex with histidyl-tRNA. Because of the altered kinetics of derepression of our mutants, the phosphoribosyltransferase from yeast was studied to examine (a) whether histidyl-tRNA binds to it and (b) whether the histidyl-tRNA synthetase is bound to it. Studies similar to those described by Goldberger gave no evidence for the binding of histidyl-tRNA^{His} to partially purified phosphoribosyltransferase from yeast. Other studies showing that the histidyl-tRNA synthetase is normal in a number of different *his1* (phosphoribosyltransferase) mutants make it unlikely that the synthetase and the phosphoribosyltransferase are the same protein. Because of the lack of evidence for involvement of the enzyme from yeast with potential regulatory molecules, the role of this enzyme in repression is not clear. It is hoped that further studies on the control elements involved in gene expression in yeast will help to clarify the altered derepression of *his1* mutants.

ACKNOWLEDGMENT

This work was supported by grant GM 15408-06 from the National Institutes of Health.

REFERENCES

1. Umbarger, H. E. (1969). Regulation of amino acid metabolism. *Ann. Rev. Biochem.* **38**:323-370.
2. Beckwith, J., and Zipser, D. (1970). *The Lactose Operon,* Cold Spring Harbor Laboratory.
3. Umbarger, H. E. (1971). Metabolite analogues as genetic and biochemical probes. *Advan. Genet.* **16**:119-140.
4. Gross, S. R. (1969). Genetic regulation mechanisms in fungi. *Ann. Rev. Genet.* **3**:395-424.
5. Metzenberg, R. L. (1972). Genetic regulatory systems in *Neurospora. Ann. Rev. Genet.* **6**:111-132.
6. Surdin, Y., Sly, W., Sirc, J., Bordes, A. M., and de Robichon-Szulmajster, H. (1965). Properties and genetic control of the amino acid permeases in yeast. *Biochim. Biophys. Acta* **107**:546-566.
7. Grenson, M., Mousset, M., Wiame, J. M., and Bechet, J. (1966). Système d'accumulation des acides aminés chez *Saccharomyces cerevisiae:* propriétés et contrôle génétique. *Biochim. Biophys. Acta* **127**:323-338.
8. Fink, G. R. (1965). Gene enzyme relationship in histidine biosynthesis in yeast. *Science* **146**:525-527.

9. Sheppard, E. C. (1964). Mutants of *Salmonella typhimurium* resistant to feedback inhibition by L-histidine. *Genetics* **50:**611-623.

10. Ramos, F., Thuriaux, P., Wiame, J. W., and Bechet, J. (1970). The participation of ornithine and citrulline in the regulation of arginine metabolism in *Saccharomyces cerevisiae. Europ. J. Biochem.* **12:**40-47.

11. Bussey, H. (1970). Simple selection for end product inhibitor sensitive mutants in yeast. *J. Bacteriol.* **101:**1081-1082.

12. Nelson, O. E. (1969). Genetic modification of protein quality in plants. *Advan. Agron.* **21:**171-194.

13. Kovach, J. S., Berberich, M. A., Venetianer, P., and Goldberger, R. F. (1969). Repression of the histidine operon: Effect of the first enzyme on kinetics of repression. *J. Bacteriol.* **97:**1283-1290.

14. Kovach, J. S., Phang, J. M., Ference, M., and Goldberger, R. F. (1969). Repression of the histidine operon. II. The role of the first enzyme in control of the histidine system. *Proc. Natl. Acad. Sci. (USA)* **63:**481-488.

15. Brenner, M., and Ames, B. N. (1971). The histidine operon and its regulation. In Vogel, H. J. (ed.), *Metabolic Pathways,* Vol. 5, Academic Press, New York, pp. 349-387.

16. Kovach, J. S., Phang, J. M., Blasi, F., Barton, R., Ballesteros-Olmo, A., and Goldberger, R. F. (1970). Interaction between histidyl tRNA and the first enzyme for histidine biosynthesis. *J. Bacteriol.* **104:**787-792.

17. Vogel, T., Meyers, M., Kovach, J., and Goldberger, R. (1972). Specificity of interaction between the first enzyme of histidine biosynthesis and aminoacylated histidine transfer ribonucleic acid. *J. Bacteriol.* **112:**126-130.

Plant Tissue and Cell Structure:
Genetic Aspects

8

Defined Mutants in Higher Plants

Peter S. Carlson, Rosemarie D. Dearing, and Brenda M. Floyd

Biology Department
Brookhaven National Laboratory
Upton, New York, U.S.A.

This chapter briefly reviews work on mutant selection using somatic cells of higher plants and then describes experiments designed to recover agriculturally useful variants. Mutants of *Nicotiana tabacum* were recovered which were resistant to an analog of methionine. These plants were found to be much less susceptible to damage by the pathogen *Pseudomonas tabaci*, which produces a toxin that is an analog of methionine. Several mutants show a specific increase in the level of free methionine.

INTRODUCTION

Defined biochemical mutants have occupied a central role in the elucidation of gene function and regulation in prokaryotes and lower eukaryotes. Major advances have come from these organisms primarily because mutant selection schemes have permitted large-scale isolation of known biochemical lesions. Similar advances in the genetic analysis of higher eukaryotes, both animal and plant, have been retarded by a paucity of biochemical variants and by the lack of ·a technique for the rapid selection of biochemically defined mutants.

The principles of genetic organization derived from studies of biosynthetic pathways in microbial organisms will not provide an adequate explanation of the genetic architecture of higher eukaryotes. The cell of a higher eukaryotic organism is a very different kind of biological entity than are cells of lower forms. The cell of a higher organism must respond to many different kinds of stimuli and is subject to distinct limitations and constraints in its specialization as part of larger biological unit. However, the basic experimental approach of molecular genetics, that of generating and recovering defined mutant types, is not limited to analyzing biochemical pathways in microbial organisms and can play a central role in the analysis of any biological process. The problem, then, is to develop methods for the isolation and characterization of mutant lesions blocked in known biological processes.

Somatic cells from higher plants cultured *in vitro* offer several unparalleled advantages for a genetic analysis of biochemical, physiological, and developmental processes. Besides the advantages of working with large populations of relatively homogeneous cells, haploid cells from a number of species can be readily obtained, cultured, and regenerated into whole organisms. The possibility of regenerating whole plants from single cultured cells is of tremendous importance for the analysis of defined genetic lesions and for identifying mutants which are blocked in distinct developmental processes.

Because the selection and characterization of auxotrophic mutants have been extensively studied in lower forms, the first attempts at mutant selection focused on recovering nutritionally deficient clones from plant cell cultures (3). The selective technique employed for the recovery of auxotrophic mutants in haploid *Nicotiana tabacum* L. cell cultures was modeled after a system designed by Puck and Kao (8) for use with mammalian somatic cell cultures. A mixed population of auxotrophic and wild-type cells can grow, but auxotrophs cannot. The cells are then exposed to a compound, such as 5-bromodeoxyuridine (BUdR), which kills only dividing cells by being incorporated into their DNA and rendering them light sensitive. In a typical experiment, a large population of single haploid cells is treated with a mutagen and grown on a minimal medium for several cell generations. This serves to deplete the pool of growth-limiting metabolite present in the individual mutant cell and halt its growth. Nonmutant cells continue to grow and divide on the minimal medium. This mixed population of cells is exposed to BUdR. Growing cells incorporate BUdR into their DNA and are subsequently killed by exposure to near-visible light. The nondividing mutant cells do not incorporate BUdR and so are not killed by the light. Auxotrophs are then recovered by culturing them on a nutritionally supplemented medium which permits their growth into callus masses. The individual masses are isolated and their nutritional requirements determined. There is little or no restriction on the auxotrophic types which can be recovered, since auxotrophs for nucleic acid bases, vitamins, and amino acids have been observed.

Whole plants have been regenerated from the mutant calluses, and the morphologies of several of them are shown in Fig. 1. Note that the rate of growth of the auxotrophic mutant plants is much slower than that of nonmutant sister plants. The growth characteristics and color of all the auxotrophic plants differ from those of the wild type. The characteristics of the hypoxanthine-re-

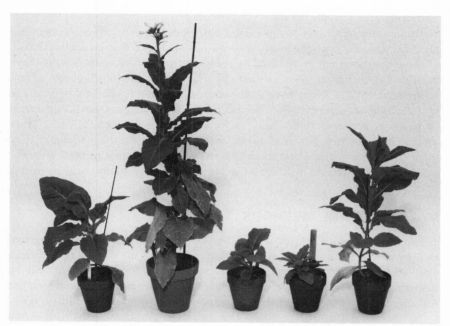

Fig. 1. Auxotrophic mutant plants of Nicotiana tabacum. Right to left: Wild-type haploid (2 months), hypoxanthine-requiring mutant (6 months), lysine-requiring mutant (6 months), lysine-requiring shoot grafted onto a wild-type stock (4 months), lysine-requiring mutant supplemented with lysine (4 months).

quiring mutants shown in Fig. 1 are distinct from the wild type in that the mutant plant demonstrates a reduction in internode length. Leaves of the mutant plant are reduced in size, more elongate in morphology, and yellow-green in color. The distinctive characteristics of the lysine-requiring mutant plant include a more yellowish leaf color and a slightly altered leaf shape. When lysine-requiring plants are supplemented with an exogenous supply of lysine, or when mutant shoots are grafted onto a wild-type base, the growth characteristics of the mutant plants resemble those of the wild type (Fig. 1). It is interesting to note that there are no distinct phenotypic traits associated with these auxotrophic plants which separate them from a variety of other types of biochemically undefined "morphological mutants" in plants. The phenotype of the mutant plants gives no external clue as to the nature of the underlying genetic lesion. Both of these mutants are transmitted as single Mendelian factors.

The work which will be described more fully here was initiated to determine if selective systems can be designed to recover agriculturally useful mutants. These experiments were designed to pose two questions: (a) Is it possible to select mutants of a higher plant which have an altered response to a pathogen by recovering cells resistant to the toxin produced by that pathogen? (b) Is it possible to increase selectively the level of a nutritionally important component in a plant by selecting mutants resistant to a toxic analog of that component? Both of these questions can be resolved by recovering and analyzing mutants of *Nicotiana tabacum* which are resistant to the methionine analog methionine sulfoximine (MSO). It has been demonstrated by Braun (1) that toxin produced by *Pseudomonas tabaci*, the bacterial pathogen which causes the wildfire disease of tobacco, is a structural analog of methionine. Braun observed that MSO, though not the true bacterial toxin, would elicit an identical response from tobacco leaves and that mutants of *Chlorella vulgaris* resistant to MSO were also resistant to the toxin. Methionine is also an essential amino acid in human nutrition.

MATERIALS AND METHODS

Haploid plants of *Nicotiana tabacum* cv. Havana Wisconsin 38 were generated by anther culture, and the haploid composition of the tissue was confirmed cytologically. Haploid protoplasts were isolated from leaf mesophyll cells by stripping the lower epidermis from sterilized, young, expanding leaves. Stripped leaf pieces were placed in an enzyme solution consisting of 4% cellulase (Onozuka SS, All Japan Biochemicals Co. Ltd.), 0.4% macerozyme (All Japan Biochemicals Co. Ltd.), and 0.6 M mannitol at pH 5.7. Flasks containing leaf pieces in the enzyme solution were evacuated briefly and returned to standard atmospheric pressure to facilitate penetration of the enzyme solution. Flasks were incubated for 12–16 hr at 21°C, after which the protoplasts were harvested by low-speed centrifugation. Medium used for the regeneration was that described by Nagata and Takebe (7). Populations of single haploid cells from *in vitro* cultures of *N. tabacum* were obtained and plated as previously described (3). Cell density when plating protoplasts and cultured cells was always greater than 2×10^3 cells/ml.

After isolation, protoplasts or cells were treated with 0.25% ethyl methanesulfonate for 1 hr, washed twice in fresh medium, and plated. The cultures were permitted to grow for 2 weeks, overlaid with an equal volume of medium containing 10 mM MSO, and incubated for 3 months. Surviving calluses were recovered and placed on medium containing no MSO. Each callus was grown for several months, divided, and retested for resistance to 10 mM MSO. Those calluses which retained resistance were diploidized and regenerated into whole plants for further genetic and physiological analysis.

RESULTS AND DISCUSSION

An analysis of approximately 2.7×10^7 viable protoplasts yielded 33 presumptive MSO-resistant calluses. From approximately 1.9×10^7 viable cells from *in vitro* cultures, 19 presumptive mutant calluses were recovered. Most of these presumed mutants were unstable in expression of the MSO resistance. After further growth of the calluses on medium lacking MSO, 49 of the 52 presumed mutants were found to segregate tissue which was no longer MSO resistant. The phenotype of the unstable tissue exhibits many characteristics common to presumed mutants recovered from animal cell cultures (5). Further work was focused on the three remaining resistant calluses, which were labeled Nos. 1, 2, and 3. Callus 1 was recovered from cultured cells, while calluses 2 and 3 were recovered from protoplasts. Diploid plants were regenerated from each of the three calluses, and their chromosomal composition was confirmed cytologically. Each mutant plant was crossed to a wild type to give an F_1 progeny. The F_1 progeny were self-fertilized to yield an F_2 generation. One hundred F_2 seedlings from each of the three crosses were germinated under sterile conditions and tested for resistance to MSO. The results are presented in Table I. The pattern of transmission of mutant 1 is complex, perhaps best described by the ratio expected from two recessive loci with additive effects and segregating independently yielding a 9:3:3:1 ratio. The patterns of transmission of mutants 2 and 3 appear simpler and best explained by single semidominant loci yielding a 1:2:1 ratio. Since the mutants were derived from mutagenic treatment and there is the possibility of extensive genetic damage, the ratios must be considered preliminary. Crosses between mutants 2 and 3 indicate that they are possibly allelic. Since these two mutants were derived from protoplasts isolated in two different experimental series, they must be derived from two different mutational events.

Figure 2 demonstrates the reaction of the leaves upon infection by *P. tabaci* or application of MSO. After infection with *P. tabaci,* the susceptible plant forms chlorotic halos that surround a brown necrotic spot at the site of inoculation. MSO causes a similar reaction except that the necrotic spot is not as pronounced. Infection of all three homozygous mutant plants and a variety of *N. tabacum* carrying a naturally occurring genetic resistance (Burley 21) (4) does

Table I. Growth of F_2 Seedlings on Medium Containing 10 mM Methionine Sulfoximine

Mutant No.	No growth	Slight growth	Normal growth
1	59	37	4
2	31	51	18
3	36	42	22

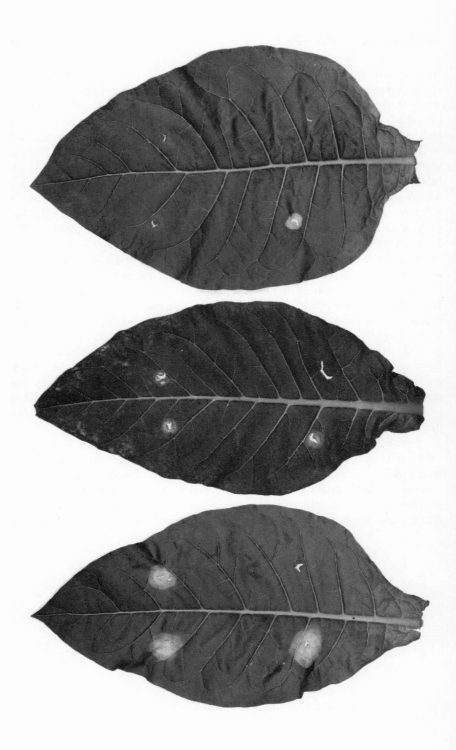

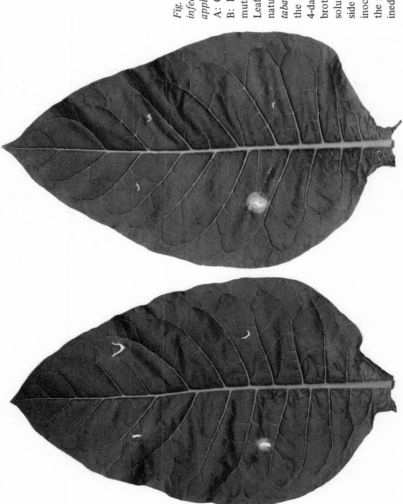

Fig. 2. Reaction of tobacco leaves to infection by Pseudomonas tabaci and to application of methionine sulfoximine. A: Control leaf from a wild-type plant. B: Leaf from mutant 1. C: Leaf from mutant 2. D: Leaf from mutant 3. E: Leaf from cv. Burley 21, which carried a naturally occurring resistance to *P. tabaci*. Each leaf was infected twice in the apical region with 0.1 ml of a 3- to 4-day-old culture of *P. tabaci* in nutrient broth. One-tenth milliliter of a 0.1 mM solution of MSO was applied to the left side of the basal portion of the leaf. Uninoculated nutrient broth was applied to the right basal region. Leaves were examined for their reaction after 6 days.

not lead to production of the characteristic chlorotic halo. Leaves of mutant 1 do show a definite necrotic spot after infection. Mutants 2 and 3 show small dark areas at the site of infection with *P. tabaci.* Burley 21 is unaffected by infection. The small dark areas on mutants 2 and 3 are similar to the blackfire disease caused by *Pseudomonas angulata.* This observation is quite striking, since *P. angulata* is considered by many plant pathologists (6) to be a variety of *P. tabaci* which does not produce toxin. All three mutant types are susceptible to infection by *P. angulata,* while Burley 21 is resistant. Under the experimental conditions used in this work, mutants 2 and 3 are distinctly more resistant to the effects of infection by *P. tabaci* than is the wild-type variety from which they were selected. The naturally occurring resistance of Burley 21 is superior to that of the mutants.

The levels of free amino acids in fully expanded leaves of wild-type and mutant tobacco are presented in Table II. Mutants 2 and 3 both show specific increases in the level of free methionine.

The answer to both questions posed in this work is affirmative. Mutants of agricultural importance can be recovered by selecting at the level of single cells.

CONCLUSIONS

We have reached the stage in the development of experimental techniques wherein the scientist interested in higher organisms and their biological processes can utilize the rigorous logical framework developed by molecular geneticists.

Table II. Concentrations of Certain Free Amino Acids in Tobacco Leaves[a]

	Methionine	Glycine	Alanine	Proline
Havana Wisconsin 38	0.4 ± 0.2	1.3 ± 0.3	1.8 ±0.3	0.3 ± 0.1
Mutant 1	0.3 ± 0.2	1.4 ± 0.3	1.7 ± 0.5	0.4 ± 0.2
Mutant 2	1.9 ± 0.5	1.7 ± 0.5	2.0 ± 0.4	0.5 ± 0.2
Mutant 3	2.4 ± 0.6	1.2 ± 0.2	1.5 ± 0.3	0.4 ± 0.2

[a] Concentrations are in nmoles/g fresh weight. Fully expanded young leaves with veins removed were homogenized at room temperature. An equal volume of 10% trichloroacetic acid was added to the homogenate and then centrifuged. The acid-soluble supernatant was run on an amino acid analyzer. Each value was calculated from three replicates. Levels of glycine, alanine, and proline are included to demonstrate that the increases in methionine in mutants 2 and 3 are specific to that amino acid.

The techniques of induction, isolation, and analysis of defined mutant types will prove to be powerful experimental tools for both basic and applied aspects of the biological sciences.

Preliminary results from a number of different experiments have demonstrated that many of the selective techniques designed for use on microbial systems are also applicable to higher organisms. Using haploid fern spores as an experimental material, we have utilized a number of different selective screening systems with positive results. The essential component of a selective technique is its ability to ask a definite yes or no question of the plant. The individual must either live or die under a given set of conditions.

ACKNOWLEDGMENTS

This research was partially supported by the U.S. Atomic Energy Commission and partially by USPHS Grant GM 18537. We thank Drs. C. C. Litton and H. A. Skoog for providing cultures of *Pseudomonas tabaci* and *P. angulata,* and our colleagues at Brookhaven for many stimulating discussions.

REFERENCES

1. Braun, A. (1955). A study on the mode of action of the wild fire toxin. *Phytopathology* 45:659-664.
2. Carlson, P. S. (1969). Auxotrophic mutants in ferns. *Genet. Res.* 14:337-339.
3. Carlson, P. S. (1970). Induction and isolation of auxotrophic mutants in somatic cell cultures of *Nicotiana tabacum. Science* 168:487-489.
4. Clayton, E. E. (1947). A wild fire resistant tobacco. *J. Hered.* 38:35-40.
5. Harris, M. (1971). Mutation rates at different ploidy levels. *J. Cell. Physiol.* 78:177-184.
6. Lucas, G. B. (1965). *Diseases of Tobacco,* 2nd ed., Scarecrow Press, New York.
7. Nagata, T., and Takebe, I. (1971). Plating of isolated tobacco mesophyll protoplasts on agar medium. *Planta* 99:12-20.
8. Puck, T., and Kao, F. T. (1967). Genetics of somatic mammalian cells. V. Treatment with 5BUdR and visible light for isolation of nutritionally deficient lines. *Proc. Natl. Acad. Sci. (USA)* 58:1227.

9

Potential of Cell and Tissue Culture Techniques as Aids in Economic Plant Improvement

Louis G. Nickell and Don J Heinz

Experiment Station
Hawaiian Sugar Planters' Association
Honolulu, Hawaii, U.S.A.

There are many ways to increase the genetic base of a population for effective selection. Sexual reproduction is nature's own way of broadening this base. It is the most effective way, but not the only tool available to the breeder. There are ways of bypassing sex. Among these are the use of induced mutations and manipulations at the cellular level. At least six ways are being studied for potential use in manipulating plant systems at the cellular level in order to use them in "asexual plant improvement." These six approaches are (a) variation in cell and tissue culture, polyploidy, aneuploidy, and chromosomal mosaics; (b) induced mutations; (c) induced polyploidy; (d) haploid plants from pollen; (e) fusion of vegetative cells (intraspecific, interspecific, intergeneric, interfamilial); and (f) transformation. Although the potential of cell and tissue culture for crop improvement could be enormous, caution in being too optimistic prematurely is stressed.

INTRODUCTION

For many centuries, man, in one way or another, has been trying to improve, for his needs, the plants and animals that sustain him. This has been accomplished through the unconscious and, more recently, conscious selection of desirable types from variable populations. It has come to be known as improvement through "breeding." The aim of any breeding program is the manipulation of genetically variable populations for the identification of desirable cultivars. The limiting factor in some crop plants is the lack of genetic variability; however, most crops possess considerable variability. In many instances, identification of desirable higher-producing cultivars is limited by the inability to identify genetically variable yield-limiting traits combined with other desirable characteristics.

Of the many ways to increase the genetic base of a population for effective selection, the use of induced mutations and manipulation at the cellular level will be discussed in this chapter.

The use of plant cell culture techniques has grown tremendously since the demonstration in 1959 by Armin Braun (6) of Rockefeller University that an entire plant could be produced from a single cell. Braun's success lies in the fact that he was the first to put together, in the correct order, the many steps which had before that time been successfully carried out separately, both by Braun and by other investigators in the field. Since then, the totipotency of plant cells has been shown for a number of plants in laboratories throughout the world.

There are at least six techniques now being studied which may have potential in manipulating plant systems at the cellular level for use in "asexual plant improvement." Some of these approaches have been more successful than others. Some species respond easily to a given method, while others are more difficult or, to date, show even no response.

The most effective use of cell suspensions and callus tissue techniques will be realized when effective selection techniques can be coupled with directed change. Admittedly, many technical problems are associated with this approach. However, proper application of these techniques, where defined questions can be asked and selection procedures applied at the cellular level, offers real potential to the plant breeder.

VARIATION IN CELL AND TISSUE CULTURES, POLYPLOIDY, ANEUPLOIDY, AND CHROMOSOMAL MOSAICS

In our work with sugarcane, it was recognized that considerable variation existed in cell suspensions and callus tissue. The extent of this variation differed from clone to clone. It can be speculated that this variation arises from the following sources: (a) inherent variation in the original plant material, i.e., aneuploidy, polyploidy, and chromosomal mosaicism; (b) mutations caused by exposure of cells to various nutrients, auxins, and other chemicals in the media; and (c) disruption of intact tissues and organelles to form cell suspensions. Not all plants exhibit variation, but enough evidence has been presented to warrant consideration. Variation of this nature has limited use to the plant breeder, and most studies have been academic; i.e., in many instances no defined problem was to be solved other than to study cell suspensions and callus tissue systems and techniques. From these studies has arisen the real possibility of using these techniques for the improvement of plants.

Early in our work with cell cultures of sugarcane, single-cell isolations were made, using the nurse technique (67), from a callus which had been isolated from internodal tissue of sugarcane clone H50-7209. The original purpose was to establish our callus collection based on single-cell isolates. As all these individual cell isolates, in this case, were from the same callus, which had been isolated from the stalk parenchyma tissue of a vegetatively propagated clone (or variety) of sugarcane, it was natural to assume that every cell would be similar and that all the calluses developed from these cells would be similar. However, of the first five callus tissues established and examined, all were different. One was beige, two were white, and two were yellow. The two yellow calluses grew at different growth rates, as did the two white ones. After much speculation on the physiological explanation for this phenomenon, cytological examinations were made of the calluses. It was found that the cells in these five different calluses had varying chromosome numbers (37). Subsequent work with entire, intact, field-grown plants established that this clone (H50-7209) was a chromosomal mosaic, i.e., was composed of cells with different chromosome numbers. It was then logical to assume that (a) if such tissue cultures were reduced to the cellular

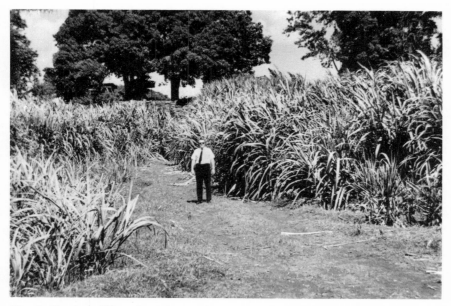

Fig. 1. Plantlets differentiated from callus tissues or cell suspensions from a number of sugarcane clones in the field for agronomic evaluation.

level in suspension culture and (b) single cells with different chromosome numbers isolated, the regeneration of plants from such cells would give plants that differed in chromosome number, and probably therefore in morphology and physiology—and growth and yield potential. This was the start of our now-extensive program in defining the use of cell and tissue culture techniques in our sugarcane improvement program (Fig. 1). Many of the plants regenerated from calluses from this chromosomal mosaic were different from the "parent" clone as well as from each other (35).

Several hundred plantlets derived from callus of H50-7209 were evaluated for agronomic characteristics. One plantlet (H69-9701) was selected on the basis of very distinct morphological, physiological (isoenzyme), and growth differences for yield testing against H50-7209. After a 2-year growth period (standard for Hawaii), H69-9701 was lower in yield, but not significantly (Table I).

Using tissue and cell culture techniques, Coleman (14) obtained variants from a sugarcane variety sensitive to mosaic virus disease which are resistant to that disease. Many of the variants appear to represent new stable genotypes with new characters such as red, albino, thick, and variegated leaves, and multi-tillered clones. Later work (Coleman, personal communication) has resulted in 116 clones from 15 varieties that have remained immune to mosaic virus disease after eight or more inoculations. The "immune" variants have been grown under field conditions favorable to mosaic spread. Some are still disease free under field conditions and are being tested to determine if they are truly immune.

Polyploidy is one of the most commonly reported nuclear variations in both normal and tumor tissues grown *in vitro* (80). Numerous articles in the literature since 1954 (97) have referred to this phenomenon, some with photographic evidence (63,64,101) and some with brief discussions (77,108), while others have presented considerable amounts of tabulated data (15,105). Most reports of polyploidy are the results of endomitosis or endoreduplication. Occasionally, however, there are cells found that do not occur in a 2, 4, 8, 16, . . . series, so another mechanism must be involved.

Partanen (81) postulated that the occurrence might result from asynchro-

Table I. Yield Comparison of H50-7209 and H69-9701[a]

Clone	Fiber % cane	Tons cane/acre	Sucrose % cane	Tons sugar/acre
50-7209	14.6	114.8 N.S.	12.0 N.S.	13.8 N.S.
69-9701	14.2	107.2	11.2	12.1
C.V.	–	4.92	9.36	9.82

[a] Six replications, 30- by 24-ft plots.

nous division of multinucleate cells, as based on observations made by Straus (101) and Mitra *et al.* (64). Reinert and Hellmann (88) demonstrated this phenomenon in cell suspensions of carrots, and Heinz (33) in a plant derived from callus tissue of sugarcane.

Until the work of Murashige and Nakano in 1966 (68), who utilized the phenomenon as a means of obtaining polyploid tobacco plants, little use was made of this means of producing polyploid horticultural and crop plants. More recently, polyploid kale plants have been selected from callus cultures (46).

One cannot conclude, however, that plant tissue cultures always will become polyploid. Many cultures have been found to remain cytologically normal (81), and others show widespread variation in chromosome number, involving the loss or gain of individual chromosomes (37, 106).

INDUCED MUTATION

Although considerable work has been carried out using radiation to obtain mutant plants, this procedure has not been outstandingly effective in many plants. One of the reasons is that, even though mutant cells can be produced by treating an entire plant or a plant part, the chances are very poor of isolating this mutant, keeping it viable, and developing a mutant plant from it. With the techniques of cell culture, this same approach becomes quite feasible. Also, the problems associated with sectors and chimeras can be overcome.

We have used both ionizing radiation and chemical mutagens. Individual

Table II. Reaction of Cell Suspensions of Sugarcane to γ-Irradiation[f]

γ rate (krad)	Clone			Progeny[d] from cross 28NG87 × H109
	H57-6466[a]	H65-8425[b]	H70-9440[c]	
2	5[e]	5	Lethal	Lethal
5	5	3	Lethal	Lethal
8	3	7	Lethal	Lethal

[a] Commercial hybrid—germ plasm from *Saccharum officinarum, S. spontaneum, S. sinense,* and *S. robustum.*

[b] *S. officinarum* × *S. spontaneum* hybrid.

[c] Complex hybrid—germ plasm from five species of *Saccharum.*

[d] 28NG87 and H109 are *S. officinarum.*

[e] Scale 1-9, 1 being best growth and differentiation, 9 very poor.

[f] From Heinz (34).

plantlets derived from irradiated callus tissue were morphologically uniform. A large number of observable mutants occurred within the plantlet population. Cell suspensions derived from four clones differing in genetic background had varying degrees of survival when exposed to 2, 5, or 8 krad of γ-irradiation from a cobalt source (Table II).

Nitsch *et al.* (76) obtained mutants of haploid tobacco plants by irradiating with a cobalt source at doses of 1500–3000 rad.

Although we have had some success with ionizing radiation, we prefer chemical mutagens because they are much easier to handle in the liquid media in which the treated cells are grown and do not require the special equipment necessary to produce radiation. Some of the chemical mutagens which we have studied include 8-ethoxycaffeine, methylmethane sulfonate, *N*-methyl-*N*-nitro-*N*-nitrosoguanidine, *N*-methyl-*N*-nitrosourea, and 1, 2, 3, 4-diepoxybutane.

Carlson (9) has devised a method for the induction and isolation of mutants in submerged cultures of tobacco haploid cells. The method is described by Carlson *et al.* in Chapter 8 of this volume.

INDUCED DOUBLING OF CHROMOSOME NUMBER WITH COLCHICINE

The use of colchicine for doubling chromosome numbers in plants is well known (16). In some plants, it is fairly easy to induce and separate polyploids; in others, it has been most difficult, if not impossible. An example of how polyploids were induced and recovered in sugarcane using cell suspensions will illustrate how this problem can be overcome.

Reports from the U.S. Department of Agriculture indicate that attempts by some of their investigators, over a number of years, to double the number of chromosomes in sugarcane clones were not successful. Grassl (26), Jagathesan (50), and others have reported no doubled plants despite attempts in their respective laboratories. Investigators at the British West Indies Central Cane Breeding Station (83, 95, 96) succeeded in doubling the chromosome number in three seedlings of *Saccharum spontaneum* from treated seed but failed in attempts with other clones using seed and asexual material.

By treating sugarcane cell suspensions with colchicine, success was achieved in doubling the chromosomal number of many cells on the first attempt, but no attempt was made to differentiate plants (61). In a subsequent study (35), cells growing in media supplemented with 2,4-D were exposed to 50 and 500 ppm of colchicine for 4 days. After a rinse with sterile water, they were transferred to solid medium without 2,4-D. Differentiation of plants was soon observed. Cytological examinations showed many of these plants to have a doubled chromosome number ($4_n \sim 224$). Some were more than doubled. In the first experiment, more than 1000 plants were differentiated from the treatment with

50 ppm colchicine, 300 of which were chlorophyll-less mutants. No plants differentiated from the 500-ppm treatment. Over 100 control (untreated) plants were differentiated; none was a chlorophyll-less mutant.

Again, considerable variation was observed in these populations. The clone used in this study is susceptible to the pathogen *Helminthosporium sacchari* and was chosen to see if resistant plantlets could be recovered at the tetraploid level. Also, a phenomenon exists in *Saccharum* such that when *S. officinarum* is pollinated by *S. spontaneum,* the full *S. officinarum* complement of chromo-somes comes through intact to many progeny of such crosses; the same thing can occur in the backcross (BC), and occasionally in BC_2. There are indications that a higher chromosome number (7) might give the potential for increased yields. With this in mind, it was thought we could double the chromosome number of sugarcane clones and then cross these with the diploids, which would produce progeny in the desired chromosome range. Unfortunately, tetraploid plantlets produced from the clone used in this study, H57-1627, rarely flower. The plantlets are reduced in vigor (Figs. 2 and 3), and the only two inflorescences obtained were sterile. Tetraploids from other clones that show the potential to flower was destroyed due to the introduction of *Ustilago scitamenea* (smut)

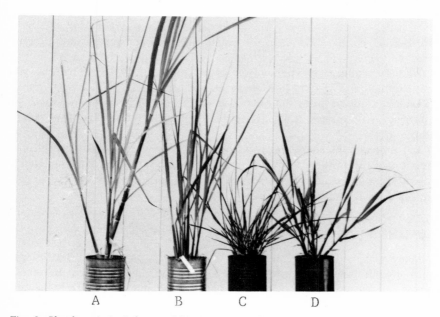

Fig. 2. Plantlets derived from colchicine-treated cell suspensions of clone H57-1627. A: Diploid. B: Tetraploid. C: Mixoploid. D: Aneuploid.

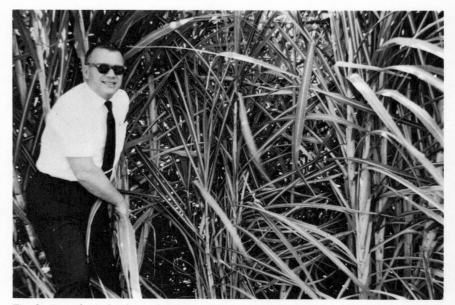

Fig. 3. Tetraploid plantlet in field surrounded by diploid plantlets differentiated from cell suspensions treated with colchicine.

into Hawaii during 1971, and all plants at the Experiment Station were destroyed (8).

We have produced polyploids from many clones, and these will be ready for study during the 1973-1974 flowering season.

Diploid plantlets from the colchicine study were screened for resistance to *H. sacchari*, with a range in highly resistant and highly susceptible plants being observed (34).

For sugarcane breeders, this technique of colchicine treating of cell cultures offers a tool that will be valuable in doubling the chromosome number of sterile progeny from inter- and intraspecific crosses. Appropriate studies are now underway and show considerable promise.

HAPLOID PLANTS FROM POLLEN

Many years of inbreeding are necessary to produce pure lines of those plants which do not breed true to type. The use of haploids to bypass the sexual process in achieving pure lines has long been known, but unfortunately the rate of natural occurrence of haploids in most plants is extremely low. Haploid organisms are desirable because mutations induced in them are readily visible and doubling their chromosomes leads directly to homozygous individuals, which breed true. The relatively recent discovery that haploid plants can be obtained from the *in vitro* culture of developing pollen is of considerable value to plant breeders. The most notable success has been in work with tobacco, pioneered by the late Dr. J. P. Nitsch and his wife (75) in France, by Tanaka and his colleagues in Japan (71, 104), and by Sunderlund and Wicks in England (102). Production of haploids directly from the pollen of *Datura* (30–32) and *Atropa belladonna* (115) also has been reported.

Production of haploid plants from pollen by going through the haploid callus stage and then embryogenesis has been reported for *Oryza* (74), *Brassica* (51), *Lilium* (94), *Lolium* (12), *Pelargonium* (1), *Arabidopsis thaliana* (29), and *Asparagus* (82).

Our attempts to obtain haploid plants from sugarcane pollen have been unsuccessful thus far.

FUSION OF VEGETATIVE CELLS

Although the isolation of protoplasts was reported as early as 1892 and fusion of isolated protoplasts from the same plant or from different plants was observed in 1937, current interest is high because of the potential of this technique for fusion of somatic cells from distantly related plants to produce new plants. After the significance placed on this approach for crop improvement by the conferees at the Rockefeller Foundation-sponsored conference on Crop Improvement Through Plant Cell and Tissue Culture in 1969 (72), an unbelievable amount of research has been carried out culminating in an international conference on protoplasts in Versailles in the summer of 1971.

Since the pioneering work of Cocking (13), protoplasts have been prepared from many plants (Table III). Many of these protoplasts have been cultured under conditions that will permit reformation of the cell wall, and plants have been developed from protoplasts of a few species: tobacco (70, 103), haploid tobacco (78), and carrot (25, 53).

Fusion of protoplasts was the next hurdle to be cleared for somatic or parasexual hybridization in plants. This was achieved by Power *et al.* (86) using sodium nitrate. Fusion, both spontaneous and induced, both intra- and interspecific, has been reported for a number of plants including *Brassica* (52), *Avena sativa* (20), *Haplopappus gracilis* (17), soybean (62), and *Torenia baillonii* and *T. fournieri* (84).

Carlson *et al.* (10) have recently demonstrated that interspecific plant hybrids can be produced by parasexual procedures. They isolated protoplasts of *Nicotiana glauca* and *N. langsdorfii*, fused protoplasts from the two species, and induced the regeneration of a hybrid plant. The somatic hybrids were recovered by using a selective screening system that depends on differential growth of the hybrid on defined culture media.

Table III. Plants from Which Protoplasts Have Been Isolated

Plant	Part	References
Agave toumeyana (agave)	Leaf meosphyll	Schmitt *et al.* (93)
Allium cepa (onion)	Root	Vreugdenhil (109) Eriksson (18) Bala Bawa and Torrey (3)
Allium fistulosum (green onion)	Leaf mesophyll	Otsuki and Takebe (79)
Arachis hypogaea (peanut)		Schenk and Hildebrandt (92)
Avena sativa (oat)	Coleoptile, leaf, root	Ruesink and Thimann (90,91) Fodil *et al.* (20) Ruesink (89)
Brassica oleracea (kale)	Root, leaf	Kameya and Takahashi (52)
Brassica rapa (turnip)	Leaf mesophyll	Otsuki and Takebe (79)
Chenopodium amaranticolor (goosefoot)	Leaf mesophyll	Otsuki and Takebe (79)
Cichorium endivia (endive)		Schenk and Hildebrandt (92)
Coleus blumei (common cultivated coleus)	Leaf mesophyll	Otsuki and Takebe (79)
Colocasia esculenta (taro)	Leaf mesophyll	Otsuki and Takebe (79)
Convolvulus arvensis (bindweed)	Root	Ruesink and Thimann (91) Bala Bawa and Torrey (3)
Crepis capillaris (hawk's-beard)		Eriksson (18)
Cryptotaenia japonica (honewort, wild chervil)	Leaf Mesophyll	Otsuki and Takebe (79)
Cucumis sativus (cucumber)	Leaf mesophyll, cotyledon	Otsuki and Takebe (79)
Daucus carota (carrot)	Root	Schenk and Hildebrandt (92) Chupeau and Morel (11) Eriksson (18) Hellmann and Reinert (38) Grambow *et al.* (25) Kameya and Uchimiya (53)
Dioscorea composita (yam)	Yam	Schmitt *et al.* (93)
Glycine max (soybean)		Schenk and Hildebrandt (92) Kao *et al.* (54,55)

Table III. (Continued)

Plant	Part	References
Gossypium hirsutum (cotton)		Keller *et al.* (57) Miller *et al.* (62) Schenk and Hildebrandt (92)
Haplopappus gracilis		Eriksson (17,18) Eriksson and Jonasson (19) Kao *et al.* (55)
Helianthus annuus (sunflower)		Schenk and Hildebrandt (92)
Hyacinthus orientalis (common hyacinth)	Leaf mesophyll	Otsuki and Takebe (79)
Lactuca sativa (lettuce)	Leaf mesophyll	Ruesink and Thimann (91) Schenk and Hildebrandt (92) Otsuki and Takebe (79)
Linum usitatissimum (flax)		Keller *et al.* (57)
Lycopersicon esculentum (tomato)	Placenta of immature fruit, leaf meosphyll	Gregory and Cocking (27, 28) Schenk and Hildebrandt (92) Otsuki and Takebe (79) Boulware and Camper (5)
Medicago sativa (alfalfa)		Eriksson (18)
Melilotus alba (white sweet clover)		Keller *et al.* (57)
Narcissus tazetta (narcissus)	Leaf mesophyll	Otsuki and Takebe (79)
Nicotiana glutinosa		Schenk and Hildebrandt (92) Schmitt *et al.* (93)
Nicotiana tabacum (tobacco)	Leaf mesophyll	Otsuki and Takebe (79) Schenk and Hildebrandt (92) Power and Cocking (85) Eriksson (18) Nagata and Takebe (69,70) Schmitt *et al.* (93) Takebe *et al.* (103) Yamada *et al.* (114)
Parthenocissus tricuspidata (Boston ivy)		Schmitt *et al.* (93)
Pelargonium hortorum (geranium)		Schenk and Hildebrandt (92)

Table III. (Continued)

Plant	Part	References
Petroselinum hortense (parsley)		Schenk and Hildebrandt (92)
Petunia species (petunia)	Leaf mesophyll	Otsuki and Takebe (79)
Phaseolus vulgaris (navy bean)		Schenk and Hildebrandt (92)
Phaseolus vulgaris (red kidney bean)		Schenk and Hildebrandt (92)
Platanus occidentalis (sycamore)		Schenk and Hildebrandt (92)
Pyrus communis (pear)		Schenk and Hildebrandt (92)
Rubus fruticosus (European blackberry)		Schmitt *et al.* (93)
Saccharum species (sugarcane)	Apical meristem, stalk parenchyma	Maretzki (58) Maretzki and Nickell (59)
Solanum nigrum (black nightshade)		Raj and Herr (87)
Spinacia oleracea (spinach)	Leaf mesophyll	Otsuki and Takebe (79) Schenk and Hildebrandt (92)
Torenia baillonii (torenia)	Petals	Potrykus (84)
Torenia fournieri (torenia)	Petals	Potrykus (84)
Triticum aestivum (wheat)		Schenk and Hildebrandt (92)
Tulipa gesneriana (garden tulip)	Leaf mesophyll	Otsuki and Takebe (79)
Vicia faba (broadbean)	Leaf mesophyll	Otsuki and Takebe (79)
Vitis vinifera (grape)		Schenk and Hildebrandt (92)
Zea mays (corn)	Root, mesocotyl, endosperm	Eriksson (18) Motoyoshi (66) Bala Bawa and Torrey (3)

TRANSFORMATION

From our point of view, the ultimate step in aiding the plant breeder would be the ability to direct transformation of cells of higher plants. This transferring of selected fragments of deoxyribonucleic acid from a donor plant to receptor cells would be akin to a form of "directed mutation"—in other words, it would allow the investigator to "call the shot." Properties of the donor species can thereby be transferred to the acceptor. The phenomenon of transformation has been successfully demonstrated in microorganisms and, to a very limited extent, in higher plants (39–45). The availability of clones with widely divergent physiological properties and morphological characteristics makes sugarcane a good prospect for successful transformation. So far, we have used two approaches toward this end, both utilizing cell suspensions (73). One of these methods requires the redifferentiation of cells to whole plants after the introduction of DNA isolated from a clone with a strong morphological marker, such as red or black stalk color, into cells obtained from a green- or yellow-stalked clone. Changes in stalk color in the population of plants from the redifferentiated cells would be an indication of possible transformed genetic material. Difficulties with redifferentiation have so far hampered this approach, because, unfortunately, the cell lines used were those which have been in culture for over 10 years and have been shown to be incapable of redifferentiation by techniques so far employed (4).

A second approach capitalizes on the differences in susceptibility of different clones to a fungal disease. We have made attempts at introducing DNA from a resistant clone of sugarcane into cells from a susceptible clone. Following a short period of continued growth, the cells are exposed to a host-specific toxin produced by *Helminthosporium sacchari* (99, 100) and cell survival was used as the criterion for transformation. So far, cells from clones with relatively low susceptibility to the toxin have been used and results showing increased resistance that might be ascribed to transformation are not convincing. However, cell suspensions from clones that are more susceptible to the eyespot toxin are now in culture and will be used in subsequent tests.

At this stage, this approach is similar to the sexual approach in that many genes are introduced. Hopefully, we will learn in the future to introduce progressively smaller units of DNA—eventually those containing the specific characteristics desired and few, if any, undesired ones.

DISCUSSION

Although tissue cultures from a number of woody plants (usually from the cambium) were isolated in the early days of plant tissue and organ culture (21, 23, 47–49, 65) and cultures have been established from many more woody trees and shrubs since that time (see ref. 22 for a review of the work carried out until that date), reports of plantlet redifferentiation from such callus tissues are scarce. Because of the interval required for generation time in the breeding of forest and crop trees, it is surprising that more effort has not been spent in the application of established techniques for this purpose. Plantlets have been obtained from callus cultures of quaking aspen (60, 110, 111, 113), European aspen (112), coffee (98), and *Eucalyptus citriodora* (2). The increasing pleas to preserve the germplasm pool of tropical rainforest trees (24) also suggest consideration of tissue culture approaches as a means to this end.

Although we have emphasized in this chapter the potential use of, as well as our own progress with, manipulation at the cellular level as it might aid in plant improvement programs, we hasten to emphasize that such approaches are of limited practical use at present. Much has to be done in the development of techniques for application to specific problems.

We have pointed out areas where these techniques can be applied directly. In those areas where crop improvement programs are just beginning or are in their infancy, we highly recommend (a) the screening of existing cultivars which might be adapted, (b) the development of a sexual breeding program utilizing available germplasm, and (c) the development of screening criteria for specific conditions and characteristics.

At present, the utilization of an asexual approach could be attempted where problems are encountered which cannot be overcome at the sexual level, and, in general, it should probably not be considered in the development of a new program. However, when the stage is reached where these techniques might be adopted, it should only be where problems are well defined and screening techniques are available at the cellular level. It is highly improbable that we will be able to select at the cellular level for higher yield until the basic physiology of a plant is much better defined than we are able to do at present.

Our present experience suggests that asexual improvement at the cellular level could be used in screening for induced disease resistance in asexually propagated plants. This would be important where high-yielding clones cannot be grown commercially because of susceptibility to a disease. Again, adequate screening techniques are required.

The ideal tool for screening would be the use of host-specific toxins, where available, or development of definitive media for selection of cells where induced resistance is based on the presence of a protein or enzyme which provides resistance. This may be possible with resistances to disease which have a simple genetic makeup.

We feel that all of the approaches discussed have some potential, ultimately. However, many are still in the research and development stage and should remain there for most countries and for most crops until the practical means of using them are established. It is clear that the proper questions need to be asked and the resultant research be aimed at answering such questions. Asexual approaches will be more applicable for some questions than for others. We would not want to underestimate the enormous potential of cell and tissue culture for crop improvement but rather to caution against too optimistic an outlook prematurely.

ACKNOWLEDGMENTS

This work is published with the approval of the Director as Paper No. 327 in the Journal Series of the Experiment Station, Hawaiian Sugar Planters' Association. Results in certain sections of this paper are from investigations supported in part with funds provided by the United States Department of Agriculture Agreements No. 12-14-100-8442 (34) and No. 12-14-100-10430(34) to the Experiment Station of the Hawaiian Sugar Planters' Association.

REFERENCES

1. Abo El-Nil, M. M., and Hildebrandt, A. C. (1971). Induction of geranium plants from anther callus. *In Vitro* 7:399.
2. Aneja, S., and Atal, C. K.(1969). Plantlet formation in tissue cultures from lignotubers of *Eucalyptus citriodora Hook. Curr. Sci. (India)* 38:69.
3. Bala Bawa, S., and Torrey, J. G. (1971). "Budding" and nuclear division in cultured protoplasts of corn, *Convolvulus,* and onion. *Bot. Gaz.* 132:240-245.
4. Barba, R., and Nickell, L. G. (1969). Nutrition and organ differentiation in tissue cultures of sugarcane, a monocotyledon. *Planta* 89:299-302.
5. Boulware, M. A., and Camper, N. D. (1972). Effects of selected herbicides on plant protoplasts. *Physiol. Plant* 26:313-317.
6. Braun, A. C. (1959). A demonstration of the recovery of the crown-gall tumor cell with the use of complex tumors of single-cell origin. *Proc. Natl. Acad. Sci. (USA)* 45:932-938.
7. Bremer, G. (1964). Some historical facts about cytological investigations of sugarcane. *Ind. J. Sugarcane Res. Develop.* 7:122-130.
8. Byther, R. S., Steiner, G. W., and Wismer, C. A. (1971). Smut found in Hawaii. Annual Report, Experiment Station, Hawaiian Sugar Planters' Association, pp. 37-39.
9. Carlson, P. S. (1970). Induction and isolation of auxotrophic mutants in somatic cell cultures of *Nicotiana tabacum. Science* 168:487-489.
10. Carlson, P. S., Smith, H. H., and Dearing, R. D. (1972). Parasexual interspecific plant hybridization. *Proc. Natl. Acad. Sci. (USA)* 69:2292-2294.
11. Chupeau, Y., and Morel, G.(1970). Obtention de protoplastes de plantes supérieures à partir de tissus cultures *in vitro. Compt. Rend. Acad. Sci. (Paris)* 270:2659-2662.
12. Clapham, D. (1971). *In vitro* development of callus from pollen of *Lolium* and *Hordeum. Z. Pflanzenzüchtg.* 65:285-292.
13. Cocking, E. C. (1960). A method for the isolation of plant protoplasts and vacuoles. *Nature* 187:927-929.
14. Coleman, R. E. (1970). New plants produced from callus tissue culture. Sugarcane Research 1970 Report, ARS, USDA, p. 38.
15. de Torok, D., and White, P. R. (1960). Cytological instability in tumors of *Picea glauca. Science* 131:730-732.

16. Eigsti, O. J., and Dustin, P. (1955). *Colchicine in Agriculture, Medicine, Biology and Chemistry,* Iowa State College Press, Ames, Ia.

17. Eriksson, T. (1965). Studies on the growth requirements and growth measurements of cell cultures of *Haplopappus gracilis. Physiol. Plant.* 18:976-993.

18. Eriksson, T. (1971). Isolation and fusion of plant protoplasts. In: *Les Cultures de Tissus de Plantes,* Coll. Internat. CNRS No. 193 (1970), Strasbourg, pp. 297-302.

19. Eriksson, T., and Jonasson, K. (1969). Nuclear division in isolated protoplasts from cells of higher plants grown *in vitro. Planta* 89:85-89.

20. Fodil, Y., Esnault, R., and Trapy, G. (1971). Fusion de protoplastes de coléoptiles d'Avoine. *Compt. Rend. Acad. Sci. (Paris)* 273:727-729.

21. Gautheret, R. J. (1948). Sur la culture indéfinie des tissus de *Salix caprea. Compt. Rend. Soc. Biol. (Paris)* 142:807.

22. Gautheret, R. J. (1959). *La Culture des Tissus Végétaux,* Masson & Cie, Paris.

23. Gioelli, F. (1938). Morfologia, istologia, fisiologia e fisiopathologia di meristemi secondari *in vitro. Att. Acad. Sci. Ferrara* 16:1-87.

24. Gomez-Pompa, A., Vazguez-Yanes, C., and Guevara, S. (1972). The tropical rain forest: A nonrenewable resource. *Science* 177:762-765.

25. Grambow, H. J., Kao, K. N., Miller, R. A., and Gamborg, O. L. (1972). Cell division and plant development from protoplasts of carrot cell suspension cultures. *Planta* 103:348-355.

26. Grassl, C. O. (1966). Comments. *ISSCT Sugarcane Breeders' Newsletter* 18:29-30.

27. Gregory, D. W., and Cocking, E. C. (1965). The large-scale isolation of protoplasts from immature tomato fruit. *J. Cell Biol.* 24:143-146.

28. Gregory, D. W., and Cocking, E. C. (1966). Studies on isolated protoplasts and vacuoles. I. General properties. *J. Exptl. Bot.* 17:57-67.

29. Gresshoff, P. M., and Doy, C. H. (1972). Haploid *Arabidopsis thaliana* callus and plants from anther culture. *Austral. J. Biol. Sci.* 25:259-264.

30. Guha, S., and Maheshwari, S. C. (1964). *In vitro* production of embryos from anthers of *Datura. Nature* 204:497.

31. Guha, S., and Maheshwari, S. C. (1966). Cell division and differentiation of embryos in the pollen grains of *Datura in vitro. Nature* 212:97-98.

32. Guha, S., and Maheshwari, S. C. (1967). Development of embryoids from pollen grains of *Datura in vitro. Phytomorphology* 17:454-461.

33. Heinz, D. J (1971). New procedures for sugarcane breeders. *Proc. Internat. Soc. Sugar Cane Technol.* 14:372-380.

34. Heinz, D. J (1972). Sugarcane improvement through induced mutations using vegetative propagules and cell culture techniques. GAO/IAEA Panel on Mutation Breeding of Vegetatively Propagated and Perennial Crops (in press).

35. Heinz, D. J, and Mee, G. W. P. (1970). Colchicine-induced polyploids from cell suspension cultures of sugarcane. *Crop Sci.* 10:696-699.

36. Heinz, D. J, and Mee, G. W. P. (1971). Morphologic, cytogenetic, and enzymatic variation in *Saccharum* species hybrid clones derived from callus tissue. *Am. J. Bot.* 58:257-262.

37. Heinz, D. J, Mee, G. W. P., and Nickell, L. G. (1969). Chromosome numbers of some *Saccharum* species hybrids and their cell suspension cultures. *Am. J. Bot.* 56:450-456.

38. Hellmann, S., and Reinert, J. (1971). Protoplasten aus Zellkulturen von *Daucus carota. Protoplasma* 72:479-484.

39. Hess, D. (1969). Versuche zur Transformation an höheren Pflanzen: Induktion und konstante Weitergabe der Anthocyansynthese bei *Petunia hybrida. Z. Pflanzenphysiol.* 60:348-358.

40. Hess, D. (1969). Versuche zur Transformation an höheren Pflanzen: Wiederholung der Anthocyan-Induktion bei *Petunia* und erste Charakterisierung des transformierenden Prinzips. *Z. Pflanzenphysiol.* 61:286-298.

41. Hess, D. (1970). Versuche zur Transformation an höheren Pflanzen: Genetische Charakterisierung einiger mutmasslich transformierter Pflanzen. *Z. Pflanzenphysiol.* 63: 31-43.

42. Hess, D. (1970). Versuche zur Transformation an höheren Pflanzen: Mögliche Transplantation eines Gens für Blattform bei *Petunia hybrida. Z. Pflanzenphysiol.* 63:461-467.

43. Hess, D. (1970). Molekulare Genetik bei höheren Pflanzen. *Ber. Deutsch. Bot. Ges.* 83:279-300.

44. Hess, D. (1971). Beseitigung der transformierenden Aktivität durch DNase. *Naturwissenschaften* 58:366.

45. Hess, D. (1972). Versuche zur Transformation an höheren Pflanzen: Nachweis von Heterozygoten in Versuchen zur Transplantation von Genen für Anthocyansynthese bei *Petunia hybrida. Z. Pflanzenphysiol.* 66:155-166.

46. Horak, J., Landa, Z., and Lustinec, J. (1971). Production of polyploid plants from tissue cultures of *Brassica oleracea* L. *Phyton* 28:7-10.

47. Jacquiot, C. (1947). Effect inhibiteur des tannins sur le dévelopment des cultures *in vitro* du cambium de certains arbres fruitiers. *Compt. Rend. Acad. Sci (Paris)* 225:434-436.

48. Jacquiot, C. (1949). Observations sur la néoformation de bourgeons chez le tissu cambial d'*Ulmus campestris* cultivés *in vitro. Compt. Rend. Acad. Sci. (Paris)* 229:529-530.

49. Jacquiot, C. (1950). Sur la culture *in vitro* de tissu cambial de Châtaignier (*Castanea vesca* Gaertn.). *Compt. Rend. Acad. Sci. (Paris)* 231:1080-1081.

50. Jagathesan, D. (1966). Comments. *ISSCT Sugarcane Breeders' Newsletter* 18:30-31.

51. Kameya, T., and Hinata, K. (1970). Induction of haploid plants from pollen grains of *Brassica. Japan. J. Breeding* 20:82-87.

52. Kameya, T., and Takahashi, N. (1972). The effects of inorganic salts on fusion of protoplasts from roots and leaves of *Brassica* species. *Japan. J. Genet.* 47:215-217.

53. Kameya, T., and Uchimiya, H. (1972). Embryoids derived from isolated protoplasts of carrot. *Planta* 103:356-360.

54. Kao, K. N., Keller, W. A., and Miller, R. A. (1970). Cell division in newly formed cells from protoplasts of soybean. *Exptl. Cell Res.* 62:338-340.

55. Kao, K. N., Gamborg, O. L., Miller, R. A., and Keller, W. A. (1971). Cell divisions in cells regenerated from protoplasts of soybean and *Haplopappus gracilis. Nature New Biol.* 232:124.

56. Katayama, Y., and Tanaka, M. (1969). Studies on the haploidy in relation to plant breeding. V. Further proposal of haploid method in plant breeding. *Zeiken Ziho.* 21:37-44.

57. Keller, W. A., Harvey, B., Gamborg, O. L., Miller, R. A., and Eveleigh, D. E. (1970). Plant protoplasts for use in somatic cell hybridization. *Nature* 226:280-282.

58. Maretzki, A. (1970). Success in preparing sugarcane protoplasts. Annual Report, Experiment Station, Hawaiian Sugar Planters' Association, pp. 64-65.

59. Maretzki, A., and Nickell, L. G. (1973). Formation of protoplasts from sugarcane cell suspensions and the regeneration of cell cultures from protoplasts. In: Protoplastes et Fusion de Cellules Somatiques Vegetales. Coll. internat. CNRS No. 212 (1972), Versailles, pp. 51-63.

60. Mathes, M. C. (1964). The *in vitro* formation of plantlets from isolated aspen tissue. *Phyton* 21:137-144.

61. Mee, G. W. P., Nickell, L. G., and Heinz, D. J (1969). Chemical mutagens–Their effects on cells in suspension culture. Annual Report, Experiment Station, Hawaiian Sugar Planters' Association, pp. 7-8.

62. Miller, R. A., Gamborg, O. L., Keller, W. A., and Kao, K. N. (1971). Fusion and division of nuclei in multinucleated soybean protoplasts. *Can. J. Genet. Cytol.* **13**:347-353.

63. Mitra, J., and Steward, F. C. (1961). Growth induction in cultures of *Haplopappus gracilis.* II. The behavior of the nucleus. *Am. J. Bot.* **48**:359-368.

64. Mitra, J., Mapes, M., and Steward, F. C. (1960). Growth and organized development of cultured cells. IV. The behavior of the nucleus. *Am. J. Bot.* **47**:357-368.

65. Morel, G. (1946). Action de l'acide pantothénique sur la croissance des tissus d'Aubépine cultives *in vitro. Compt. Rend. Acad. Sci. (Paris)* **223**:166-168.

66. Motoyoshi, F. (1971). Protoplasts isolated from callus cells of maize endosperm. *Exptl. Cell Res.* **68**:452-456.

67. Muir, W. H., Hildebrandt, A. C., and Riker, A. J. (1954). Plant tissue cultures produced from single isolated cells. *Science* **119**:877-878.

68. Murashige, T., and Nakano, R. (1966). Tissue culture as a potential tool in obtaining polyploid plants. *J. Hered.* **57**:115-118.

69. Nagata, T., and Takebe, I. (1970). Cell wall regeneration and cell division in isolated tobacco mesophyll protoplasts. *Planta* **92**:301-308.

70. Nagata, T., and Takebe, I. (1971). Plating of isolated tobacco mesophyll-protoplasts on agar medium. *Planta* **99**:12-20.

71. Nagata, K., and Tanaka, M. (1968). Differentiation of embryoids from developing germ cells in anther culture of tobacco. *Japan. J. Genet.* **43**:65-71.

72. Nickell, L. G., and Torrey, J. G. (1969). Crop improvement through plant cell and tissue culture. *Science* **166**:1068-1069.

73. Nickell, L. G., Maretzki, A., Higa, A., and Richards, G. M. (1971). Transformation attempts. Annual Report, Experiment Station, Hawaiian Sugar Planters' Association, pp. 33-34.

74. Niizeki, H., and Oono, K. (1968). Induction of haploid rice plants from anther culture. *Proc. Japan. Acad.* **44**:554-557.

75. Nitsch, J. P., and Nitsch, C. (1969). Haplöid plants from pollen grains. *Science* **163**:85-87.

76. Nitsch, J. P., Nitsch, C., and Pereau-Leroy, P. (1969). Obtention de mutants à partir de *Nicotiana* haploides issus de grains de pollen. *Compt. Rend. Acad. Sci. (Paris)* **269**:1650-1652.

77. Norstog, K. J. (1956). Growth of rye-grass endosperm *in vitro. Bot. Gaz.* **117**:253-259.

78. Ohyama, K., and Nitsch, J. P. (1972). Flowering haploid plants obtained from protoplasts of tobacco leaves. *Plant Cell Physiol.* **13**:229-236.

79. Otsuki, Y., and Takebe, I. (1969). Isolation of intact mesophyll cells and their protoplasts from higher plants. *Plant Cell Physiol.* **10**:917-921.

80. Partanen, C. R. (1963). Plant tissue culture in relation to developmental cytology. *Internat. Rev. Cytol.* **15**:215-243.

81. Partanen, C. R. (1965). Cytological behavior of plant tissues *in vitro* as a reflection of potentialities *in vivo.* In White, D. R., and Grove, A. R. (eds.), *Proceedings of the International Conference on Plant Tissue Culture,* McCutchan, Berkeley, Calif.

82. Pelletier, G., Raquin, C., and Simon, G. (1972). La culture *in vitro* d'anthéres d'Asperge (*Asparagus officinalis*). *Compt. Rend. Acad. Sci. (Paris)* **274**:848-851.

83. Phillips, A. Y. (1967). Colchicine treatment of noble canes. Thirty-fourth Annual Report BWI Central Cane Breeding Station, pp. 12-14.

84. Potrykus, I. (1971). Intra and interspecific fusion of protoplasts from petals of *Torenia baillonii* and *Torenia fournieri*. *Nature New Biol.* **231**:57-58.
85. Power, J. B., and Cocking, E. C. (1970). Isolation of leaf protoplasts: Macromolecule uptake and growth substance response. *J. Exptl. Bot.* **21**:64-70.
86. Power, J. B., Cummins, S. E., and Cocking, E. C. (1970). Fusion of isolated plant protoplasts. *Nature* **225**:1016-1018.
87. Raj, B., and Herr, J. M. (1970). The isolation of protoplasts from the placental cells of *Solanum nigrum* L. *Protoplasma* **69**:291-300.
88. Reinert, J., and Hellmann, S. (1971). Mechanism of the formation of polynuclear protoplasts from cells of higher plants. *Naturwissenschaften* **58**:419.
89. Ruesink, A. W. (1971). The plasma membrane of *Avena* coleoptile protoplasts. *Plant Physiol.* **47**:192-195.
90. Ruesink, A. W., and Thimann, K. V. (1965). Protoplasts from the *Avena* coleoptile. *Proc. Natl. Acad. Sci. (USA)* **54**:56-64.
91. Ruesink, A. W., and Thimann, K. V. (1966). Protoplasts: Preparation from higher plants. *Science* **154**:280-281.
92. Schenk, R. U., and Hildebrandt, A. C. (1969). Production of protoplasts from plant cells in liquid culture using purified commercial cellulases. *Crop Sci.* **9**:629-631.
93. Schmitt, C., Kopp, M., and Hirth, L. (1971). Aptitude de diverses souches de tissus de plantes cultivés *in vitro* à donner des protoplastes. *Compt. Rend. Acad. Sci. (Paris)* **272**:2447-2450.
94. Sharp, W. R., Raskin, R. S., and Sommer, H. E. (1972). Haploidy in *Lilium*. *Phytomorphology* (in press).
95. Sisodia, N. S. (1965). Techniques of colchicine application for chromosome doubling. Thirty-second Annual Report BWI Central Cane Breeding Station, pp. 30-31.
96. Sisodia, N. S. (1966). Colchicine for chromosome doubling. Thirty-third Annual Report BWI Central Cane Breeding Station, pp. 40-44.
97. Skoog, F. (1954). Substances involved in normal growth and differentiation of plants. *Brookhaven Symp. Biol.* **6**:1-21.
98. Staritsky, G. (1970). Embryoid formation in callus tissues of coffee. *Acta Bot. Neerl.* **19**:509-514.
99. Steiner, G. W., and Byther, R. S. (1971). Partial characterization and use of a host-specific toxin from *Helminthosporium sacchari* on sugarcane. *Phytopathology* **61**:691-695.
100. Steiner, G. W., and Strobel, G. A. (1971). Helminthosporoside, a host-specific toxin from *Helminthosporium sacchari*. *J. Biol. Chem.* **246**:4350-4357.
101. Straus, J. (1954). Maize endosperm tissue grown *in vitro*. II. Morphology and cytology. *Am. J. Bot.* **41**:833-839.
102. Sunderland, N., and Wicks, F. M. (1969). Cultivation of haploid plants from tobacco pollen. *Nature* **224**:1227-1229.
103. Takebe, I., Labib, G., and Melchers, G. (1971). Regeneration of whole plants from isolated mesophyll protoplasts of tobacco. *Naturwissenschaften* **58**:318-320.
104. Tanaka, M., and Nagata, K. (1969). Tobacco plants obtained by anther culture and the experiment to get diploid seeds from haploids. *Japan. J. Genet.* **44**:47-54.
105. Torrey, J. G. (1959). Experimental modification of development in the root. In Rudnick, D. (ed.), *Cell, Organism and Milieu,* Ronald Press, New York, pp. 189-222.
106. Torrey, J. G. (1967). Morphogenesis in relation to chromosomal constitution in long-term plant tissue cultures. *Physiol. Plant.* **20**:265-275.
107. Torrey, J. G., Reinert, J., and Merkel, N. (1962). Mitosis in suspension cultures of higher plant cells in a synthetic medium. *Am. J. Bot.* **49**:420-425.

108. Tulecke, W. (1957). The pollen of *Ginkgo biloba: In vitro* culture and tissue formation. *Am. J. Bot.* **44**:602-608.
109. Vreugdenhil, D. (1957). On the influence of some environmental factors on the osmotic behaviour of isolated protoplasts of *Allium cepa. Acta Bot. Neerl.* **6**:472-542.
110. Winton, L. L. (1968). Plantlets from aspen tissue cultures. *Science* **160**:1234-1235.
111. Winton, L. L. (1970). Shoot and tree production from aspen tissue cultures. *Am. J. Bot.* **57**:904-909.
112. Winton, L. L. (1971). Tissue culture preparation of European aspen. *Forest Sci.* **17**:348-350.
113. Wolter, K. E. (1968). Root and shoot initiation in aspen callus cultures. *Nature* **219**:509-510.
114. Yamada, Y., Koso, K., Sekiya, J., and Yasuda, T. (1972). Examination of the conditions for protoplast isolation from tobacco cells cultured *in vitro. Agr. Biol. Chem.* **36**:1055-1059.
115. Zenkteler, M. (1971). *In vitro* production of haploid plants from pollen grains of *Atropa belladonna* L. *Experientia (Basel)* **27**:1087.

10

Factors Favoring the Formation of Androgenetic Embryos in Anther Culture

C. Nitsch and B. Norreel

Laboratoire de Physiologie Pluricellulaire
CNRS
Gif-sur-Yvette, France

Guha and Maheshwari in 1966 (4) were the first to obtain haploid embryos *in vitro* by culturing anthers of *Datura*. Realizing the wide potential of these interesting results, Dr. J. P. Nitsch started to pursue the work by regenerating whole haploid plants. He obtained haploid *Nicotiana* in 1967 (3). Such plants, in his view, could be of great interest for plant breeding and genetic studies.

By culturing anthers, many authors have now obtained haploid plants from several species, which we divide into two groups:

a. Plants formed directly from pollen following a true embryogenetic development. This is the case with a large number of species of *Nicotiana* (3,12,14,20,34), *Datura* (15,20,26), and *Atropa belladonna* (37). Plate I describes the phenomenon; note the similarity between Fig. 1 (somatic embryo) and Fig. 2 (androgenetic embryo).

b. Plants regenerated from callus. A few other species have given positive results in this group: *Brassica* (9), *Oryza* (8,16), *Lycopersicon* (32), *Petunia* (30), *Lolium* (25), *Solanum nigrum* (6), *Asparagus* (28), and *Solanum tuberosum* (10).

We feel that the second system reduces the possibilities for experimentation because of the resultant changes in chromosome behavior (36) during the callus stage. For this reason, in our laboratory we try to avoid callus formation in making haploid plants.

The methods which will be described provide for (a) better yield of haploid

Plate I. Androgenesis in Nicotiana.

Zygotic (*Fig. 1*) and androgenetic (*Fig. 2*) embryos of *Nicotiana tabacum* (var. large-leaved, red-flowered) at the torpedo stage (fixative FAA, staining methyl green pyronin, ×480). The two embryos look alike except for the absence of suspensor in the adrogenetic embryo and the organization of the procambium, which seems greater in the androgenetic embryo and may be a reason why it can germinate directly without dormancy.

Fig. 3. After 4 weeks in culture on a suitable medium, numbers of embryos in all stages of development are visible (×380).

Fig. 4. Left: Diploid *Nicotiana tabacum* L.; note the presence of fruits. Right: Haploid *Nicotiana tabacum* L., derived from anther culture. The haploid plant is only slightly smaller but has no seeds.

Fig. 5. Chromosomes from a diploid *Nicotiana tabacum* L. var. *alata* (2n = 18) (×2050).

Fig. 6. Chromosomes from the corresponding haploid (n = 9) (×2050).

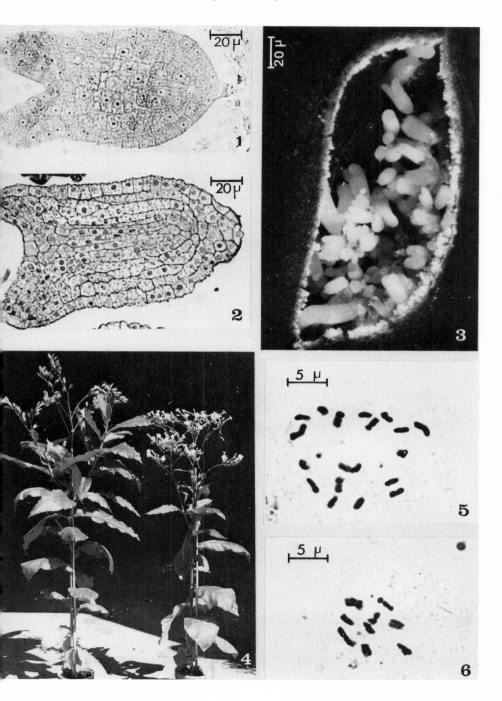

plants from pollen cultures in or outside the anther; (b) obtaining the corresponding homozygous diploids, by taking advantage of the endomitosis phenomenon which occurs in callus cultures; (c) regenerating plants from protoplasts originated from different haploids and ultimately after interspecific fusion.

BETTER YIELD OF HAPLOID PLANTS

To overcome the fact that the production of haploid plants from anther culture was restricted to only a few taxa, some authors (1, 2) have tried to produce protoplasts from pollen grains and to follow their development as somatic cells. Our aim was to simplify the system and to grow a whole plant directly from the pollen grain isolated from the anther. Our first attempt was to increase the percentage of pollen grains producing embryos inside the anther and then use this improved technique to eliminate the anther. The following results have been obtained with *Datura innoxia*.

Effect of a Trauma

Earlier work showed that to give rise to embryos the anther had to be planted just before or at the time of the first haploid division (19, 26, 27). The culture medium can be rather simple (19). When the first mitosis gave two equal nuclei instead of one vegetative and one generative, the pollen grain would give rise to an embryoid (26). Knowing of Sax's report (31) that an alteration in mitosis would initiate additional divisions in the microspore, we studied the effect of a thermic shock in our system (18).

As shown in Table I, if we pick the flower buds and keep them for 48 hr at $3°C$, we increase the percentage of anthers producing embryos to 21%, compared with 3.2% in the control.

Table I. Effect of Temperature Trauma on the Number of
Anthers Yielding Embryos in *Datura innoxia*[a]

Treatment given to the flower bud	Number of anthers planted	Number of anthers yielding embryos	Percentage of anthers yielding embryos
None	162	2	1.2
48 hr at $24°C$	218	7	3.2
48 hr at $3°C$	219	46	21

[a] The stage of the pollen in the anther is checked with acetocarmin at the start of the culture. The pollen is in mitosis.

Table II. Effect of Environmental Temperatures on the Yield of Embryos in *Datura innoxia*

Temperature at which the plant is grown	State of the pollen	Treatment given to the flower bud	Number of anthers in culture	Number of anthers producing embryos	Percentage of anthers yielding embryos
17°C	Just before mitosis	None	24	2	8
		48 hr at 3°C	24	13	54
24°C	Just before mitosis	None	76	34	45
		48 hr at 3°C	73	65	89
24°C	During mitosis	None	74	7	9
		48 hr at 3°C	60	36	60

Plate II. Effect of Cold Treatment on Pollen Culture in *Datura innoxia.*

Figs. 8–13. Microscopic study (fixative FAA; staining 8, 9, 11 hematoxylin - ruthenium red, 10, 12, 13 Feulgen - methyl green; ×3200; a.m., axes of mitosis).

8–10: No cold treatment.

8: Normal first haploid mitosis (side view of telophase; note the oblique direction of the axes of mitosis).

9: Side view of a binucleate pollen grain with vegetative and reproductive nuclei normally differentiated.

11–12: With pretreatment (48 hr at 3°C).

11: Disturbed first haploid mitosis, telophase (note that this axis of mitosis is parallel to the pollen grain wall; compare with Fig. 8).

12: Pollen grain with two equal nuclei; from their position, we can see that they originate from two mitoses similar to that in Fig. 11 (compare with Fig. 9).

10–13: Proembryos.

10: With two different types of nuclei (reproductive and vegetative).

13: All nuclei appear the same (vegetative type).

Fig. 14. Anthers of *Datura innoxia* after 3 weeks in culture (×3). Left: No cold treatment. Right: The flower bud had 48 hr at 3°C before the anthers were removed.

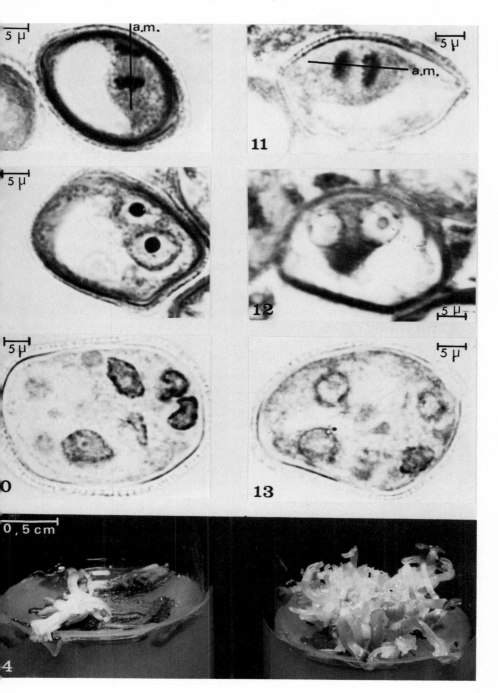

Effect of the Environment of the Mother Plant

Datura plants were grown at different temperatures in the Phytotron at Gif. In this experiment, we studied the effect of the temperature at which the plant was grown (17 or 24°C with long or short days) using flower buds in which the pollen was at a stage just before the first division or in mitosis. In each case, four out of the five stamens were planted and the last one was used for determination of the state of the pollen with acetocarmin coloration. The results are shown in Table II and may be briefly stated as follows: (a) If the plant is grown at its optimal temperature, i.e., 24°C, the pollen reacts better with (89%) or without (45%) cold treatment than if the plant is grown at 17°C (54% *vs.* 89% and 8% *vs.* 45%). (b) When the cold treatment is given to the anther just prior to the start of mitosis, it is less effective (45% *vs.* 89%) than if it is given during mitosis (9% *vs.* 60%).

Plate II shows the state of the nucleus in pollen grains having received the cold treatment (Figs. 11, 12, 13) compared with that in grains taken directly (Figs. 8, 9, 10) as well as the improvement in the number of embryos formed (Fig. 14).

In Table III, we see that the percentage of abnormal divisions is greatly enhanced by the cold treatment at the start of the culture (0 *vs.* 16%) or after 5 days in culture (1.6% *vs.* 12.2%). On the other hand, we noticed that after 5 days in culture the number of dead microspores is smaller with the cold

Table III. Effect of Temperature Treatment on the Type of Cell Division in Pollen Grains of *Datura innoxia*

Treatment given to the flower bud	Percentage of grains with two different nuclei (1 vegetative, 1 reproductive)	Percentage of grains with two nuclei identical	Percentage of dead grains	Number of grains studied
At the start of culture				
None	18.8	0	0	579
48 hr at 3°C	21	16.7	0	370
After 5 days in culture				
None	1.1	1.6	92.6	668
48 hr at 3°C	3.9	12.2	62.2	511

treatment (62.2%) than with no treatment (92.6%). The cold temperature seems to protect the microspore, perhaps by stopping the course of mitosis while the anther is adjusting to its new environmental conditions.

With the appropriate environmental treatments, we now obtain a larger number of embryos. Changes in day length were not found to affect the number of embryos appreciably.

Culture of Pollen Grains Isolated from the Anther

Having greatly improved the number of anthers and the number of micro-spores giving rise to plantlets, we then tried to culture the pollen outside the anther, which makes it possible to follow the development of the embryos during different treatments. Experimentation is not possible if the pollen is cultured in the anther or on a nurse callus (32, 29).

By adding to the usual medium of Halperin (i.e., macro elements (5) completed with 10^{-4} M Fe EDTA, 100 μg/liter IAA, 2 gr/liter glutamine, 2% sucrose) a water extract of anthers giving embryos at a concentration of one anther/ml (18), we could obtain, in liquid culture, the development of micro-spores into plantlets.

Plate III shows the different stages of the embryos—globular, heart-shaped, and torpedo (Figs. 15, 16)—obtained in such cultures. The plantlets were transferred after 8 weeks' growth to a very simple medium without auxin or sugar to enhance root development (Fig. 17) and then transplanted to pots in the greenhouse. Mr. P. Debergh, in our laboratory, has also obtained very satisfactory results, at least as far as the globular stage, using the same method with *Lycopersicum*.

CONVERSION OF THE HAPLOID TO THE CORRESPONDING HOMOZYGOUS DIPLOID PLANT

Most geneticists obtain diploid plants by using colchicine. The treatment has to be repeated several times, and, in our hands, the technique is not always reliable. Since the plants studied regenerate easily from callus, we made use of the phenomenon of endomitosis, which occurs in callus cultures, to obtain the corresponding diploid. This method was first used by Murashige and Nakano (13).

In previous work (22), we were able to show that by producing a callus from the haploid tobacco plant and keeping it in culture under known conditions the level of ploidy in the cell could be changed. The effect of different auxins and cytokinins was studied (17), and it was shown that a high concentration of IAA (10^{-5} M) enhances the endomitosis. When no cytokinin is added to the medium, the occurrence of endomitosis is reduced. Benzyladenine seems to be the

Plate III. Embryo Formation in a Culture of Microspores Isolated from the Anther (*Datura innoxia*).

Fig. 15. After 6 weeks in culture, numerous embryos are evident (×1.5).

Fig. 16. Stages of embryo development from isolated microspore (globular, heart-shaped, and torpedo) (×40).

Fig. 17. Plantlet transferred from the dish of Fig. 15 to a solid medium after 8 weeks in culture (×3).

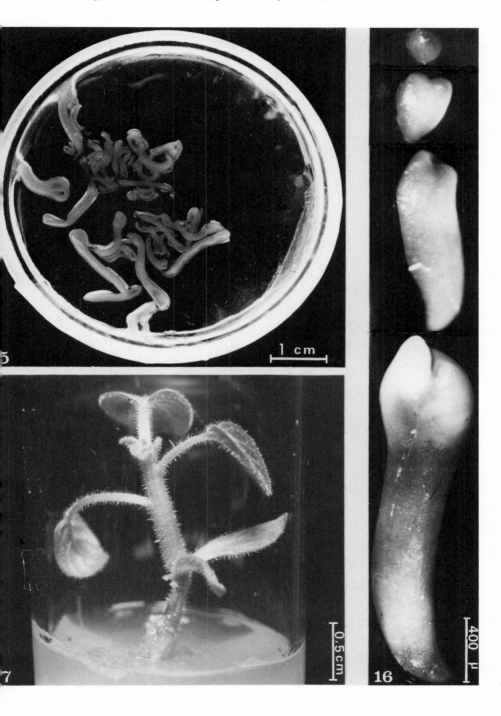

Plate IV. Regeneration of a Whole Plant from a Haploid Protoplast Derived from Leaves of
Nicotiana tabacum.

    Fig. 18. Isolated protoplasts (×450).

    Fig. 19. First division of a protoplast (×450).

    Fig. 20. Regenerated flowering plant.

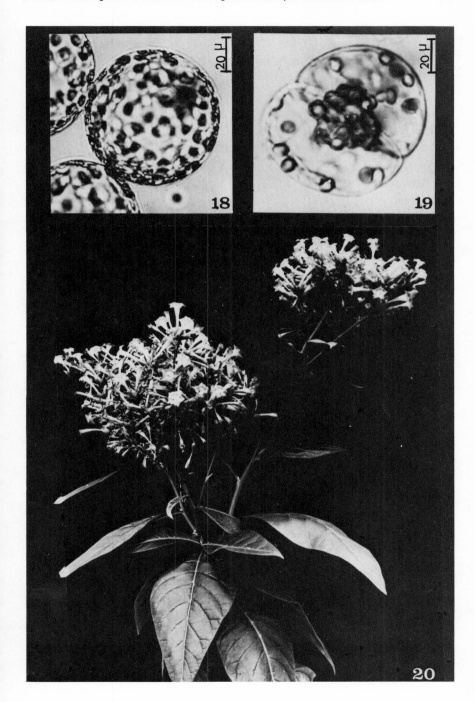

cytokinin which most favors the diploidization of the cells. These results confirm the work of Torrey (35).

Thus, now having a callus with diploid cells, following the work of Skoog and Tsui (33) it was easy to regenerate diploid plants which were homozygous and fertile.

CULTURE OF HAPLOID TOBACCO PROTOPLASTS AND REGENERATION TO COMPLETE PLANTS

The possibility of growing microspores isolated from the anther in liquid medium makes it experimentally feasible to pursue studies of mutation. Mutagenic treatments given to the microspores give more homogeneous results than treatments of a pluricellular mass. Moreover, starting with haploid material, mutation can be readily observed (23).

The aim of Dr. J. P. Nitsch in this work was to produce new plants by (a) fusing two protoplasts of new mutants, thinking that haploid protoplasts would be easier to fuse than diploids, and (b) regenerating new plants from these protoplasts.

In our laboratory, to date, we have had more success in the second part than in the first. Starting with protoplasts isolated from leaves of haploid tobacco, Nitsch and Ohyama (24) were able to regenerate the whole plant from them. Plate IV illustrates a few steps of the experimentation with haploid *Nicotiana tabacum* (Red var.). Our aim is now to be able to use the same technique starting with fused protoplasts. So far, except for the brilliant work of Carlson, fused protoplasts do not seem to differentiate as easily as nonfused protoplasts.

CONCLUSION

It has been shown that the percentage of anthers yielding embryos can be greatly increased by low-temperature treatment of the flowers. The number of live pollen grains is also increased in this way, and a specific modification of the culture medium allows the growth of isolated pollen grains outside the anther. Thus haploid entire plants can be regenerated from this material as can the corresponding diploids.

We hope that this new technique of producing haploid plants from pollen grains outside the anther will permit us to obtain haploid plants of more species, especially, perhaps, plants containing inhibitory substances in the anthers. With this method, work on mutations will have a wider range. After the brilliant work of Ledoux and Huart (11) on barley and Hess (7) on *Petunia,* which shows the possibility that DNA extracted from bacteria can penetrate into higher plants and even replicate there, we may hope for a very exciting future for plant breeders.

REFERENCES

1. Bhojwani, S. S., and Cocking, E. C. (1972). Isolation of protoplast from pollen tetrads. *Nature New Biol.* **239**:29-30.

2. Binding, H. (1972). Isolated protoplast from orchids pollen. EMBO, Tübingen, unpublished.

3. Bourgin, J. P., and Nitsch, J. P. (1967). Obtention de *Nicotiana* haploïdes à partir d'étamines cultivées *in vitro. Ann. Physiol. Vég.* **9**:377-382.

4. Guha, S., and Maheshwari, S. C. (1966). Cell division and differentiation of embryos in the pollen grains of *Datura in vitro. Nature* **212**:97-98.

5. Halperin, W., and Wetherell, D. F. (1965). Ammonium requirement for embryogenesis *in vitro. Nature* **205**:519-520.

6. Harn, C. (1971). Studies on anther culture in *Solanum nigrum. Sabrao Newsletter* **3**:39-42.

7. Hess, D. (1969). Versuche zur Transformation an höheren Pflanzen: Wiederholung der Anthocyan. Induktion bei *Petunia* und erste Charakterisierung des transformierenden Prinzips. *Z. Pflanzenphysiol.* **61**:286-298.

8. Iyers, R. D., and Raina, S. K. (1972). The early ontogeny of embryoids and callus from pollen and subsequent organogenesis in anther cultures of *Datura metel* and rice. *Planta (Berl.)* **104**:146-156.

9. Kameya, T., and Hinata, K. (1970). Induction of haploid plants from pollen grains of *Brassica. Japan. J. Breeding* **20**:82-87.

10. Kohlenbach, Z., and Geier, T. (1972). Embryonen aus *in vitro* kultivierten Antheren von *Datura meteloides* Dun., *Datura wrigtii* Regel, und *Solanum tuberosum* L. *Pflanzenphysiologie* **67**:161-165.

11. Ledoux, L., and Huart, R. (1969). Fate of exogenous bacterial deoxyribonucleic acids in barley seedlings. *J. Mol. Biol.* **43**:243-262.

12. Melchers, G., and Labib, G. (1970). Die Bedeutung haploider höherer Pflanzen für Pflanzenphysiologie und Pflanzenzüchtung. *Ber. Deutsch. Bot. Ges.* **83**:129-150.

13. Murashige, T., and Nakano, R. (1966). Tissue culture as a potential tool in obtaining polyploid plants. *J. Hered.* **57**:115-118.

14. Nakata, K., and Tanaka, M. (1968). Differentiation of embryoids from developing germ cells in anther culture of tobacco. *Japan. J. Genet.* **43**:65-71.

15. Narawanaswamy, S., and Chandy, L. P. (1971). *In vitro* induction of haploid, diploid and triploid androgenetic embryoids and plantlets in *Datura metel* L. *Ann. Bot.* **35**:535-542.

16. Niizeki, H., and Oono, K. (1968). Induction of haploid rice plant from anther culture. *Proc. Japan. Acad.* **44**:554-557.

17. Nitsch, C. (1971). Transformations génétiques obtenues au moyen de cultures *in vitro*. 96e *Congr. Soc. Sav. (Toulouse) Sciences* **4.**

18. Nitsch, C., and Norreel, B. (1972). Effet d'un choc thermique sur le pouvoir embryogène du pollen de *Datura innoxia* cultivé dans l'anthère et isolé de l'anthère. *Compt. Rend. Acad. Sci. (Paris)* **276(1)**:303-306.

19. Nitsch, J. P. (1969). Experimental androgenesis in *Nicotiana. Phytomorphology* **19**:389-404.

20. Nitsch, J. P. (1970). La production *in vitro* d'embryons haploïdes: Résultats et perspectives. *Coll. Internat. CNRS (Strasbourg)*, pp. 281-294.

21. Nitsch, J. P., and Nitsch, C. (1970). Obtention de plantes haploïdes à partir de pollen. *Bull. Soc. Bot. France* **117**:339-360.

22. Nitsch, J. P., Nitsch, C., and Hamon, S. (1969). Production de *Nicotiana* diploides à

partir de cals haploides cultivés *in vitro. Compt. Rend. Acad. Sci. (Paris)* 269(D):1275-1278.

23. Nitsch, J. P., Nitsch, C., and Péreau-Leroy, M. P. (1969). Obtention de mutants à partir de *Nicotiana* haploïdes issus de grains de pollen. *Compt. Rend. Acad. Sci. (Paris)* 269(D):1650-1652.

24. Nitsch, J. P., and Ohyama, K. (1971). Obtention de plantes à partir de protoplastes haploïdes cultivés *in vitro. Compt. Rend. Acad. Sci. (Paris)* 273:801-804.

25. Nitzsche, W. (1970). Herstellung haploider Pflanzen aus *Festuca-Lolium* Bastarden. *Naturwissenschaften* 57:199-200.

26. Norreel, B. (1970). Etude cytologique de l'androgenèse expérimentale chez *Nicotiana tabacum* et *Datura innoxia. Bull. Soc. Bot. France* 117:461-478.

27. Norreel, B. (1971). La néoformation d'embryons *in vitro* chez *Daucus carota, Nicotiana tabacum* et *Datura innoxia.* Thèse 3ème cycle, Université Paris VI, 66 pp., 33 planches (non publié).

28. Pelletier, G., Raquin, C., and Simon, G. (1972). La culture *in vitro* d'anthères d'asperge (*Asparagus officinalis*). *Compt. Rend. Acad. Sci. (Paris)* 274:848-851.

29. Pelletier, G., and Durran, V. (1972). Recherche de tissus nourriciers pour la réalisation de l'androgenèse expérimentale chez le *Nicotiana tabacum. Compt. Rend. Acad. Sci. (Paris)* 275:35-37.

30. Raquin, C. (1970). Production de *Petunia* haploïdes par culture d'anthères *in vitro.* D.E.A. D'Amélioration des Plantes, Faculté des Sciences d'Orsay.

31. Sax, K. (1935). The effect of temperature on nuclear differentiation in microspore development. *J. Arnold Arbor.* 19:301-310.

32. Sharp, W. R., Raskin, R. S., and Sommer, H. E. (1972). The use of nurse culture in the development of haploid clones in tomato. *Planta (Berl.)* 104:357-361.

33. Skoog, F., and Tsui, C. (1948). Chemical control of growth and bud formation in tobacco stem segments and callus cultured *in vitro. Am. J. Bot.* 35:782-787.

34. Sunderland, N., and Wicks, F. M. (1971). Embryoid formation in pollen grains of *Nicotiana tabacum. J. Exptl. Bot.* 22:213-226.

35. Torrey, J. G. (1961). Kinetin as trigger for mitosis in mature endomitotic plant cells. *Exptl. Cell Res.* 23:281-299.

36. Torrey, J. G. (1967). Morphogenesis in relation to chromosomal constitution in long-term plant tissue cultures. *Physiol. Plant.* 20:265-275.

37. Zenkteler, M. (1971). *In vitro* production of haploid plants from pollen grains of *Atropa belladonna. Separatum Experiantia* 27:1087.

Plant Hormonal Mechanisms

11

Cytokinins in Regulation of Plant Growth

Folke Skoog

Institute of Plant Development, Birge Hall
University of Wisconsin
Madison, Wisconsin, U.S.A.

The extension of principles governing gene-controlled protein biosynthesis in prokaryotes as a basic regulatory mechanism common to all growth and developmental processes in eukaryotes, also, is now generally accepted. The question, then, is, what factors are involved in modulating the expression of genetic potentials in cells with an identical genome so as to permit development of functional, multicellular organisms? In the case of plants, it is clear that environmental factors, temperature, light, and inorganic nutrients influence differentiation and development in striking, specific ways, but, as in animals, it is recognized that endogenous growth factors, or hormones, mediate these effects and more generally serve to regulate the expression of genetic potentials. Furthermore, in plants as in animals, several categories of such substances exist, and changing balances in activity between them may modulate metabolism and bring about morphogenesis and functional changes characteristic of normal ontogeny. In this context, I wish to discuss the group of substances referred to as cytokinins.

DEFINITION AND BIOASSAYS

Cytokinins have been arbitrarily defined (76) in terms of their capacity to promote cell division (cytokinesis) and continuous growth *in vitro* of callus tissue under specified conditions, in the same manner as does kinetin (6-furfurylaminopurine), the first substance of this type to be identified (60). This terminology is analogous to the use of "auxin" as a generic name for substances which promote cell elongation in specific test systems in the same manner as does indole-3-acetic acid, the first of its kind to be identified. Cytokinins, like

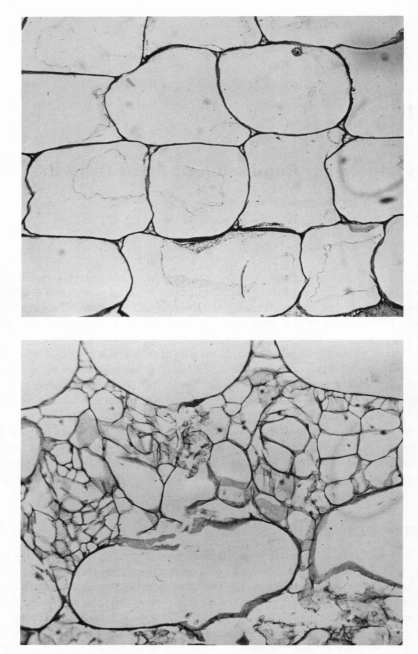

Fig. 1. Effect of cytokinin on cell division and growth of excised tobacco tissue.
Top: without; bottom: with 100 μg/liter kinetin in the nutrient medium.

auxins and gibberellins, exert regulatory functions in all phases of plant development. Sometimes the effects of these three kinds of substances appear to be from opposing actions of one against another, but more generally the three act synergistically, and each one appears to be essential for growth.

Tissue cultures of several plant species (tobacco, soybean, carrot, etc.) have been used to measure growth responses. Other responses such as expansion of excised leaf tissue, release of inhibited lateral buds, biosynthesis of various pigments, and retention of chlorophyll also have been utilized for bioassays of cytokinin activity (53,73). The effects of cytokinin on cell division in excised tobacco pith tissue are illustrated in Fig. 1, and relationships between the cytokinin concentration and yield of tobacco callus, as in a typical bioassay, are presented in Fig. 2.

Cytokinins have been reported to promote growth of animal cells. Most notable are lymphocyte cultures, in which cytokinin-active ribonucleosides may accelerate early stages and inhibit late stages of the cell cycle. There are also reports of positive cytokinin effects on the growth of microorganisms, including bacteria, algae, yeasts, and other fungi. So far, however, only plant systems have been utilized for bioassays or detailed physiological studies.

Recent reviews of cytokinins and their effects include the following: Gaspar and Xhaufflaire (26), Hall (28), Kende (38), Leonard (48), Letham (53a), Skoog and Armstrong (72), Skoog and Schmitz (74), Skoog (71), and Steward and Krikorian (77).

NATURAL OCCURRENCE AND PROPERTIES OF CYTOKININ-ACTIVE ADENINE DERIVATIVES

The chemistry of cytokinins, including syntheses, structure/activity relationships, identification of naturally occurring species, and aspects of their metabolism, has been reviewed by Leonard (48).

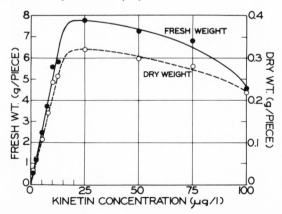

Fig. 2. Effect of cytokinin concentration on growth of tobacco tissue cultures.

Table I. Naturally Occurring and Some Related Cytokinins

Substance: chemical name [synonym and/or abbreviation]	Structure:			Source				Number in Fig. 4
	R_1	R_2	R_3	Bacteria	Fungi	Higher plants	Animals	
6-(3-Methyl-2-butenylamino)purine [N^6-Δ^2-isopentenyladenine; 2ip, or i^6 Ade]	(isopentenyl)	H	H	+	+	+	?	2
6-(3-Methyl-2-butenylamino)-9-β-D-ribofuranosylpurine [N^6-(Δ^2-isopentenyl)adenosine; 2iPA, i6Ado, or i^6 A]	"	H	Rib^a	+	+	+	+	6
6-(3-Methyl-2-butenylamino)-2-methylthiopurine [ms2iP or $ms^2 i^6$ Ade]	"	H_3CS	H	?	+	?		4
6-(3-Methyl-2-butenylamino)-2-methylthio-9-β-D-ribopuranosylpurine [ms2iPA or $ms^2 i^6$ A]	"	H_3CS	Rib	+	+	+		8
6-(4-Hydroxy-3-methyl-trans-2-butenylamino)purine [zeatin, t-io^6 Ade]	(hydroxy OH)	H	H		+	+		1
6-(4-Hydroxy-3-methyl-trans-2-butenylamino)-9-β-D-ribofuranosylpurine [ribosylzeatin; t-io^6 A]	"	H	Rib		+	+		5
6-(4-Hydroxy-3-methyl-trans-2-butenylamino)-2-methylthiopurine [mszeatin; t-$ms^2 io^6$ Ade]	"	H_3CS	H		+	?		3

Compound	Structure	(2)	(9)			Ref.
6-(4-Hydroxy-3-methyl-*trans*-2-butenylamino)-2-methylthio-9-β-D-ribofuranosylpurine [msribosylzeatin]; *t*-ms² io⁶ A]	⟋⟍OH	H₃CS	Rib	+	+	7
6-(4-Hydroxy-3-methyl-*cis*-2-butenylamino)purine [*cis*-zeatin; *c*-io⁶ Ade]	⟋OH	H	H	+	?	III^b
6-(4-Hydroxy-3-methyl-*cis*-2-butenylamino)-2-β-D-ribofuranosylpurine [ribosyl-*cis*-zeatin *c*-io⁶ A]	"	H	Rib	+?	+?	XII^b
6-(4-Hydroxy-3-methyl-*cis*-2-butenylamino)-2-methythiopurine [ms*cis*-zeatin; *c*-ms² io⁶ Ade]	"	H₃CS	H	?		
6-(4-Hydroxy-3-methyl-*cis*-2-butenylamino)-2-methylthio-9-β-D-ribofuranosylpurine [msribosyl-*cis*-zeatin; *c*-ms² io⁶ A]	"	H₃CS	Rib	+?	+	
6-(3-Methylbutylamino)purine [N⁶-isoamyladenine; H₂iP; or H₂i⁶ Ade]	⟋⟍	H	H		+?	10
6-(3-Methylbutylamino)-9-β-D-ribofuranosylpurine [N⁶-isoamyladenosine; H₂iPa; or H₂i⁶ A]	"	H	Rib			14
6-(3-Methylbutylamino)-2-methylthiopurine [msH₂iP, or ms²H₂i⁶ Ade]	"	H₃CS	H			12
6-(3-Methylbutylamino)-2-methylthio-9-β-D-ribofuranosylpurine [msH₂iPA or ms²H₂i⁶ A]	"	H₃CS	Rib			16
6-(4-Hydroxy-3-methylbutylamino)purine [dihydrozeatin; H₂io⁶ Ade]	⟋⟍OH	H	H	+	+	9
6-(4-Hydroxy-3-methylbutylamino)-9-β-D-ribofuranosylpurine [ribosyldihydrozeatin]; H₂io⁶ A	"	H	R	+	+	13

Table I. (Continued)

Substance: chemical name [synonym and/or abbreviation]	Structure: R₁	R₂	R₃	Source Bacteria	Fungi	Higher plants	Animals	Number in Fig. 4
6-(4-Hydroxy-3-methylbutylamino)-2-methylthiopurine [msdihydrozeatin; ms²H₂io⁶Ade]	$\sim\!\!\sim$OH							11
6-(4-Hydroxy-3-methylbutylamino)-2-methylthio-9-β-D-ribofuranosylpurine [msribosyldihydrozeatin; ms²H₂io⁶A]	"							15
6-(3-Hydroxy-3-methylbutylamino)purine [30HiP]ᶜ	OH	H	H	?		?	?	
6-(3-Hydroxy-3-methylbutylamino)-9-β-D-ribofuranosylpurine [30HiPA]ᶜ	"	H	Rib	?	?	?	?	
6-Furfurylaminopurine [kinetin]ᶜ	(furfuryl)	H	H	?	?	?	?	

[a] Ribosyl.
[b] Number of the compound in Fig. 7.
[c] Not generally accepted as naturally occurring.

Known naturally occurring cytokinins which are adenine derivatives and some closely related substances which also may be expected to occur in nature are listed in Table I, together with synonyms, abbreviations, and current information on their distribution in organisms. A set of 16 of these compounds, representing the possible combinations of the four main modifications of N^6-Δ^2-isopentenyladenine (2iP) found in naturally occurring cytokinins, were synthesized and compared for activity in the tobacco bioassay as shown in Figs. 3 and 4 (68).

6-(3-Methyl-2-Butenylamino)purine

6-(3-Methyl-2-butenylamino)purine (2iP) (No. 2 in Figs. 3 and 4) may be considered as the archetype of all cytokinins of the isopentenyladenine type. It was first synthesized by Leonard and coworkers in 1961 and has served as a reference standard in the isolation of naturally occurring cytokinins. It was itself isolated in 1966, both as a main cytokinin present as a free base in *Corynebacterium fascians* cultures (35,41) and as the ribonucleotide (odd base) adjacent to the anticodon in yeast $tRNA_{I+II}^{Ser}$ (82,83). It has since been identified (as the ribonucleoside, 2iPA, No. 6 in Fig. 4) in tRNA hydrolysates from a broad spectrum of organisms including bacteria, fungi, higher plants, and animals. 2iPA is the only cytokinin so far characterized from animal sources (beef and rat liver tRNA) and insects (*Drosophila* $tRNA^{Ser}$; Armstrong *et al.*, unpublished).

Zeatin

Zeatin, the *trans*-4-hydroxyl derivative of 2iP (No. 1 in Fig. 4) identified by Letham *et al.* (54), is the most active cytokinin of this group. It has been isolated repeatedly either as the free base or as the riboside, mainly the *cis*-isomer, in tRNA from plant material. The enhancement of activity by the 4-hydroxyl group holds also for derivatives with saturated side chain and/or additionally substituted as shown in Fig. 4. Hydroxyl substituents at other positions lower cytokinin activity (51).

Formal modification of zeatin as an exogenous cytokinin by deoxidation, hydrogenation, methylthiation, or ribosidation leads to systematic decreases in biological activity, and combinations of these modifications generally lead to additive or greater losses in activity. The depressive effect of 2-methylthiation on growth-promoting activity is in contrast with its reported enhancement of tRNA-ribosomal binding (see below). In this context, the marked decrease in growth-promoting activity brought about by ribosidation was also unexpected. However, testing of substituted 8-aza-9-deaza purines (pyrazolo[4,3-d] pyrimidines) suggests that the ribosyl moiety is not necessary for promotion of cell division and growth by exogenous cytokinins (33).

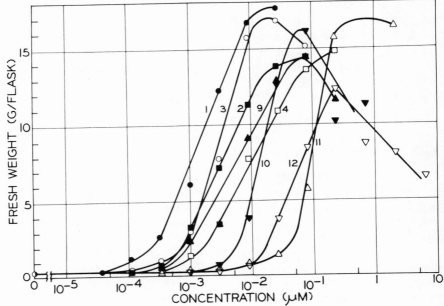

Fig. 3.

Scheme I.

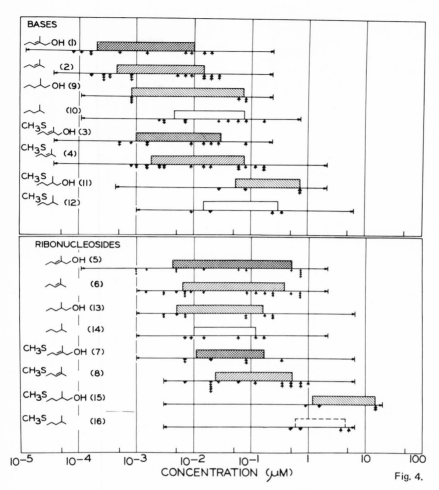

Fig. 3. Comparison of effectiveness of eight N^6-isopent(en)yladenines in promoting growth of tobacco callus. The compounds are numbered as in Scheme I and Fig. 4. From Schmitz *et al.* (68); reprinted with permission of the publishers of *Phytochemistry*.

Fig. 4. Summary of cytokinin activities of some naturally occurring and closely related N^6-isopent(en)yl adenine and adenosine derivatives in the tobacco bioassay. The compounds are numbered as in Scheme I and Fig. 3. For easy reference, the substituents at the N^6-position and the methylthio group at the 2-position are shown also in the margin. The baselines represent the tested concentration ranges, and the bars represent the average values of the concentration ranges over which growth increases as a nearly linear function of the $\log_{10}$ of the concentration of added cytokinin. The arrows underneath the baselines represent start and end points of the linear growth response in individual experiments. Chain structure is indicated by shading of the bars as follows: open bars, isopentyl group; right-to-left hatched bars, Δ^2-isopentenyl group; left-to-right hatched bars, OH-substituted group. The bar outlined with a broken line indicates that no concentration achieved the full growth response. From Schmitz *et al.* (68); reprinted with permission of the publishers of *Phytochemistry*.

A few notable exceptions have been found to the general rule that disubstitution or other modification of zeatin leads to a decrease in growth-promoting activity. 2-Chlorozeatin and 6-(3-chlorobutenylamino)purine are the most active synthetic cytokinins so far tested in the tobacco bioassay. Esters of zeatin also tend to be distinctly more active than zeatin itself, probably by serving to release the free base gradually in the course of the bioassay (Fig. 5) (67). Some 8-substituted adenine derivatives or related compounds are also more active than their parent compounds (ref. 46 and Leonard *et al.*, unpublished).

Zeatin Isomers

The stereoselective synthesis of *cis*-zeatin (52,65) has made possible the synthesis, identification, and comparison of biological activities of geometric and position isomers of zeatin. Zeatin extracted as the free base from plant sources

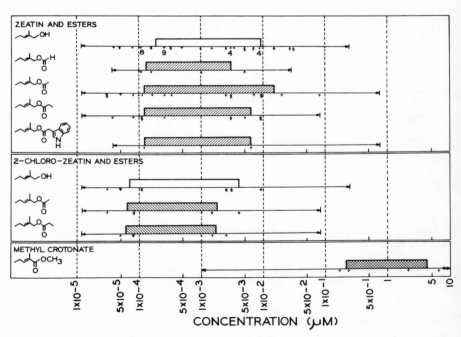

Fig. 5. Comparison of activities of esters of zeatin and 2-chlorozeatin in the tobacco bioassay. Presentation of data is as in Fig. 4. The tested compounds in order from the top are zeatin, *trans*-methoxyzeatin, *trans*-ethoxyzeatin, *trans*-propoxyzeatin, zeatin indole-3-acetate, 2-chlorozeatin, 2-chloro-*trans*-methoxyzeatin, 2-chloro-*trans*-ethoxyzeatin, and zeatin-methylcrotonate. From Schmitz *et al.* (67); reprinted with permission of the publishers of *Phytochemistry*.

so far has been exclusively the *trans*-isomer (53*a*, 54), while the ribonucleoside isolated from plant tRNA hydrolysates has been reported to be the *cis*-isomer (3,29,30). tRNA hydrolysates from *Pisum* shoots, however, have yielded both the *cis*- and *trans*-isomers of ribosylzeatin (81) and also the two corresponding 2-methylthio derivatives (Vreman *et al.*, unpublished). As shown by tests of synthetic preparations in Figs. 6 and 7, zeatin (II) is nearly 50 times as active as *cis*-zeatin (III) in the tobacco bioassay, but both are highly effective cytokinins. Similarly, a marked difference in activity is found between the *trans*- and *cis*-isomers of isozeatin (V and III) and between each pair of corresponding ribonucleosides (XI and XII; XIV and XV). The data show further that shifting the methyl group from the 3- to the 2-position in the side chain, as in isozeatin (V), or its removal, as in norzeatin (VIII), markedly decreases biological activity. Cyclization of the chain, as in cyclic norzeatin (IX), practically eliminates cytokinin activity.

Dihydrozeatin

Dihydrozeatin has been isolated from seeds of lupin (43) and beans (45). As shown by the relative activities in Figs. 6 and 7 and in Fig. 4, hydrogenation of the side chain decreases the activity of zeatin but increases that of *cis*-zeatin (compare compound IV with II and III in Fig. 7). The same holds for the corresponding ribonucleosides (compare compound XIII with XI and XII in Fig. 7). It should be noted, however, that IV and XIII represent mixtures of (±) enantiomers in unknown proportions, of which the (−) form, isolated from lupins, must be much the more active on the basis of available information for related pairs of isomers (44). In tests of activity based on growth and greening of excised *Cucumis* cotyledons, dihydrozeatin has been found to be closely comparable to zeatin (Tahbaz *et al.*, unpublished). It should be noted that hydrogenation results in a more drastic loss in activity in 2-methylthiozeatin than in zeatin (compare differences between compounds 3 and 11 and between 1 and 9 in Fig. 4), and this holds also for the corresponding pairs of ribonucleosides (compare 7 and 15 *vs.* 5 and 13 in Fig. 4). Hydrogenation of the side chain in 2iP and its ribonucleoside decreases the activity more than in the corresponding zeatin derivatives (compare difference between 2 and 10 with that between 6 and 14 in Fig. 4). The same holds for the 2-methylthiated derivatives, except that in this case the hydrogenated 2iP derivatives are somewhat more active than the corresponding zeatin derivatives (compare compound 11 with 12 and 15 with 16 in Fig. 4).

6-(3-Hydroxyisopentylamino)purine

6-(3-Hydroxyisopentylamino)purine, the isomer of dihydrozeatin, and its derivatives are included in Table I because even though they are not accepted as

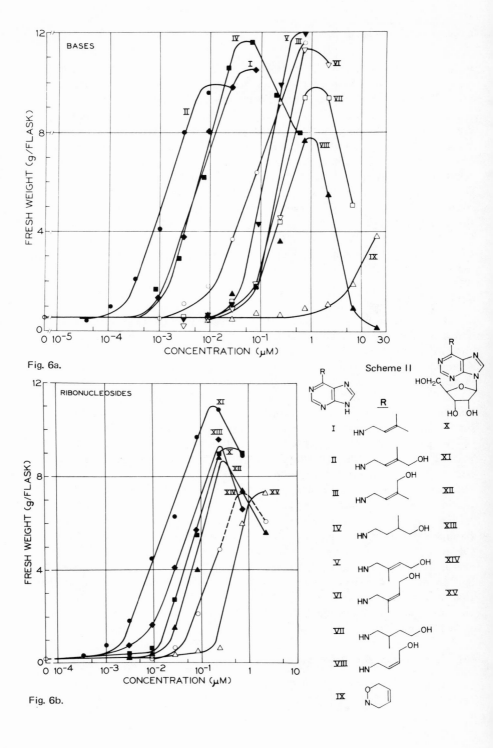

Fig. 6a.

Fig. 6b.

Scheme II

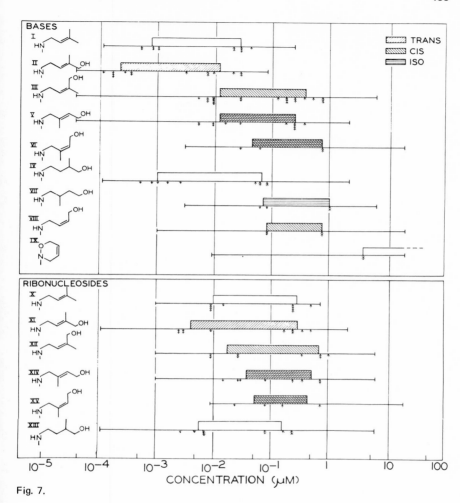

Fig. 7.

Fig. 6. Cytokinin activities of geometric and position isomers of zeatin and ribosylzeatin. The compounds are numbered as in scheme II and Fig. 7. Concentration curves from single experiments. Data from Schmitz *et al.* (69); reprinted with permission of the publishers of *Plant Physiol.*

Fig. 7. Summary of cytokinin of activities of trans-, cis-, iso-, and nor-zeatins and dihydro-zeatins. The compounds are numbered as in scheme II and Fig. 6. For easy reference, the substituents at the 6-position are indicated also in the margin, and the bars are shaded to distinguish between kinds of isomers. The data are presented as described in Fig. 4. Data from Schmitz *et al.* (69); reprinted with permission of the publishers of *Plant Physiol.*

bona fide natural constituents they readily arise as artifacts derived from 2iP or its derivatives. 6-(3-Hydroxyisopentylamino)purine is a hundredfold less active than zeatin (50), but the two compounds are sufficiently alike to prevent their separation by common isolation procedures. Thus the diagnosis of zeatin by most of the current chromatographic and other methods short of rigorous chemical identification may in fact be misleading or totally in error, especially if

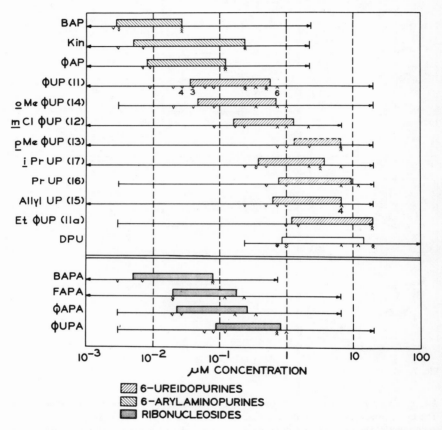

Fig. 8. Comparison of cytokinin activities of N,N¹-diphenylurea, 6-ureidopurines, and 6-arylaminopurines. The compounds are, in order from the top, BAP, 6-benzylaminopurine; Kin, 6-furfurylaminopurine; φAP, 6-phenylaminopurine; φUP, 6-phenylureidopurine; oMeφUP, 6-o-tolylureidopurine; mClφUP, 6-m-chlorophenylureidopurine; pMeφUP, 6-p-tolylureidopurine; iPrUP, 6-isopropylureidopurine; PrUP, 6-n-propylureidopurine; Ally1UP, 6-allylureidopurine; EtφUP, 6-N-ethyl-N'-phenylureidopurine; DPU, N,N'-diphenylurea; and BAPA, etc., the 9-β-D-ribofuranosyl derivatives of the first four listed purines. Presentation of data is as described in Figs. 4 and 6. From McDonald *et al.* (59); reprinted with permission of the publishers of *Phytochemistry*.

acid conditions which enhance the hydration of 2iP are employed. It seems likely that 6-(3-hydroxyisopentylamino)purine and its derivatives will in fact be found to occur naturally.

Kinetin

Kinetin (6-furfurylaminopurine), often considered to be an artifact, is included in Table I because it can be derived from deoxyadenosine and other nucleic acid constituents (see ref. 73). Its presence in tissues in trace amounts is not unlikely, and it may not be without functional significance.

Other Cytokinins

The list of naturally occurring cytokinins presented in Table I may be far from complete. For example, the cytokinin-active 2-methylthio derivatives found in tRNA of both bacteria and plants may be only one of several kinds of 2-substituted adenines that may occur in free or combined form. An unusual, known example is a cytokinin-active ribonucleoside (apparently the 2-mercapto derivative, HS2iPA) which occurs instead of ms2iPA in tRNA of a "methylation-defective" *Escherichia coli* mutant (Armstrong *et al.*, unpublished). Similarly, 8-substituted and 2,8-disubstituted derivatives which are active may be found in nature.

Other substances with activities similar to that of kinetin or the above N^6-isopent(en)yladenine derivatives in promoting cell division and growth may be classified as cytokinins. These include N,N^1-diphenylurea, isolated from coconut milk by Steward and coworkers (70), and a large number of synthetic urea derivatives all containing a —NH—CO—NH— ring moiety which apparently is the component structure essential for their biological activity (10). Relative activities of selected 6-phenylureidopurine derivatives as compared with kinetin and BAP in the tobacco bioassay are shown in Fig. 8. While diphenylurea may satisfy the cytokinin requirement in the tobacco bioassay, apparently it is inactive in the soybean bioassay (17).

BRIEF SURVEY OF MORPHOLOGICAL AND PHYSIOLOGICAL EFFECTS

As stated above, cytokinins are involved in all phases of metabolism, and they influence plant metabolism in many ways. Only a few biochemical and morphogenetic effects will be considered here. (For a more detailed review, see refs. 72 and 74.)

RNA and DNA Synthesis

At the cellular level, the first observed effect of cytokinin and auxin treatments on tobacco pith tissue was enhanced DNA and RNA synthesis followed by or associated with mitosis and cell division (13). Both hormones (kinetin and IAA) were required for continuous nucleic acid synthesis and for growth, but a 20% increase in DNA, obtained by treatments with kinetin alone, did not result in cell division or growth. Marked stimulation of nucleic acid biosynthesis also has been reported for other tissues.

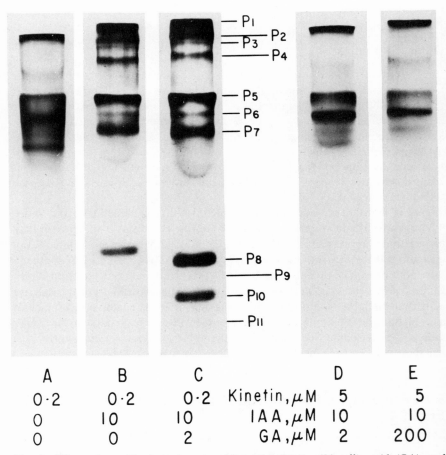

Fig. 9. Effect of combined treatments with auxin (IAA), gibberellic acid (GA), and cytokinin (kinetin) on peroxidase isozymes in tobacco callus tissue. Data kindly furnished by Dr. T. T. Lee.

General Enhancement of Anabolism

More or less specific enhancement of the biosynthesis of particular products by cytokinin treatments has been reported for numerous, both structural and catalytic, cell constituents, including starch, lignin, pectin, and other carbohydrate polymers, chlorophyll and other pigments, as well as various proteins, specific enzymes, and isozymes. Effects of combined treatments with cytokinins, gibberellins, and IAA on the contents of peroxidase isozymes in tobacco tissue obtained by T. T. Lee are shown in Fig. 9. It may be seen that the presence and the intensity of specific bands vary with the concentration as well as with the presence and absence of cytokinins and other hormones. In general, cytokinins tend to bring about a stable, highly polymerized state of the cytoplasm. They promote the formation and retention of chloroplasts and other plastids, and they are required in relatively high concentration for survival of protoplasts *in vitro*. (For a survey of cytokinins in relation to protein biosynthesis, see ref. 71.)

Induction of Organ Formation

Morphogenetic effects of cytokinins are illustrated by the effect of 2iP and IAA on growth and organ formation in tobacco callus cultures (Fig. 10). Also in this case, both cytokinin and auxin may be said to be generally required from exogenous sources for growth to occur. Furthermore, the types of growth and differentiation depend on the concentrations and proportions of the two hormones in the nutrient medium. High cytokinin/auxin ratios lead to bud formation and low ratios to root formation (only faintly visible in lower left corner of this figure). Intermediate ratios lead to growth of undifferentiated callus. Cell size and other properties of the callus also will vary with the proportions of the two hormones. However, the effectiveness of the hormone treatments depends on other factors, including temperature and light, levels of specific inorganic nutrients, and other organic growth factors. Thus high light intensity, high phosphate levels, and added tyrosine tend to promote budding, whereas added gibberellic acid prevents budding and promotes growth of undifferentiated callus. It may be seen in Fig. 10 that no growth was obtained in the absence of exogenous 2iP, but growth did occur in the absence of IAA when 2iP was provided in 1 μM or higher concentrations. This can be accounted for by an effect of high cytokinin concentrations on auxin biosynthesis.

It has been shown in the case of both auxin and thiamine, which are normally required from exogenous sources, that their endogenous content in the cultures is quantitatively related to the concentration of added cytokinin. A continuous supply of cytokinin at levels considerably higher than required for growth in their presence is needed for their biosynthesis (55). In each case, the

2 i P (μM)

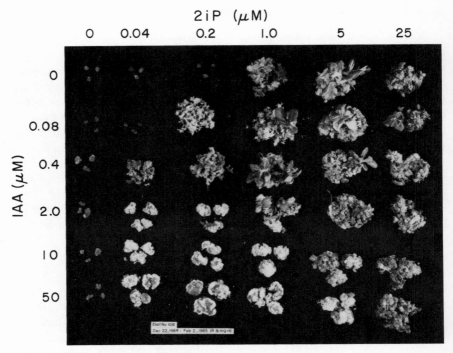

Fig. 10. Effects of serial combinations of cytokinin (2iP) and auxin (IAA) concentrations on growth and organ formation by tobacco callus cultures. Experiment by H. Q. Hamzi and J. Rogozinska; growth period Dec. 22, 1964 to Feb. 2, 1965.

dependence on high cytokinin levels for adequate biosynthesis has been demonstrated in more than 20 successive transfers over a 2-year period. In the case of thiamine, *de novo* synthesis in response to cytokinin treatment was demonstrated (15). Presumably this holds also for auxin.

Shifting Patterns of Metabolic Activity and Growth

In the intact plant, cytokinins are powerful correlation agents. They function in some manner as a key factor in the regulatory mechanism that determines which parts of a plant will stay alive and develop and which parts will mature and die. Presumably this regulation is exerted via effects on nucleic acid and protein metabolism, but one of its important aspects is the control of translocation and accumulation of inorganic nutrients and assimilates (61,66). Both exogenous and endogenous cytokinins have striking effects on the distribution patterns of metabolic activity, especially nitrate reduction and amino acid biosynthesis, and on the changes of these patterns with the age of the plant (47). Cytokinin applied to the stem end of a decapitated plant can replace the function of the terminal bud in attracting and maintaining the flow of assimilates and nutrients. It would appear that rapid action sustaining or modifying physical properties of membranes and more indirect influences on biosynthesis of various metabolites are involved in this process.

Release of Apical Dominance

In the release of apical dominance by treatment of lateral buds with exogenous cytokinin, it has been shown (14) that induction of growth in the treated lateral is preceded by an increase in auxin production in it and a concomitant decrease in the terminal bud. This quantitative shift in biosynthesis and subsequent growth results in branching or, when complete, in the development of a new main axis.

Regulation of Leaf Growth and Form

The regulation of leaf growth and form is another case of apparent interaction of growth factors, especially between cytokinins and gibberellins. The former promote the growth of laminar tissue and inhibit that of vascular tissue; the latter have the opposite effects. It is thus possible to modify both the size and the shape of leaves by exogenous combinations of the two hormones either by addition to the medium of *in vitro* cultures (19) or by spraying young shoots (78).

The two hormones also have opposite effects on the growth of stems. Gibberellins strikingly promote elongation, and cytokinins tend to retard this process. This inhibiting effect is said to result from altering the orientation of microfibril deposition in the cell wall.

Senescence

Senescence has been investigated more than any other developmental phase with reference to cytokinin regulation of protein biosynthesis (4). Early work suggested that cytokinins might act directly via influences on amino acid accumulation, which in turn, through mass action, would prevent protein breakdown (61). Recent evidence suggests that *de novo* synthesis of specific proteins is a prerequisite for senescence. Thimann and coworkers (56) stress the key role of certain hydrolases which contain serine or similarly acting amino acids in their "active centers," and which are inhibited by cytokinins. The enhancement of senescence by these amino acids and its prevention by cytokinin could thus be accounted for.

General Mode of Action

From the evidence now available, it may be deduced that regardless of the mode of action at the molecular level, one role of cytokinins in regulating plant development (organ formation, apical dominance, growth and form of leaves, senescence, etc.) is the quantitative regulation of *in vivo* synthesis of various cell constituents, especially of the growth factors (exemplified by auxin and thiamine), which tend to become limiting for growth of plant cells.

CYTOKININ ORIGIN AND SITE OF ACTION

Cytokinin Biosynthesis

The origin of cytokinins is not clear, but it has been proposed that the free cytokinins (bases, ribonucleosides, and ribotides) are released by degradation of tRNA (28). These presumably could then be converted to glycosides, which also are present.

Evidence has been presented for enzyme-catalyzed formation of cytokinins in tRNA from mevalonate or isopentenyl pyrophosphate as substrate in both *in vivo* and *in vitro* systems of microorganisms and higher plants (5,21,28,63,80). The last reference includes enzymatic thiomethylation of the 2iPA moiety in *E. coli* tRNA to ms2iPA. However, the report that mevalonate may be substituted for exogenous cytokinin in cytokinin-dependent tobacco callus cultures (12) was not confirmed (58). Possibly mevalonate can be utilized more effectively by tissue cultures which have lost their exogenous cytokinin requirement.

A striking demonstration of the difference in biosynthetic capacity of cytokinin-dependent and -independent strains of tobacco callus is the utilization of adenine as a substrate for cytokinin synthesis (18). The cytokinin autotrophic tissue extracted with alcohol yielded cytokinin-active compounds separating on Sephadex LH-20 columns in regions corresponding to ribosylzeatin, zeatin, and 2iP, and when supplied with ^{14}C-adenine yielded peaks of radioactive components, detectable within 2 hr, corresponding to zeatin and 2iP. No corresponding peaks of activity were obtained from cytokinin-dependent tissues supplied with ^{14}C-adenine and assayed in the same manner (see Fig. 11). The minimum concentration of the major cytokinin in the autotrophic tissue, which corresponds to zeatin, was estimated therefore to be approximately 0.02 μg/kg (i.e., about 10^{-10} M). In another autotrophic strain of Wisconsin No. 38 callus, 2iPA was identified by Dyson and Hall (16) as the main cytokinin present in "free" form and in quantities up to 10 μg/kg of tissue (i.e., about 3×10^{-8} M). In each instance, the total level of cytokinin-active free bases and nucleosides was judged adequate for optimal growth of the tissue on the basis of its own lack of an exogenous requirement and by comparisons with that of cytokinin-dependent

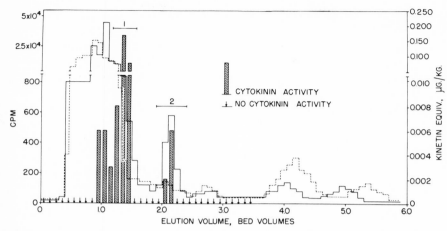

Fig. 11. *Cytokinin biosynthesis in cytokinin autotrophic tobacco callus supplied with* ^{14}*C-8-adenine.* Solid line represents radioactivity, and vertical bars indicate cytokinin activity in profile from Sephadex LH20 column eluted with 25% EtOH. Tissue was grown for 5 hr in the presence of ^{14}C-8-adenine—extracted with 70% EtOH, chromatographed twice on Dowex 50-X4(H$^+$) column eluted with H$_2$O followed by 1 N NH$_4$OH. The dried final NH$_4$OH eluate was extracted with ethyl acetate and chromatographed on a Sephadex LH20 column. The broken line represents the distribution of radioactivity in the Sephadex LH20 profile of cytokinin-dependent tobacco callus tissue treated with ^{14}C-8-adenine and extracted in the same manner. No cytokinin activity was found in this profile. Horizontal bars 1 and 2 correspond to elution volumes of zeatin and 2iP, respectively. Data from Einset and Skoog (18); reprinted with permission of the publishers of *Proc. Natl. Acad. Sci. (USA)*.

tissue. The latter, in each case, was estimated to contain maximum levels of about 10^{-10} M zeatin equivalents of free cytokinin.

The incorporation of ^{14}C-adenine into cytokinin was delayed as compared with its incorporation into RNA and was inhibited by concentrations of actinomycin D which inhibited the latter, but more compelling evidence that free cytokinin arises from degradation of tRNA is lacking.

In intact plants, the content and capacity for cytokinin synthesis vary with the tissue. There is evidence that cytokinins may be preferentially synthesized in roots and be transported to the shoots. Relatively high levels are restricted to meristems, but biosynthetic capacity may be repressed rather than absent in tissues which have an exogenous cytokinin requirement for growth.

In tumor cells of genetic or crown gall origin, this biosynthetic capacity is considered to be derepressed (9). The question of what cytokinin is present in crown gall tissue is not settled. Some investigators are finding zeatin and its closely related derivatives. Wood and Braun (see ref. 9) report a different kind of cell division factor, therefore called "cytokinesin." The crown gall bacterium itself (*Agrobacterium tumefaciens*) in culture appears to produce 2iP at least as a major cytokinin component. An exceptionally rich source of free cytokinin is *Corynebacterium fascians*, which in culture gives rise to thousandfold higher concentrations of 2iP and other cytokinins than are found in higher plants, and, apparently for this reason, is a plant pathogen responsible for witches broom. The labial glands of *Stigmella*, a leaf miner which produces galls, are another enormously rich source of cytokinin (62).

Localization in tRNA

Unfractionated RNA preparations which have been thoroughly tested generally have contained cytokinin activity. The only known exceptions are a virus RNA and one of three tested tRNA preparations from *Mycoplasma.*

In tRNA preparations, cytokinin activity is restricted to a relatively small portion which is retained longer than the rest on benzoylated DEAE-cellulose columns. When this portion has been further fractionated, the cytokinin activity has been found only in tRNA species which respond to codons starting with uridine.

I ST	2 ND LETTER				3 RD
LETTER	U	C	A	G	LETTER
U	PHE	SER	TYR	CYS	U
	PHE	SER	TYR	CYS	C
	LEU	SER	C.T.	C.T.	A
	LEU	SER	C.T.	TRY	G
C	LEU	PRO	HIS	ARG	U
	LEU	PRO	HIS	ARG	C
	LEU	PRO	GLN	ARG	A
	LEU	PRO	GLN	ARG	G
A	ILEU	THR	ASN	SER	U
	ILEU	THR	ASN	SER	C
	ILEU	THR	LYS	ARG	A
	MET (C.I.)	THR	LYS	ARG	G
G	VAL	ALA	ASP	GLY	U
	VAL	ALA	ASP	GLY	C
	VAL	ALA	GLU	GLY	A
	VAL (C.I.)	ALA	GLU	GLY	G

Fig. 12. Distribution of cytokinin-containing tRNA species from E. coli on the genetic code. Striped codons correspond to tRNA species known to contain cytokinins (ms2iPA and/or 2iPA). Boxed-in codons correspond to tRNA species known to contain a 6-threoninecarbamoylpurine (derivative).

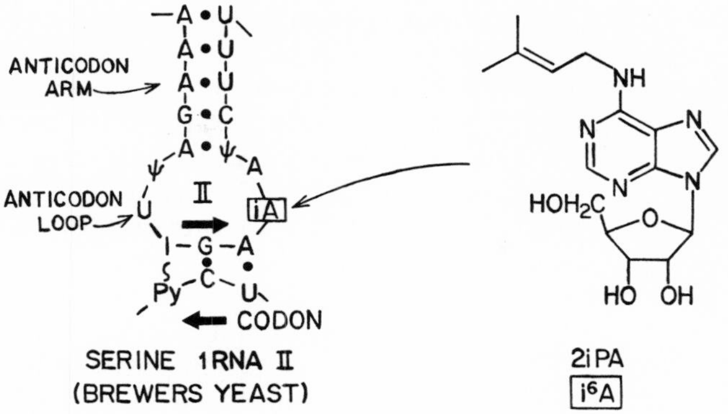

Fig. 13. Anticodon section of serine tRNA from brewer's yeast (82,83). From Leonard (48).

In the case of *E. coli,* activity has been demonstrated for at least one tRNA species corresponding to each of the six amino acids (Phe, Leu, Ser, Tyr, Cys, and Trp) for which there are codon assignments starting with uridine (see Fig. 12) (1,6). The same distribution has been reported for 2iPA in *Lactobacillus acidophilus* tRNA (64).

In yeast, tRNA species coding for four of the six amino acids of the U-codon group contain cytokinin-active bases (1), but tRNA ^{Phe} and apparently tRNA ^{Trp} instead contain base Y. This is a more highly modified purine derivative which becomes active in the tobacco bioassay only after it has been heated (32).

In tissues of higher organisms studied so far, cytokinin activity seems to be restricted to fewer tRNA species, mainly tRNA ^{Ser} and possibly one or two others, also of the U-codon group (2).

It is clear from the work on *E. coli,* furthermore, that also in microorganisms there are species of tRNA devoid of a cytokinin-active base which respond to codons starting with uridine. In fact, there is no evidence that any codon is utilized exclusively by cytokinin-containing tRNA species.

In all cases where the position of the cytokinin base in tRNA has been established, it has been located next to the 3'-end of the anticodon, as illustrated in Fig. 13; so also is base Y (see ref. 72).

In no case has cytokinin activity been reported for tRNA species in any other than the U-codon group. An interesting analogy exists, however, in that in *E. coli* there are tRNA species for most if not all the codons starting with adenine which contain 6-threoninecarbamoylpurine instead of a 6-isopentenyl-aminopurine as the odd base adjacent to the 3'-end of the anticodon (37). The resemblance of 6-threoninecarbamoylpurine, especially in the form of lactones, to phenylurea derivatives and particularly to phenylureidopurines which are active in the tobacco bioassay (Fig. 8) is of interest with regard to its possible functions.

Information on the unique or random association of a given cytokinin with any given tRNA species and/or specific codon is still rudimentary. The relative contents and distribution of 2iPA and ms2iPA in hydrolysates from highly purified preparations of cytokinin-containing tRNA species in *E. coli* are shown in Table II. It may be seen that each cytokinin is present in tRNA species with different amino acid assignments, i.e., responding to different codons. Furthermore, as both cytokinins are represented in tRNA species for each of four amino acids, tRNA species with different cytokinins can respond to the same codon, at least in the case of $tRNA_{UUG}^{Leu}$ and $tRNA_{UGG}^{Trp}$. The proportions of the two cytokinins differ with the amino acid assignment and change with age of the culture. For example, the marked increase in $tRNA^{Phe}$ in the late stages of growth may account for a relative increase in total 2iPA content observed at that time.

No functional significance has been established for the presence of several cytokinins in the tRNA of an organism. The possibility is being examined that different cytokinins may be associated with tRNA in different organelles. A

Table II. Distribution of Cytokinin-Containing Ribonucleosides in *E. coli* tRNA Species

tRNA sample	Coding properties	Specific aminoacyl acceptor activity (pMoles/A$_{260}$ unit)	Estimated cytokinin ribonucleosides (μg/mg tRNA)	
			1[a]	2[b]
Phe	UUY	1050	1.6	0.2
Leu	UUG	1550	0.03	2.0
Ser$_4$	UCR	1400	—	2.0
Tyr	UAY	1650	—	2.2
Cys	UGY	860	0.2	9.5
Trp$_2$	UGG	1400	0.01	2.4

Data from Bartz *et al.* (6).

[a] 6-(3-Methyl-2-butenylamino)-9-β-D-ribofuranosylpurine.

[b] 6-(3-Methyl-2-butenylamino)-2-methylthio-9-β-D-ribofuranosylpurine.

model for such behavior is the distribution of base Y, which is present in cytoplasmic tRNA^{Phe} of both *Neurospora* and *Euglena* but absent from tRNA^{Phe} in mitochondria of the former and in chloroplasts of the latter organism (20). What if any cytokinins occur in tRNA species present exclusively in organelles is not known, but *Euglena* tRNA does contain 2iPA and at least two other cytokinin-active ribonucleosides (Swaminathan *et al.*, unpublished).

Function in tRNA

The strategic location of the cytokinin next to the anticodon in tRNA suggests that it plays a specific role in the functioning of this macromolecule in protein biosynthesis. Reports are agreed that cytokinins, like all but one known ribonucleotide in the anticodon loop, do not significantly affect the aminoacyl acceptor activity of the tRNA molecule. Several kinds of experiments, on the other hand, indicate that the cytokinin component does improve the binding of the tRNA to the ribosome-mRNA complex. Reductions down to about half the control values have been reported for mild treatments of yeast tRNA^{Ser} with KMnO$_4$ or iodine (21,36,42) which remove or modify the side chain of 2iPA (see ref. 48). From treatments of yeast tRNA^{Tyr} with bisulfite followed by mild alkali, which modify both the uridine at the 5'-end and the 2iPA at the 3'-end of the anticodon, Furuichi *et al.* (25) deduce that only the treatments which include modification of the 2iPA decrease ribosomal binding and that modification specifically of the 2iPA results in a 65% loss in the efficiency of the binding of the tRNA to the ribosome-mRNA complex. Such treatments have no effect on the aminoacyl acceptor activity of the tRNA.

Gefter and Russell (27), utilizing a phage-induced tyrosine suppressor mutant strain of *E. coli*, distinguished three species of tRNA^{Tyr} responding to the UAG codon which differ only in that one contains unsubstituted adenine, the second 2iP, and the third ms2iP as the base of the nucleotide adjacent to the 3'-end of the anticodon. The relative ribosome-binding efficiencies of the three tRNA^{Tyr} species were found to be in the proportions 14:54:100, values which are in good agreement with the relative effectiveness of the three species in *in vitro* tests of suppression. They found, furthermore, that the tRNA species with the unmodified adenine base perhaps failed to discriminate between the CAG and UAG codons. Thus the cytokinin-active bases in tRNA enhance the efficiency of ribosomal binding and may increase the specificity of codon recognition.

The general conclusion may be drawn that the cytokinin-active bases in tRNA species of the U-codon group do function in protein biosynthesis. It seems logical to assume that 6-threoninecarbamoylpurine in tRNA species of the A-codon group functions in an analogous manner.

Incorporation of Cytokinin into tRNA

The question arises whether or not cytokinins exert their growth regulatory function(s) as constituents of specific tRNA species. If so, it should be possible to demonstrate the incorporation of exogenous cytokinins into tRNA as a prerequisite for activity in growth promotion. There have been reports for (23,24) as well as against (39) the incorporation of cytokinins into tRNA, based on radioactivity measurements on nucleic acid hydrolysate fractions from tissue cultures supplied with isotope-labeled 6-benzylaminopurine (BAP), but this evidence is far from conclusive. In a study of cytokinins in tRNA of cytokinin-dependent tobacco callus grown with synthetic BAP as the exogenous source (11), five cytokinin-active ribonucleoside fractions were separated by chromatography of tRNA hydrolysate from approximately 40 kg of tissue. Four of these correspond to the ribonucleosides of zeatin, 2iP, mszeatin, and ms2iP, which are normally found in plants. The first three, but not the fourth, ms2iPA, were present in quantities sufficient for rigorous characterization by mass spectrometry. The fifth active fraction was also identified by high- and low-resolution mass spectra, ultraviolet absorption spectra, and chromatographic properties as the riboside of BAP (6-benzylamino-9-β-D-ribofuranosylpurine, BAPA).

By utilizing BAP doubly labeled with ^{3}H in the benzene ring and ^{14}C at the 8-position, and with different proportions of the two isotopes in repeat experiments, the radioactivity in the nucleosides was found mainly in the BAPA fraction, and the ratio of ^{3}H/^{14}C remained the same in this fraction as in the BAP used as the exogenous source (see Table III). It is clear, therefore, that the isolated ribonucleoside contained the 6-BAP molecule incorporated intact and did not arise from side-chain transfer of the benzyl group in 6-BAP to adenine in tRNA.

As the radioactivity in BAPA was not lowered significantly by prior incubation of the tRNA preparation with unlabeled BAPA and its ribotide at denaturing temperatures, the BAPA appears to have been covalently bound. However, the incorporation was at a low level, providing for only a minute fraction of the estimated content of cytokinin-active ribonucleosides, and has not been pinned to a locus in specific tRNA species. Hence it may be nonspecific and without functional significance for growth. Of special interest in this connection is a BAP complex found to accumulate in soybean callus tissue supplied with BAP and to persist as a cytokinin-active entity throughout or even beyond the growth period of these cultures (17). Such a complex might give rise to BAPA in the above experiments with tobacco tissue.

Other Functions of Cytokinins in RNA

Alternative mechanisms of a regulatory function of cytokinins in RNA metabolism have been reported. It has been suggested that free cytokinins may interfere with the binding of cytokinin-containing tRNA species in the ribo-some-mRNA complex (7). Relatively higher affinities in ribosome-binding tests of the biologically highly active cytokinins are cited in support of this view, but the critical experiment of competitively removing or excluding tRNA species from the ribosome complex was not performed. Birmingham and Maclachlan (8) have suggested a growth regulatory function of cytokinins in conjunction with auxins in terms of the inhibition and promotion, respectively, of microsomal ribonuclease activity by the two types of hormones.

Recent success in elucidating hormone action in terms of cyclic AMP and membrane function and progress in isolating protein receptors for steroid hor-mones have stimulated work on cytokinin-protein complexes. Of special interest is a kinetin-protein complex reported to act specifically at the gene transcription level in promoting RNA synthesis (57). Interactions at this level between cytokinins and specific tRNA species in association with suppressor proteins might provide a mechanism of extreme sensitivity and specificity for regulating growth and morphogenesis.

CYTOKININ ANTAGONISTS

The development of competitive cytokinin antagonists is one approach to locating sites of cytokinin action that also might be useful in extending the study of cytokinins to biological systems which normally do not have an exogenous cytokinin requirement. Many substances, especially auxins, gibberel-lins, and abscisic acid (ABA) are known to "interact" indirectly with cytokinins, as evidenced by influences on growth and development, but until recently no substance closely related structurally to the highly cytokinin-active purine deriv-atives was known to serve as an antimetabolite interfering specifically and reversibly in cytokinin metabolism. 6-Methylaminopurine, a weak cytokinin which in high concentrations also lowers the response to more active cytokinins, is an exception to this (41).

On the basis of the decreases in cytokinin activity known to result from modifications of the purine ring, especially the exchange of 8-CH and 9-N (33), modifications of the 6-side chain, and introduction of additional substituents, potent cytokinin antagonists have been developed (34). The effects of three structural modifications in 2iP which convert it to 3-methyl-7-(3-methyl-butylamino)pyrazolo[4,3-d] pyrimidine (compound 6 in Table III) are illustrated in Fig. 14. By comparing the micromolar concentrations (on the bottom line) required for equivalent growth, and proceeding from bottom to top, one can gauge the separate effects of the following modifications of 2iP: saturation of the side chain, exchange of 8—CH and 9—N, this exchange plus methylation of the CH, the exchange plus saturation of the side chain, and the combination of all three modifications.

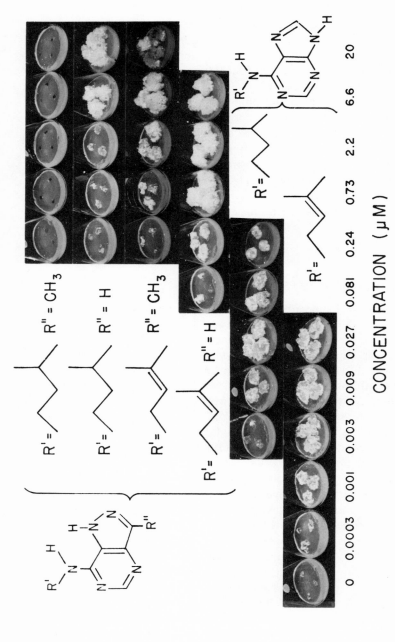

Fig. 14. Loss in biological activity from formal modifications of 2iP leading to anticytokinin potency. The bottom row represents growth of tobacco callus, obtained with increasing concentrations of 2iP. Proceeding upward are shown the effect of saturating the side chain, the exchange of C-9 and N-9 atoms, and the addition of the methyl substituent (R''). The top row shows the lack of growth-promoting activity of 3-methyl-7-(3-methylpentylamino)pyrazolo[4,3-d]pyrimidine (compound 6 in Table III), which incorporates all three modifications. From Skoog et al. (75); reprinted with permission of the publishers of Phytochemistry.

Table III. Relation of the Structure of 7-Substituents to Biological Activity of Pyrazolo[4,3-d]pyrimidine Derivatives

Compound No.	R'' =	R' =	Number C atoms in R'	Range tested[a] (μM)	Cytokinin activity Min. conc. (μM) for Detection	Cytokinin activity Min. conc. (μM) for Maximum growth	Antagonist activity against 0.003 μM 2iP Min. conc. (μM) for Detection	Antagonist activity against 0.003 μM 2iP Min. conc. (μM) for Lethal dosage
XIV	H	HN	5	0.009–20	1.0	20	N.A.[b]	—
XV	H	HN	5	0.001–20(3)	0.08	1.0	N.A.	—
XVI	Me	HO	0	0.08–20	N.A.	—	N.A.	—
I	Me	S	1	0.24–20	N.A.	—	N.A.	—
XIII	Me	HN	5	0.08–20(4)	0.24	6.6	N.A.	—
XI	Me	HN	2 × 4	0.24–20	N.A.	—	N.A.	—
IX	Me	HN	6	0.73–20	N.A.	—	N.A.	—
VII	Me	HN	5	0.73–20	N.A.	—	6.6	N.R.[c]
IV	Me	HN	4	0.24–20	2.2	7[d]	6.6	N.R.
II	Me	HN	2	0.73–20	N.A.	—	2.2	N.R.
XII	Me	HN—OH	10	0.24–20	N.A.	—	3.0	N.R.
X	Me	HN	7	0.03–6.6	N.A.	—	0.2	2.2
III	Me	HN	4	0.03–6.6	N.A.	—	0.1	0.73
VI	Me	HN	5	0.009–20(4)	N.A.	—	0.1	0.73
VIII	Me	HN	6	0.009–20	N.A.	—	0.03	0.5
V	Me	HN	5	0.009–20(3)	N.A.	—	0.03	0.2

From Skoog et al. (75); reprinted with permission of the publishers of Phytochemistry.

[a] All values are averages of two tests except as indicated by superior numbers in parentheses. Testing was done between April 1970 and December 1971.

[b] Not active.

[c] Not reached.

[d] Only slight growth stimulation.

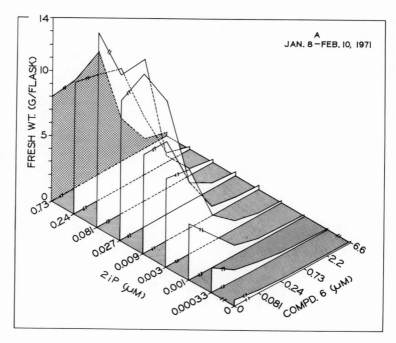

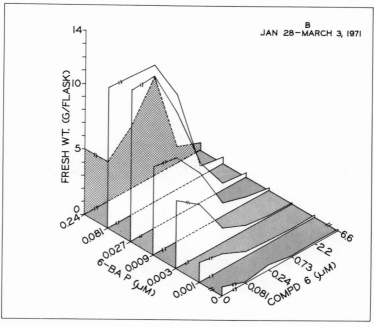

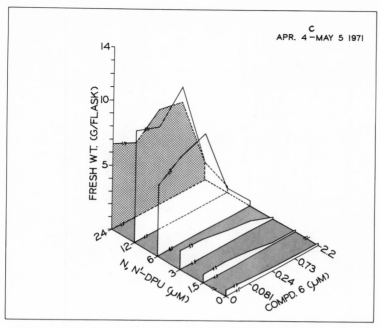

Fig. 15. Yields of tobacco callus. Cultured on media with serial combinations of cytokinin antagonist and either 2iP (A) BAP (B), or diphenylurea, DPU (C). From Skoog *et al.* (75); reprinted with permission of the publishers of *Phytochemistry.*

No combination of two modifications eliminates cytokinin activity entirely, but the combination of all three results in a cytokinin antagonist lethal to tobacco callus. Its anticytokinin potency, measured by comparison of its effect in serial combinations with 2iP, is illustrated in Fig. 15. Note that the antagonist counteracts 2iP both in its low, growth-promoting concentration range and in its superoptimal, growth-retarding range, where the action of the antagonist, therefore, may serve to promote growth. A similar interaction between antagonist and 2iP, in medium with low IAA conducive to bud formation, is shown in Fig. 16. The antagonist is similarly counteracted by other cytokinins in concentrations which reflect their relative activities in the tobacco bioassay, as, for example, by BAP in approximately tenfold or diphenylurea in greater than a hundredfold higher concentrations than of 2iP (see Fig. 15B,C).

Concentrations of antagonist higher than about 1 μM, which tend to be lethal, are not effectively counteracted by any concentration of 2iP or other tested cytokinins, but the tolerance (range of effective reversal) can be more

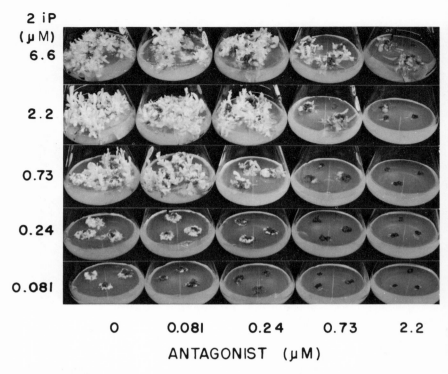

2 iP
(μM)
6.6

2.2

0.73

0.24

0.081

0   0.081   0.24   0.73   2.2
ANTAGONIST (μM)

Fig. 16. Effect of serial combinations of cytokinin antagonist and 2iP on growth and budding on media with low (0.01 μM) IAA. From Skoog et al. (75); reprinted with permission of the publishers of Phytochemistry.

than doubled by addition of adenine in concentrations which do not affect yields in treatments without or with low concentrations of antagonist.

No evidence for a reversal of the growth inhibition comparable to that obtained with 2iP was observed in experiments in which either gibberellic acid or IAA was used as a variable in serial combinations with the antagonist.

Abscisic acid (ABA), an effective natural inhibitor of plant growth known to be counteracted by cytokinins in some systems (40,79), was compared with the antagonist in the tobacco assay (see Fig. 17). On a molar basis, the antagonist is the more effective inhibitor. It should be noted that the compact callus produced in the presence of ABA suggests that cell expansion rather than cell division was curtailed, while the loose, watery tissue produced in the presence of the cytokinin antagonist indicates that cell division had become limiting. Furthermore, when tested in serial combinations with the antagonist, in the presence of 0.003 μM 2iP, ABA neither increased nor counteracted the effect of the antagonist.

It appears, therefore, that the anticytokinin action of the effective 7-substituted 3-methylpyrazolo[4,3-d]pyrimidines is both more drastic and more specific than that of ABA. All these results suggest that the antagonist does in fact exert a highly specific anticytokinin action when supplied in low dosages, but in high dosages it probably interferes also in other phases of purine metabolism.

Further study of modifications which affect antagonist activity of pyrazolo[4,3-d]pyrimidine derivatives (75) has revealed remarkable specificity in the structural requirements of the 7-side chain which both compares and contrasts with the specificity in the N^6-side-chain requirements for cytokinin activity of adenine derivatives (see Table III). Similarities include restriction of high potency to derivatives with side chains 4–6 C atoms long. The optimum is 5, and either shortening or lengthening the chain beyond the 4–6 C atom range markedly decreases activity. Cyclization of the chain, or in the case of antagonists, the addition of rings, practically eliminates biological activity.

In contrast, both the *n*-pentyl and *n*-hexyl groups are more effective than the isopentenyl group in conferring antagonist activity on the pyrazolo[4,3-d]pyrimidines. Also, the *n*-butyl group is relatively effective, but it is striking that a second butyl group at the 7-position renders the compound inactive. The marked quantitative differences in anticytokinin activity of pyrazolo[4,3-d]pyrimidine derivatives stemming from changes in detailed structure of the side chain at the 7-position would seem to reflect a unique role of this chain at a specific receptor site. Further work has shown that the effectiveness of modifications in the side chain is closely dependent on specific substituents at other positions, as well as on the overall configuration of the antagonist molecule (Hecht *et al.,* unpublished).

In preliminary tests with various plants, the antagonist (compound 6 in

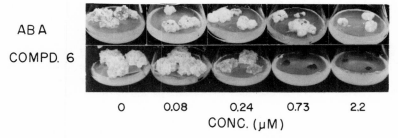

Fig. 17. Comparison of the inhibiting effects of abscisic acid (ABA) and cytokinin antagonist (compound 6) on growth of tobacco callus on medium with 0.003 μM 2iP. From Skoog et al. (75); reprinted with permission of the publishers of Phytochemistry.

Table III) has been shown to stop germination of seeds and to kill seedlings, but there is no evidence that these effects are reversible by treatments with cytokinins. In fact, in some tests 2iP was equally injurious. In *Cucumis* cotyledons, the antagonist effectively prevents both the greening and the expansion which are promoted by cytokinins, and it strikingly hastens senescence (Tabhaz *et al.,* unpublished). It appears, therefore, that cytokinin antagonists may be useful in studies of growth regulation and the role of cytokinins in this process.

ACKNOWLEDGMENTS

The author is grateful to students and colleagues at the University of Wisconsin and to Professor N. J. Leonard and his coworkers at the University of Illinois for having contributed the major part of the material presented here. Special acknowledgment is due Drs. D. J. Armstrong and R. Y. Schmitz, University of Wisconsin, and Dr. T. T. Lee, Canadian Department of Agriculture, London, Ontario, for biochemical and physiological data, and Professor S. M. Hecht, Massachusetts Institute of Technology, for cytokinin antagonists. Work done at the University of Wisconsin has been supported in part by NSF research grants GB-25812 and GB-35260X. Work done at the University of Illinois has been supported in part by NIH Research Grant GM-05829.

REFERENCES

1. Armstrong, D. J., Burrows, W. J., Skoog, F., Roy, K. L., and Söll, D. (1969). Cytokinins: Distribution of tRNA species of *E. coli. Proc. Natl. Acad. Sci. (USA)* **63**:834-841.
2. Armstrong, D. J., *et al.* (unpublished).
3. Babcock, D. F., and Morris, R. O. (1970). Quantitative measurement of isoprenoid nucleosides in transfer nucleic acid. *Biochemistry* **9**:3701-3705.
4. Back, A., and Richmond, A. E. (1971). Interrelations between gibberellic acid, cytokinins, and abscisic acid in retarding leaf senescence. *Physiol. Plant.* **24**:76-79.
5. Bartz, J. K., and D. Söll, (1972). *Biochemie* **54**:31.
6. Bartz, J., Söll, D., Burrows, W. J., and Skoog, F. (1970). Identification of the cytokinin-active ribonucleosides in pure *E. coli* tRNA species. *Proc. Natl. Acad. Sci. (USA)* **67**:1448-1453.
7. Berridge, M. W., Ralph, R. K., and Letham, D. S. (1970). *Biochem. J.* **119**:75.
8. Birmingham, C., and Maclachlan, G. A. (1971). Generation and suppression of ribonuclease activity after treatments with auxin and cytokinin. *Plant Physiol.* **49**:371-375.
9. Braun, A. C. (ed.) (1972). Plant tumor research. *Prog. Exptl. Tumor Res.* **15**:1-235.
10. Bruce, M. I., and Zwar, J. A. (1966). Cytokinin activity of some substituted ureas and thioureas. *Proc. Royal Soc. Ser. B* **165**:245-265.
11. Burrows, W. J., Skoog, F., and Leonard, N. J. (1971). Isolation of four cytokinin-active ribonucleosides from tRNA of cytokinin dependent tobacco tissue supplied with 6-benzylaminopurine. *Biochemistry* **10**:2189-2194.
12. Chen, C.-M., and Hall, R. H. (1969). Biosynthesis of N^6-(Δ^2-isopentenyl)adenosine in the tRNA of cultured tobacco pith tissue. *Phytochemistry* **8**:1687-1695.

13. Das, N. K., Patau, K., and Skoog, F. (1958). Autoradiographic and microspectrophotometric studies of DNA synthesis in excised tobacco pith tissue. *Chromosoma* 9:606-617.

14. Davidson, D. R. (1971). PhD. thesis, University of Wisconsin, 101 pp.

15. Dravniecks, D. E., Skoog, F., and Burris, R. H. (1969). Cytokinin stimulation of *de novo* thiamine synthesis in tobacco cultures. *Plant Physiol.* 44:866-870.

16. Dyson, W. H., and Hall, R. H. (1972). N^6-(Δ^2-Isopentenyl)adenosine: Its occurrence as a free nucleoside in an autonomous strain of tobacco tissue. *Plant Physiol.* 50:616-621.

17. Dyson, W. H., Fox, J. E., and McChesney, J. D. (1972). Short term metabolism of urea and purine cytokinins. *Plant Physiol.* 49:506-513.

18. Einset, J. W., and Skoog, F. (1973). Biosynthesis of cytokinins in autotrophic tobacco callus. *Proc. Natl. Acad. Sci. (USA)* 70:650-660.

19. Engelke, A. L., Hamzi, H. Q., and Skoog, F. (1973). Cytokinin-gibberellin regulation of shoot development and leaf form in tobacco plantlets. *Am. J. Bot.* 60:491-495.

20. Fairfield, S. A., and Barnett, W. E. (1971). *Proc. Natl. Acad. Sci. (USA)* 68:2972.

21. Fittler, F., and Hall, R. H. (1966). Selective modification of yeast seryl tRNA and its effect on acceptance and binding functions. *Biochem. Biophys. Res. Commun.* 25:441-446.

22. Fittler, F., Kline, L. K., and Hall, R. H. (1968). Biosynthesis of N^6-(Δ^2-isopentenyl) adenosine. The precursor relationship of acetate and mevalonote to the Δ^2-isopentenyl group of the transfer ribonucleic acid of microorganisms. *Biochemistry* 7:940-944.

23. Fox, J. E. (1966). Incorporation of a kinin, N^6-benzyladenine into soluble RNA. *Plant Physiol.* 41:75-82.

24. Fox, J. E., and Chen, C. M. (1967). Characterization of labeled ribonucleic acid from tissue grown on ^{14}C-containing cytokinins. *J. Biol. Chem.* 242:4490-4494.

25. Furuichi, Y., Wataya, Y., Hayatsu, H., and Ukita, T. (1970). *Biochem. Biophys. Res. Commun.* 41:1185.

26. Gaspar, T., and Xhaufflaire, A. (1968). Les cytokinines. *Ann. Biol.* 7:39-87.

27. Gefter, M. L., and Russell, R. L. (1969). Role of modifications in tyrosine transfer RNA. A modified base affecting ribosome binding. *J. Mol. Biol.* 39:145-157.

28. Hall, R. H. (1970). N^6-(Δ^2-Isopentenyl)adenosine: Chemical reactions, biosynthesis, metabolism and significance of the structure and function of tRNA. In Davidson, J. N., and Cohn, W. E. (eds.). *Prog. Nucleic Acid Res. Mol. Biol.* 10:57-86.

29. Hall, R. H., and Srivastava, B. I. S. (1968). Cytokinin activity of compounds obtained from soluble RNA. *Life Sci.* 7:7-13.

30. Hall, R. H., Csonka, L., David, H., and McLennan, B. (1967). Cytokinins in soluble RNA of plant tissues. *Science* 156:69-71.

31. Hecht, S. M., Leonard, N. J., Schmitz, R. Y., and Skoog, F. (1970). Cytokinins: Synthesis and growth promoting activity of 2-substituted compounds in the N^6-isopentenyl adenine and zeatin series. *Phytochemistry* 9:1173-1180.

32. Hecht, S. M., Bock, R. M., Leonard, N. J., Schmitz, R. Y., and Skoog, F. (1970). Cytokinin activity in tRNA^{Phe}. *Biochem. Biophys. Res. Commun.* 41:435-440.

33. Hecht, S. M., Bock, R. M., Schmitz, R. Y., Skoog, F., Leonard, N. J., and Occolovitz, J. (1971). Question of the ribosyl moiety in the promotion of growth by exogenously added cytokinin. *Biochemistry* 10:4224-4228.

34. Hecht, S. M., Bock, R. M., Schmitz, R. Y., Skoog, F., and Leonard, N. J. (1971). Bytokinins: The development of a potent antagonist. *Proc. Natl. Acad. Sci. (USA)* 68:2608-2610.

35. Helgeson, J. P., and Leonard, N. J. (1966). Cytokinins: Identification of compounds isolated from *Corynebacterium fascians*. *Proc. Natl. Acad. Sci. (USA)* **56**:60-63.
36. Hirsch, R., and Zachau, H. G. (1970). *Z. Physiol. Chem.* **351**:563.
37. Ishikura, H., Yamada, Y., Murao, K., Saneyoshi, M., and Nishimura, S. (1969). The presence of N-[9-β-D-ribofuranosyl purin-6-ylcarbamoyl] threonine in serine, methionine and lysine tRNAs from *E. coli*. *Biochem. Biophys. Res. Commun.* **37**:990-996.
38. Kende, H. (1971). The cytokinins. *Internat. Rev. Cytol.* **31**:301.
39. Kende, H., and Tavares, J. E. (1968). On the significance of cytokinin incorporation into RNA. *Plant Physiol.* **43**:1244-1248.
40. Khan, A. A. (1971). Cytokinins' permissive role in seed germination. *Science* **171**:853-859.
41. Klämbt, D., Thies, G., and Skoog, F. (1966). Isolation of cytokinins from *Corynebacterium fascians*. *Proc. Natl. Acad. Sci. (USA)* **56**:52-59.
42. Kline, L. K., Fittler, F., and Hall, R. H. (1969). *Biochemistry* **8**:4361.
43. Koshimizu, K., Kusaki, T., Mitsui, T., and Matsubara, S. (1967). Isolation of a cytokinin (−)-dihydrozeatin from immature seeds of *Lupinus luteus*. *Tetrahedron Letters* **14**:1317-1320.
44. Koshimizu, K., Kobayashi, A., Fujita, T., and Mitsui, T. (1968). Structure activity relationships in optically active cytokinins. *Phytochemistry* **7**:1984-1994.
45. Krusnuk, M., Witham, F. H., and Tegley, J. R. (1971). Cytokinins extracted from pinto bean fruit. *Plant Physiol.* **48**:320-324.
46. Kulaeva, O. N., Cherkasov, V. M., and Tretyakova, G. S. (1968). Effect of modification of the structure of cytokinins on their physiological activity. *Dokl. Akad. Nauk. Uz. SSR.* **178**:1204-1207.
47. Kursanov, A. L. (1963). Metabolism and transport of organic substances in the phloem. *Advan. Bot. Res.* **1**:209-274.
48. Leonard, N. J. (1973). The chemistry of cytokinins. In *Symposium on Chemistry and Biochemistry of Plant Hormones,* Syracuse, N.Y., Academic Press (in press).
49. Leonard, N. J., and Playtis, A. J. (1972). The synthesis of *cis* and *trans* isozeatin. *An. Real. Soc. Espan. Fis. Quim.* **68**:821.
50. Leonard, N. J., Hecht, S. M., Skoog, F., and Schmitz, R. Y. (1968). Cytokinins: Synthesis of 6-(3-methyl-3-butenylamino)-9-β-D-ribofuanosylpurine (3iPA) and the effect of side chain saturation on the biological activity of isopentylaminopurine and their ribosides. *Proc. Natl. Acad. Sci. (USA)* **59**:15-21.
51. Leonard, N. J., Hecht, S. M., Skoog, F., and Schmitz, R. Y. (1969). Cytokinins: Synthesis, mass spectra and biological activity of compounds related to zeatin. *Proc. Natl. Acad. Sci. (USA)* **63**:175-182.
52. Leonard, N. J., Playtis, A. J., Skoog, F., and Schmitz, R. Y. (1971). A stereoselective synthesis of *cis*-zeatin. *J. Am. Chem. Soc.* **93**:3056-3058.
53. Letham, D. S. (1967). Regulators of cell division in plant tissue. V. A. comparison of the activities of zeatin and other cytokinins in five bioassays. *Planta* **74**:228-242.
53 a. Letham, D. S. (1967). Chemistry and physiology of kinetin-like compounds. *Ann. Rev. Plant Physiol.* **18**:349-364.
54. Letham, D. S., Shannon, J. S., and McDonald, T. R. (1964). The structure of zeatin, a (kinetin-like) factor inducing cell division. *Proc. Chem. Soc. Lond.,* pp. 230-231.
55. Linsmaier, E. M., and Skoog, F. (1966). Thiamine requirement in relation to cytokinin in "normal" and "mutant" strains of tobacco callus. *Planta* **72**:146-154.
56. Martin, C. C., and Thimann, K. V. (1972). Role of protein synthesis in the senescence of leaves. II. The influence of amino acids on senescence. *Plant Physiol.* **50**:432-437.
57. Matthysse, A. G., and Abrams, C. (1970). *Biochim. Biophys. Acta* **199**:511.
58. McChesney, J. D. (1970). *Can. J. Bot.* **48**:2357.

59. McDonald, J. J., Leonard, N. J., Schmitz, R. Y., and Skoog, F. (1971). Cytokinins: Synthesis and biological activity of phenylureidopurines. *Phytochemistry* **10**:1429-1439.
60. Miller, C. O., Skoog, F., Okumura, F. S., von Saltza, M. H., and Strong, F. M. (1956). Isolation, structure and synthesis of kinetin, a substance promoting cell division. *J. Am. Chem. Soc.* **78**:1375-1380.
61. Mothes, K. (1964). The role of kinetin in plant regulation. In *Regulateurs Naturels de la Croissance Végétale,* CNRS, Paris, pp. 131-140.
62. Mothes, K. (1969). Oral Report to Twelfth International Botany Congress, Seattle, Wash. (See Engelbrecht, L. (1971) Cytokinin activity in larval infected leaves. *Biochem. Physiol. Pflanzeri* **162**:9-27).
63. Peterkofsky, A. (1968). Incorporation of mevalonic acid into the N^6-($\triangle^2$-isopentenyl) adenosine of transfer ribonucleic acid in *Lactobacillus acidophilus. Biochemistry* **7**:472-482.
64. Peterkofsky, A., and Jesensky, C. (1969). The localization of N^6-($\triangle^2$-isopentenyl) adenosine among the acceptor species of transfor ribonucleic acid of *Lactobacillus acidophilus. Biochemistry* **8**:3798-3809.
65. Playtis, A. J., and Leonard, N. J. (1971). The synthesis of ribosyl-*cis*-zeatin and thin layer chromatographic separation of the *cis* and *trans* isomers of ribosylzeatin. *Biochem. Biophys. Res. Commun.* **45**:1-5.
66. Pozsár, B. I., and Kiraly, Z. (1966). Phloem transport in rust infected plants and the cytokinin-directed long-distance movement of nutrients. *Phytopathol. Z.* **56**:297-309.
67. Schmitz, R. Y., Skoog, F., Hecht, S. M., and Leonard, N. J. (1971). Cytokinins: Synthesis and biological activity of zeatin esters and related compounds. *Physochemistry* **10**:275-280.
68. Schmitz, R. Y., Skoog, F., Hecht, S. M., Bock, R. M., and Leonard, N. J. (1972). Comparison of cytokinin activities of naturally occurring ribonucleosides and corresponding bases. *Phytochemistry* **11**:1603-1610.
69. Schmitz, R. Y., Skoog, F., Playtis, A. J., and Leonard, N. J. (1972). Cytokinins: Synthesis and biological activity of geometric and position isomers of zeatin. *Plant Physiol.* **50**:702-705.
70. Shantz, E. M., and Steward, F. C. (1955). Identification of compound A from coconut milk. *J. Am. Chem. Soc.* **77**:6351-6354.
71. Skoog, F. (1973). A survey of cytokinins and cytokinin antagonists. In Goodwin, (ed.), *Proceedings of the IUBC Symposium on Nitrogen Metabolism in Plants, Leeds, 1972* (in press).
72. Skoog, F., and Armstrong, D. J. (1970). Cytokinins. *Ann. Rev. Plant Physiol.* **21**:359-384.
73. Skoog, F., and Leonard, N. J. (1969). Sources and structure/activity relationships of cytokinins. In Wightman, F., and Setterfield, G. (eds.), *Biochemistry and Physiology of Plant Growth Substances,* Runge Press, Ottawa, pp. 1-18.
74. Skoog, F., and Schmitz, R. Y. (1972). Cytokinins. In Steward, F. C. (ed.), *Plant Physiology: A Treatise,* Vol. VIB, Academic Press, New York, pp. 181-213.
75. Skoog, F., Schmitz, R. Y., Bock, R. M., and Hecht, S. M. (1973). Cytokinin antagonists: Synthesis and physiological effects of 7-substituted 3-methylpyrazolo[4,3-*d*] pyrimidines. *Phytochemistry* **12**:25-37.
76. Skoog, F., Strong, F. M., and Miller, C. O. (1965). Cytokinins. *Science* **148**:532-533.
77. Steward, F. C., and Krikorian, A. D. (1971). *Plants, Chemicals and Growth,* Academic Press, New York.
78. Tronchet, A. (1968). Quelques effets de la kinétine et de l'acid gibbérellique sur la

forme et la structure anatomique des feuilles de *Coleus blumei. Ann. Sci. Univ. Besançon 3ᵉ Sér. Bot.* **5**:3-8.

79. van Overbeek, J. (1966). Plant hormones and regulators. *Science* **152**:721-731.
80. Vickers, J. D., and Logan, D. M. (1970). N^6-(Δ^2-Isopentenyl)adenosine: A heterologous system for *in vitro* synthesis in *E. coli* B transfer RNA. *Biochem. Biophys. Res. Commun.* **41**:741-747.
81. Vreman, H. J., Skoog, F., Frihart, C. R., and Leonard, N. J. (1972). Cytokinins in *Pisum* transfer ribonucleic acid. *Plant Physiol.* **49**:848-851.
82. Zachau, H. G., Dütting, D., and Feldman, H. (1966). Nucleotide sequences of two serine-specific tRNAs. *Angew. Chem.* **78**:392; *Internat. Ed. Engl.* **5**:422.
83. Zachau, H. G., Dütting, D., and Feldman, H. (1966). The structures of two serine transfer ribonucleic acids. *Z. Physiol. Chem.* **347**:212-235.

12

Environmental and Hormonal Control in Seedlings

Jochen Kummerow

Laboratorio de Botánica
Instituto de Ciencias Biológicas
Universidad Católica de Chile
Santiago, Chile

The ever increasing urge for intensive and highly productive agriculture demands from biological research the answers to numerous new or scarcely investigated questions. Besides the more spectacular problems of genetic research, the use of foliar fertilizers, the intensive application of herbicides and insecticides, etc., there are many other unresolved problems. The work on such problems may not provoke another "green revolution" but may help our understanding of the physiology of development, a field of considerable practical importance.

The purpose of this chapter is to focus attention on some of these less spectacular problems and to show within limited space some of the unanswered questions of the physiology of plant development, paying special attention to seedling development. We emphasize that development, beginning with the emergence of the radicle from the germinating seed until flowering and fruiting of the mature plant, is a continuous process. Therefore, discussing only a single developmental step with beginning and end arbitrarily fixed may be considered too artificial because early or late stages of development must also be taken into account. Without any doubt, the first step of development, germination, has long received the most intensive attention. The results of an immense number of individual research papers dealing with the physiology of germination have been compiled by several authors, e.g., Mayer and Poljakoff-Mayber (13).

Our objective here is the control of some developmental steps of the seedling plant by environmental conditions. This raises the question of how to define a "seedling plant." Morphologically, the seedling may be described as a plant somewhere between the emergence of the radicle out of the seed coat and a stage where the first foliar leaves have developed. Such a descriptive definition seems unsatisfactory for our purpose because we are interested in the physiology of development. Therefore, we will consider as a seedling the new plant until the transition from the heterotrophic to the completely autotrophic stage is accomplished. During this transition phase, the relative sensitivity of the seedlings to heat and frost, drought and fungus infection is maximal. The seedlings have to pass through this critical phase by fast growth; not only is a rapid leaf size increment necessary to expose a maximum area for photosynthesis, but also the fast-growing root system uses part of the reserve material.

As long as favorable climatic and edaphic conditions enhance seedling development, there does not seem to be a major problem. But as soon as climatic difficulties appear, stress situations may build up and seedling development is retarded. This seems important when we consider the ample use of highly productive varieties of cultivated plants not always completely adapted to the regions into which they have been introduced. Normally, the seedling plant overcomes all these difficulties, and it is attractive to study how the endogenous control factors, influenced by environmental conditions, ensure the necessary harmony of development. A better understanding of this harmony could yield important information on seedling responses to stress conditions. Since we cannot offer a complete picture of these extremely complex processes, we shall show with a few examples how environmental conditions and endogenous factors control seedling development.

LIGHT

Quite independent from its role in photosynthesis, light can strongly influence the pattern of seedling development. Downs and Borthwick (3) kept seedlings of *Catalpa bignonioides* growing continuously for a year under 16-hr photoperiods. The plants were 3 m tall at the year's end. Others, grown for a year under 8-hr photoperiods, were only 5 cm tall. The intensity of the artificial light used to extend the natural photoperiod need not be high. The effect is definitely of a photoperiodic nature and not related to total available light. Results are quite different, however, depending on whether incandescent or fluorescent lamps are used. Stem elongation is retarded with fluorescent lamps, although the number of nodes is not reduced. Without doubt, we have here a striking example of morphogenesis independent of photosynthesis.

The photomorphogenetic responses of the seedling plants of *Sinapis alba* have been analyzed in detail by Mohr (15). The morphogenesis of a seedling grown in light is entirely different from that of a dark-grown one. In the presence of light, hypocotyl growth is very limited (a "reasonable" reaction), and, correspondingly, the cells of the hypocotyl are shorter than those of dark-grown seedlings. With light, a certain percentage of hypocotyl epidermal cells differentiate into hairs and the subepidermal layer synthesizes abundant anthocyanins. We will not continue this listing of photoresponses of the *Sinapis* seedlings but rather ask what control mechanism is responsible for these phenomena. The action spectra for the induction of these photoresponses coincide with the absorption spectra of the phytochrome system (19). The red range of the spectrum (500–700, maximum 660 nm) promotes induction, and the dark red (700–800, maximum 730 nm) reverses this effect. This means that a photoresponse can be induced at 600 nm and canceled at 730 nm. But these well-known facts do not tell us the mechanism of action of the phytochrome system. Mohr (15), drawing on considerable experimental evidence, suggested a system of differential gene activation. This system is based on the assumption of active, inactive, and potentially active genes. A potentially active gene could be induced to activity by the active phytochrome P730. This step would initiate specific mRNA synthesis, resulting ultimately in enzyme synthesis. These enzymes would catalyze the conversion of a precursor to a final product, e.g., anthocyanin, in the subepidermal layer of the *Sinapsis* seedling.

As was mentioned above, good experimental evidence supports this theory. Nevertheless, another possibility may explain the mode of action of the phytochrome system. Haupt (for literature review, see refs. 1 and 8), studying the light-induced and phytochrome-controlled chloroplast movement in the green alga *Mougeotia,* came to the conclusion that the phytochrome is likely to be localized in the outer cytoplasm layer, probably in the plasmalemma. Changes in permeability, membrane potential, and transport, as well as control of enzyme synthesis, are considered as primary processes caused by phytochrome P730.

It may be recalled that the photoperiodic action of the seedling plant as well as other photoresponses is under the control of the phytochrome system. This may operate by means of differential gene activation, but it could also be that changes in the structure of cytoplasmic membrane systems, e.g., plasmalemma, are in some way responsible for the observed phenomena. Finally, it may be observed that these two theories do not exclude each other and could well operate simultaneously in controlling seedling development in the daily rhythm of light and dark.

TEMPERATURE

The necessity of a low-temperature treatment to overcome the dormancy of seeds (stratification) is well known. It may be emphasized that low temperatures are also of decisive importance for the normal seedling development of many temperate climate species.

Seeds of *Rhodotypos kerrioides* were collected in late summer (6). At this season, the seeds still had not gone through any period of postmaturation. The embryos were separated from their seed coats and placed in germination chambers under a temperature regime of 25°C. After 1 week, about 15% of the naked embryos started growth. When elongation of the hypocotyls became visible, the seedlings were transplanted and further observed. All the seedlings were dwarfed and showed extremely limited elongation of their stems. The internodes remained short, and the leaves appeared thick and dark green. This situation contrasted with that of the seedlings from normally cold-treated embryos, which showed extended internodes and light-green leaves. Similar observations have been made with seeds and seedling plants from many other species. This very specific growth inhibition resulting from lack of low-temperature treatment can be nullified in many cases by use of gibberellic acid (for literature review, see ref. 20). In the case of *Paeonia suffruticosa,* it has been possible to replace the 8-week 5°C treatment of the seeds with gibberellic acid, but this cannot be considered a rigid rule extending to other species. Embryos of a single species and even variety may show differences of cold requirements depending on local climatic conditions, the meteorological situation during harvest or even the preharvest season, and storage conditions after harvesting. The receptive organ for this cold effect seems to be the shoot apex, whereas the leaves do not play a major role in this relation. But it is possible that the low temperatures induce the response only in dividing cells, and the high sensitivity of the shoot apices may result from the high frequency of cell divisions in this organ. But all this still does not explain the mode of action. An important key for understanding lies in the work of Phinney and West (17), who treated seedling plants of a single-gene dwarf mutant of corn with gibberellic acid simply by dropping the solutions into the axils of primary leaves as soon as they emerged from the coleoptiles. Under this treatment, the plants became undistinguishable from normal tall corn plants. The mutation apparently has been the loss of the plant's ability to synthesize its own gibberellins. Gibberellic acid is known to induce *de novo* synthesis of specific proteins (for literature review, see ref. 5), and it may be that gibberellic acid triggers specific enzyme synthesis necessary for elongation growth in the corn dwarf mutants.

This situation we have just considered shows neatly how an environmental factor, low temperature in our case, may direct, via hormonal control, growth of seedling plants.

PRECONDITIONING

The importance of water for plant growth need not be stressed. Nevertheless, there exists an interesting complex of questions that will be briefly discussed. Repeated drying and subsequent soaking of plants is well known to produce greater drought resistance in certain plant species. Based on these observations,

Henckel and his collaborators (for literature review, see ref. 9) developed the concept of "presowing hardening of plants against drought." The basic idea is that soaking and redrying seeds or caryopses before sowing improves the drought-resistance qualities of the plants developing from these seeds. By means of such a pretreatment, fundamental physiological changes are said to be induced in the soaked seeds, and these changes are responsible for the adaptation of the growing seedling against environmental stress. It is even claimed that these changes can be transmitted to following plant generations. Müller-Stoll and Rammelt (16) made a comprehensive study of these problems; first, because the questions are of the greatest agricultural importance and, second, because the results of Henckel's group have found opposition (4). Growth intensity, water content, and osmotic values of seedling plants, transpiration, respiration, phosphatase and catalase activity, as well as ethanol-soluble purines and pyrmidines, were analyzed in relation to the presowing hardening of cereal grains. The authors could not confirm any of the claims of Henckel. Increases in water content or osmotic values did not occur in "hardened" seedlings. There was no significant difference in the transpiration rates of plants grown from "hardened" and control caryopses. In brief, all the parameters investigated have not shown any signs that the presowing seed treatment by Henckel's method does induce a physiological advantage to the seedlings as compared with plants grown from untreated control seeds.

Seeds can be preconditioned to modify future development, as reported by Highkin and Lang (10). These authors observed a significant difference in the final height and other parameters of vegetative growth of pea plants depending on the germination temperature. This effect seems similar to vernalization, where a low-temperature treatment of the vegetative plant induces the flowering. The data of Highkin and Lang make it clear that high temperatures (23°C) applied to a sensitive seedling stage can have inductive influence on vegetative growth characteristics.

CORRELATIVE INHIBITION

The functions of the different growth regulators in relation to apical dominance, especially auxins, cytokinins, and gibberellins, have been repeatedly analyzed (11, 18). Even if the precise mode of action still needs further clarification, there exists general agreement that the critical point is not the absolute concentration of one or several growth regulators but rather a harmonious combination of concentrations of all the plant hormones involved.

The effects of phytohormones on lateral bud development are complex. Gibberellins promote and auxin inhibits bud growth initiation on decapitated stems, and cytokinins antagonize in this case the action of auxin. However, with nondecapitated plants, the situation may be different. Cytokinins stimulate the arrested axillary buds to initiate their growth. Auxin, given additionally, enhances this cytokinin effect instead of antagonizing it.

These observations seem to bear only a very marginal relation to our basic question, since it remains open just how far environmental factors are involved with this control system. However, environmental factors probably are involved. Gregory and Veale (7) express this issue clearly in stating that "nutrition is the main factor in correlative inhibition." McIntyre (14) decapitated flax seedlings at the epicotyl level and showed that one of the two shoots produced at the cotyledonary nodes tends to inhibit the growth of the other. This inhibition is due primarily to competition between the shoots for a limited mineral nutrient supply. Interesting also is the interaction of gibberellic acid and kinetin on apical dominance in tomato (2). Both the growth regulators combined were applied to the leaf axils of decapitated plants which had been treated on the cut surface with auxin. Actually, the expected promotion of lateral bud growth was observed but was dependent on the nitrogen level in the culture medium.

DISCUSSION

Several apparently arbitrarily chosen processes related to seedling development have been briefly described. Phytochromes, endogenous growth regulators in their complex and still not fully understood relationships, the very polemical technique of presowing hardening of seeds, and an example of correlative inhibition have been mentioned. But all these examples, as different as they are, made one basic rule very clear: all the different endogenous growth-regulating systems respond to environmental factors whether they are external or internal. Obviously enough, a phytochrome system becomes senseless without the daily light-dark periodicity. Enzyme synthesis does not start without the low-temperature triggering in the case of low-temperature stratification. Henckel's presowing hardening method for obtaining more drought-resistant and more highly productive plants could not be verified under Central European and Israelian conditions. But it should not be excluded that the phenomena described by Henckel could have agronomical value under different climatic conditions. Ultimately, the process of vernalization and also the influence of high germination temperature on future seedling and mature plant development seem to be similar processes: the environmental factor "temperature" acts during a sensitive phase of germination, but the effect becomes visible at a much later stage of development. It may be stressed that in no case are we suggesting that heritable developmental changes are produced by temperature and humidity treatments, even if this has been suggested by Henckel's school. But we cannot exclude the action of a selective factor.

The interest in the problem of correlative inhibitions is reflected by an increasing amount of work done in this field. Historically, this complex problem has been considered to be a result of competitive forces (12). Later, the hormonal factors came more and more into focus (11). But during the last years the importance of the principle of competition for a limited supply of mineral nutrients came again into the foreground (14). Thus there is good reason to claim that an environmental factor, the mineral nutrition, has a controlling function over this very specific detail of seedling development. An understanding of the capacity of regenerative forces in plants is of the utmost importance and depends to a great degree on the understanding of correlative bud inhibition. Empirically, these phenomena have been known for thousands of years (e.g., the pruning of grapes in ancient Babylonia), but only recently have we begun to get some insight into the causal relations.

The research of the coming years will have to concentrate on the relations between directing environmental factors and controlling endogenous mechanisms. The seedling plant is the ideal research object, and results obtained with it may have great potential for increasing yields of agricultural plants.

REFERENCES

1. Briggs, W. R., and Rice, H. V. (1972). Phytochrome: Chemical and physical properties and mechanism of action. *Ann. Rev. Plant Physiol.* **23**:293-334.
2. Catalano, M., and Hill, T. A. (1969). Interaction between gibberellic acid and kinetin in overcoming apical dominance, natural and induced by IAA in tomato (*Lycopersicum esculentum* Mill. cultivar Potentate). *Nature (Lond.)* **222**:985-986.
3. Downs, R. J., and Borthwick, H. A. (1956). Effects of photoperiod on growth of trees. *Bot. Gaz.* **117**:310-326.
4. Evenari, M. (1964). Hardening treatment of seeds as a means of increasing yields under conditions of inadequate moisture. *Nature (Lond.)* **204**:1010-1011.
5. Filner, P., Wray, J. L., and Varner, J. E. (1969). Enzyme induction in higher plants. *Science* **165**:358-367.
6. Flemion, F. (1933). Physiological and chemical studies of after-ripening of *Rhodotypos kerrioides* seeds. *Contr. Boyce Thompson Inst.* **5**:143-159.
7. Gregory, F. G., and Veale, J. A. (1957). A reassessment of the problem of apical dominance. *Symp. Soc. Exptl. Biol.* **10**:1-20.
8. Haupt, W. (1965). Perception of environmental stimuli orienting growth and movement in lower plants. *Ann. Rev. Plant Physiol.* **16**:267-290.
9. Henckel, P. A. (1964). Physiology of plants under drought. *Ann. Rev. Plant Physiol.* **15**:363-386.
10. Highkin, H. R., and Lang, A. (1966). Residual effect of germination temperature on the growth of peas. *Planta (Berl.)* **68**:94-98.
11. Letham, D. S. (1969). Cytokinins and their relation to other phytohormones. *BioScience* **19**:309-316.
12. Loeb, J. (1924). *Regeneration,* McGraw-Hill, New York.
13. Mayer, A. M., and Poljakoff-Mayber, A. (1963). *The Germination of Seeds,* Pergamon Press, Oxford-London-New York-Paris.
14. McIntyre, G. J. (1968). Nutritional control of the correlative inhibition between lateral shoots in the flax seedling (*Linum usitatissimum*). *Can. J. Bot.* **46**:147-155.

15. Mohr, H. (1969). *Lehrbuch der Pflanzenphysiologie,* Springer-Verlag, Berlin-Heidelberg-New York.
16. Müller-Stoll, W. R., and Rammelt, R. (1970). Über den Einfluss von Vorquellung und Rücktrocknung der Caryopsen vor der Aussaat auf die Entwicklung und einige Stoffwechselprozesse von Getreidepflanzen. *Kulturpflanze* **18:**133-167.
17. Phinney, B. O., and West, C. A. (1960). In Rudnick, D. (ed.), *Developing Cell Systems and Their Control,* Ronald Press, New York.
18. Sachs, T., and Thimann, K. V. (1964). Release of lateral buds from apical dominance. *Nature (Lond.)* **201:**939-940.
19. Siegelman, H. W., Turner, B. C., and Hendricks, S. B. (1966). The chromophore of phytochrome. *Plant Physiol.* **41:**1289-1292.
20. Vegis, A. (1965). Die Bedeutung von physikalischen und chemischen Aussenfaktoren bei der Induktion und Beendigung von Ruhezuständen bei Organen und Geweben höherer Pflanzen. In *Handbuch der Pflanzenphysiologie,* Vol. XV/2, Springer-Verlag, Berlin-Heidelberg-New York, pp. 534-637.

13

Factors Affecting Flowering of Coffee

Paulo de T. Alvim

Centro de Pesquisas do Cacau
Itabuna, Bahia, Brazil

Two distinct processes should be considered when studying the relation between environmental factors and the flowering of coffee: flower-bud initiation and flower opening or anthesis. These two processes are controlled by different environmental factors. With most coffee varieties, it has been experimentally demonstrated that flower-bud initiation is a typical response to short days (10,19), one exception being the variety *semperflorens* which produces flower buds under any photoperiodic condition (22). Anthesis, on the other hand, depends primarily on rainfall distribution and appears to be a response to rain following a period of moisture stress (3). This chapter will review the present knowledge concerning the external and internal factors controlling flower opening, or the transition from dormancy to bud break.

THE FLOWER BUD

The development of the inflorescence and flower buds of coffee has been studied, for example, by van der Muelen (23) and Newton (17). The buds are always formed in the axil of the leaves and are arranged in a series, in contrast to most plants where the buds occur singly. As many as five buds may be formed in each leaf axil. The largest bud is nearest the stem, with the smallest bud nearest the petiole of the subtending leaf. The primordium is apparently laid down in the node of the branch tip at the same time that the growth is occurring with the leaves separating from the terminal bud.

Whether an inflorescence or a vegetative shoot will originate from an axillary bud cannot be ascertained until the bud reaches a certain stage of development.

At this stage, if conditions conducive to flowering prevail, there is a flattening of the apical growing point, which subsequently divides into two flower-bud primordia. These may develop into lateral dome-shaped growing points which produce additional lateral flower buds, resulting in an inflorescence with two pairs of opposite and decussate flower buds. The four buds may or may not develop into flowers, depending on the external conditions and on the position of the inflorescence in the leaf axil. According to Mes (13), the number of flower buds per inflorescence in one leaf axil is four or fewer. Three or four inflorescences, each with four flower buds in any one leaf axil, were found only under the most favorable conditions for growth.

In other studies, shoot growth of certain buds in the series has been induced by pruning back the branch. Based on this procedure, it has been estimated that floral determination after bud initiation could take up to 1 month.

Once the flower buds are differentiated, they grow rather slowly for a period of about 2 months up to a length of about 6–8 mm. At this stage, the buds stop growing for a period lasting from a few weeks to several months, depending on the rainfall distribution. As will be seen later, this check in growth is not a simple case of quiescence or imposed rest, i.e., a state of rest caused by unfavorable external growth conditions such as low temperature or water deficit as Mes (15) and Rees (21) suggested, but rather appears to be a case of true dormancy in which growth is checked by unfavorable internal conditions.

THE FLOWERING PATTERN

Tropical plants can be grouped into four flowering periodicity classes: everflowering, nonseasonal flowering, seasonal flowering, and gregarious flowering (4).

Everflowering species produce flowers continuously throughout the year (examples are *Hibiscus* spp., *Ficus* spp., and *Carica papaya*). Nonseasonal flowering species also have flowers throughout the year but not continuously on the same plant; there is a variation from plant to plant and sometimes even from branch to branch (examples, *Spathodea campanulata, Michelia champaca,* and *Cassia fistula*). Seasonal flowering species occur in areas with a periodical dry season or variation in day length. Some nonseasonal flowering species become seasonal when they are growing under such conditions (4). In gregarious flowering species, all individual plants flower simultaneously over extended areas and within short periods. From one day to the next all the plants bloom, and, depending on the climatic pattern of the region, this sudden blooming can be seasonal or nonseasonal. Coffee is a typical gregarious flowering species, and other well-known examples are certain epiphytic orchids such as *Dendrobium crumenatum* or "pigeon orchid" (9) and *Zephyranthes rosea.*

In equatorial regions with no well-defined alternations between wet and dry periods and with an inductive photoperiod throughout the year, the coffee trees flower at any time of the year and at odd intervals, varying from 2 to several weeks. Because of the repeated flowering over several months, the numbers of harvests and consequently the costs of production are greatly increased in these regions. Morales *et al.* (16) found that in some regions of Colombia, where flowering occurs practically every month, the picking operation accounted for 58% of the total labor cost in a coffee farm. In Costa Rica, where there are over 12 or 15 flowerings in a year, harvesting amounted to 41% of the total labor cost.

In southern Brazil (latitude 20–25°S), there are usually two or three flowerings at the beginning of the rainy season (normally between September and November), and as a rule there is only one harvest at most farms during May or June. Two factors contribute to this flowering pattern in Brazil: long summer days (over 13 hr) which inhibit flower-bud initiation for 3 or 4 months, and well-defined wet and dry seasons.

TEMPERATURE RELATIONS

Studies carried out by Went (22) and Mes (13) under controlled environmental conditions showed that the initiation and growth of coffee flower buds are greatly affected by temperature. Various alternating temperature regimes were used in these experiments under an 8-hr photoperiod. The results indicated that the number of flower buds tended to decrease when the plants were submitted to relatively high temperatures.

With a regime of 23°C during the day and 17°C at night, inflorescences with four flower buds were common, and up to three such inflorescences were found in one leaf axil. At 26–20°C and 30–24°C, the number of flower buds per inflorescence decreased to between three and one. In young plants (13 months old) only one bud, or occasionally two, was produced per inflorescence, while more buds were formed per tree at temperature combinations which included a 23°C night temperature, such as 26–23°, 23–23°, and 20–23°C. There was no flower-bud differentiation at combinations of 30–23° and 30–17°C.

The rate of bud growth, both before and after bud break, increased with higher temperatures. At 30–24°, anthesis occurred in 8 days, at 26–20° in 10 days, at 23–24° in 9 days, and at 23–17°C in about 11 days after bud break (14).

Plants grown under relatively high temperatures produced many flower buds which did not develop into normal flowers; some dried up, but the majority showed the floral atrophy known as "star flowers." Mes (13) pointed out that the production of star flowers not only is the result of high temperature but also may be caused by unfavorable growth conditions. Porteres (20) conclusively showed that inadequate water supply or drought predisposes the coffee trees to floral atrophy. By means of irrigation, he was able to reduce the percentage of star flowers from 57% to 5% with an irrigation equivalent to 20 mm of rainfall, and to nearly 0% with the application of more water. The effect of high temperature on floral atrophy, as reported by Mes (13) and others, could be a response to moisture stress caused by higher transpiration rates.

Some authors believe that a temperature drop following rain plays a decisive role in breaking flower-bud dormancy in coffee (21,22). The effect of a temperature drop associated with rains has been described as breaking flower-bud dormancy in other gregarious flowering species such as the orchid *Dendrobium crumenatum* (9). Apparently, however, no one has ever been able to demonstrate experimentally that cooling can actually break this dormancy in coffee. By submerging branches with dormant flower buds in water at different temperatures, I (1) obtained better flowering at 35° than at 25°C, the percentage of opened buds being 65.5 and 46.5%, respectively. Water at 15°C caused only 3.5% of the buds to open. It would appear from these results that low temperature actually neutralizes the effect of watering on bud break.

C. M. Franco (personal communication) enclosed coffee branches with dormant flower buds in cold boxes (polystyrene boxes with ice at the bottom) where temperature was kept at 13–18°C or about 15–20°C below the outside temperature. The experiments were carried out under field conditions during the normal flowering season (September to October), and the plants were protected from rainfall by a plastic roof. The treatments were repeated several times for 2–8 hr. All branches flowered at the same time as plants growing in the surrounding field; in no case did the cold treatment effectively induce bud break.

Went (22) observed flowering 2 weeks after coffee trees had been transferred from an alternating temperature of 30–24°C to one of 23–17°C. These results are sometimes presented as evidence in favor of the cold-stimulus process (13). Since Went's experiments were carried out without any control of atmospheric humidity, it is difficult to say whether flowering was actually a response to temperature drop or to an increase in the internal water potential of the plants as a result of lower transpiration losses in the cooler environment.

WATER RELATIONS

It has been known for many years that coffee flowering is closely related to rainfall distribution. In Haiti, Arndt (6) observed that flower buds seem to mature during the dry season and that the flowers open 8 days "after the first rain subsequent to the winter dry season." It has been reported elsewhere that flowering occurs in Kenya from 9 to 15 days after the onset of rainy seasons and in southern India 9 days after the first substantial showers. Hacquart (12) and Porteres (20) also observed that coffee flowering after rain usually occurs when the rain is preceded by a dry period. Piringer and Borthwick (19), in their studies of photoperiodic reactions with potted coffee seedlings, observed that "all plants on which flower buds were induced could be repeatedly stimulated to bloom by alternate periods of drying and watering. When water was withheld from the plants for several days and then copiously applied, anthesis occurred within approximately two weeks." Although these studies imply that rain or irrigation is only effective in breaking dormancy when preceded by a period of moisture deficiency, none of these studies gave particular attention to the role played by moisture stress in the mechanism of bud break. Piringer and Borthwick (19) simply concluded that their results were in "agreement with reports that rain is one of the controlling factors for coffee flowering."

Mes (15) stated that coffee flower buds do not have a true dormancy, but rather an imposed dormancy, or quiescence, in which growth is stopped because of moisture deficiency. According to this theory, bud break induced by rainfall would simply be a response to water uptake by the buds. This hypothesis was refuted (3) by experimentally demonstrating that moisture stress is a necessary prerequisite for bud break and that dormancy can be prolonged for an indefinite period provided the plants are irrigated at frequent intervals. It is true that an increase in the water potential of the plant brought about by either rain, irrigation, or artificial moisture of the buds is also necessary for flower opening, but these treatments had no effect if the plants were not previously submitted to moisture stress. This fact seems to indicate that coffee flower buds, and possibly other buds of gregarious flowering species, go through two phases of rest: (a) a true dormancy, under the control of a growth inhibitor (or inhibitors), the concentration of which decreases during drought, thus putting the buds in a ready-to-grow state, and (b) a quiescence or imposed dormancy which persists after the true dormancy is over because of inadequate water supply. In other words, moisture stress is necessary to release the dormant phase, but water uptake is necessary to release the quiescent phase.

It is important to mention that my experiments on dormancy release by moisture stress were carried out in the desert coastal region of Peru, where transpiration rates are relatively low due to the reduced solar irradiation and where the water potential of the plants is predominantly controlled by the available soil moisture. Under conditions favoring high transpiration rates, moisture stress can be prevented neither by frequent irrigation nor, apparently, by growing the plants in nutrient solution. In my opinion, this fact could account for Franco's (11) observation that coffee plants in a nutrient solution at Campinas, Brazil, blossomed at the same time as the coffee in the surrounding field. It would also explain the results with *Coffea rupestris* in Nigeria by Rees (21), who observed some flowering, particularly following rains, in plants which were kept watered during the dry season.

Van der Veen (24) expressed the opinion, based on experiments in Indonesia with *Coffea canefora* grown in nutrient solution, that the period of water stress needed for bud break could be minimal "but all the same it was necessary for flowering." When the nutrient solution was cooled in the morning by adding pieces of ice, "the plants wilted more or less at 10 or 11 a.m. but recovered in the afternoon when the solution warmed up again to the normal temperature. A week later the plants were flowering abundantly, while the control plants retained their flower buds in a dormancy condition." Since no mention is made of rainfall during the period when these observations were made, it is assumed that in this particular case flower opening was induced by moisture stress alone without the need for subsequent rain. This apparently does not happen with field-grown plants, where flowering occurs only after rain or irrigation following a dry period. There are, however, some indications that an increase in relative humidity might also induce flowering. According to Professor J. F. Carvajal (personal communication), coffee plants grown under greenhouse conditions in Costa Rica often flower at the same time as plants grown in the open, usually 10 days after rain has followed a dry spell. Since plant water potential is affected by relative humidity (5) and greenhouse temperature varies only slightly with rain, it seems probable that the rise in relative humidity rather than a cold shock controlled bud break.

In 1960, I suggested that under tropical conditions water stress has an effect comparable to the chilling which breaks the dormancy of some temperate zone plants. The term "hydroperiodism" was proposed for this peculiar type of plant-water relation in which a transition from dryness to wetness plays a decisive role not only in the flowering but also in the growth-flush mechanism of some species (4,5).

HORMONE RELATIONS

It is well established that dormancy and the opening of flower buds in coffee, as in any plant, are controlled by hormones. Flower anthesis following rain, irrigation, or submersion of branches in water is not simply the result of the physical process of water uptake or of releasing moisture tension in the flower bud, as suggested by Mes (15). Several arguments (1) have been presented against this hypothesis and have demonstrated experimentally the possibility of inducing flowering by spraying the buds with an aqueous solution of gibberellic acid (GA_3). Several other hormones and chemical products have been tested by various authors without any success. These included indolacetic acid; indolebutyric acid; napththaleneacetic acid; 2,4-dichlorophenoxyacetic acid; 2,4,5-trichlorophenoxypropionic acid; 2,4,6-trichlorophenoxyacetic acid; transcinhamic acid; maleic hydrazide; naphthaleneacetamide; ethylene chlorohydrine; thiourea; sugar; and many other substances (1). The effectiveness of gibberellic acid in inducing flowering of coffee was confirmed by Pagaez (18), van der Veen (24), and Browning (7). Browning also found that bud break could be induced by cytokinin, although the response was not as pronounced as with GA_3. I have suggested (1) that rain or irrigation might increase the concentration of gibberellic acid in the flowering buds and have demonstrated that its effectiveness in breaking flower-bud dormancy is definitely greater when the plants are in a condition of moisture stress (3). It was also suggested that water stress removes a growth inhibitor responsible for bud dormancy (2). Spraying with GA_3 during the rainy season in Costa Rica gave disappointing results (J. Leon, personal communication), apparently due to the absence of moisture stress. Gibberellic acid sprays have no effect on star (abortive) flowers of very small size, but the larger star flowers, which generally have the corolla slightly opened at the extremity and the stigmas exposed, react to GA_3 like normal buds and produce fruits of normal appearance (1).

It is now generally believed that abscisic acid (ABA) is a growth inhibitor associated with the mechanism of bud dormancy in temperate trees. Van der Veen (24) demonstrated that coffee flower buds treated with 200 ppm ABA in lanolin paste remained dormant for several months and then deteriorated or developed into star flowers. Watering following a period of drought, which caused opening of untreated buds after 10 days, had no effect on the ABA-treated buds.

Browning *et al.* (8) recently demonstrated the presence of ABA in coffee flower buds collected before and after bud break caused by rain. The yield of ABA as estimated by bioassay was $0.1-0.16$ $\mu g/g$ dry weight for the dormant flower buds and $0.04-0.09$ $\mu g/g$ dry weight for the buds collected 2 days after rain. They concluded that ABA accounts for about 75% of the inhibitory activity in the acidic extract.

Browning (7) also demonstrated that the concentration of GA in the flower buds increased significantly after bud break. The increase preceded the stage when the buds started to take up water rapidly and expand. Browning believed that bud break in response to rainfall or irrigation involved the release of free GA from a bound, inactive form rather than a *de novo* synthesis of GA. Thus the hypothesis implicating GA in the mechanism of bud break would appear to be well supported, but more data are needed on the changes of the ABA concentration in dormant buds collected at different times during a dry period before we can determine whether ABA levels in the buds actually decrease as a consequence of moisture stress. Other investigators have found an increase in the absolute amount of ABA in wheat leaves which have been detached and allowed to wilt. The suggestion is that moisture stress in the field may increase the ABA content of plant tissue. As pointed out by Browning *et al.* (8) and Browning (7), this evidence does not preclude the possibility that the amount of ABA in dormant coffee flower buds is lower after the tree has been exposed to drought. The inhibitor responsible for bud dormancy is thought to originate in the leaves, and reduced translocation during water stress might decrease its movement from the leaves to the flower buds.

CONCLUSIONS AND SUMMARY

Additional research is obviously needed in order to understand the physiological processes underlying the relation between environmental factors and coffee flowering. Among the problems deserving particular attention are measurements of ABA concentration in relation to internal water potential, the responses of dormant buds to different temperature treatments, and the effect of relative humidity on dormancy and bud break.

Based on the evidence described in this review, the following hypothesis is tentatively suggested to explain the mechanism of flower opening in coffee and possibly in other gregarious flowering species sensitive to hydroperiodism or the transition from dryness to wetness:

a. Conditions favoring constant high water potential, such as frequent irrigation and low transpiration rates, keep flower buds dormant apparently because of a relatively high concentration of ABA (7,24).

b. Moisture stress, caused by either low soil moisture or high transpiration rates, reduces ABA concentration in the flower buds, possibly because of reduced translocation from the leaves to the flower buds.

c. True dormancy terminates because of reduced ABA concentration, but quiescence or imposed dormancy persists as a result of inadequate water supply or low internal water potential.

d. Rain, irrigation, or an increase in atmospheric humidity raises the water potential of the buds.

e. Increase in water potential stimulates conversion of gibberellin from a bound to a free form (7).

f. Buds start growing toward anthesis.

Day length and rainfall distribution are the main external factors controlling flowering of coffee. Bud differentiation is induced by short days (photoperiodism), whereas bud anthesis is associated with rainfall *following a dry period* or a sequence from a dry to a wet period. The term "hydroperiodism" is used to refer to this effect of changing moisture status on flowering behavior.

In regions where coffee is continuously exposed to inductive photoperiods, such as occur near the equator, flower-bud differentiation occurs throughout the year and blooming is regulated only by rainfall distribution. In the coffee regions of Brazil (latitude 20–25°S), flowering is controlled by rainfall distribution as well as by seasonal changes in day length.

Treatments to prevent internal water deficit, such as frequent irrigation, have proven effective in imposing flower-bud dormancy, particularly in regions with high relative humidity or low evaporating power of the air such as in Lima, Peru. When conditions are favorable for high transpiration rates, frequent irrigation might not be completely effective in preventing bud break due to internal water deficit.

Recent studies indicate that dormancy release by hydroperiodism is associated with an increase in the gibberellin - abscisic acid ratio in the flower buds. The following hypothesis is tentatively suggested to explain the hormonal relation between flowering and internal moisture status: moisture stress decreases ABA translocation into the flower buds, thus rendering the buds "ready to grow"; subsequent release of moisture stress increases GA concentration, thus inducing bud growth (anthesis).

REFERENCES

1. Alvim, P. de T. (1958). Estimulo de la floración y fructificación del cafeto por aspersiones con ácido giberélico. *Turrialba* **8(2)**:64-72.
2. Alvim, P. de T. 1960). Physiology of growth and flowering in coffee. *Coffee (Turrialba)* **2(6)**:57-62.
3. Alvim, P. de T. (1960). Moisture stress as a requirement for flowering of coffee. *Science* **132(3423)**:354.
4. Alvim, P. de T. (1964). Tree growth periodicity in tropical climates. In *Formation of Wood in Forest Trees,* Academic Press, New York, pp. 479-495.
5. Alvim, P. de T., Machado, A. D., and Vello, F. (1972). Physiological responses of cacao to environmental factors. Fourth International Cocoa Research Conference, Trinidad and Tobago, January 9-18.
6. Arndt, C. H. (1929). Configuration and some effects of light and gravity on *Coffea arabica* L. *Am. J. Bot.* **16(3)**:173-178.
7. Browning, G. (1971). The hormonal regulation of flowering and cropping in *Coffea arabica.* Ph.D. Thesis, University of Bristol.
8. Browning, G., Hoad, G. V., and Gaskin, P. (1970). Identification of abscisic acid in flower buds of *Coffea arabica* L. *Planta (Berl.)* **94(3)**:213-219.
9. Coster, C. (1926). Periodische Bluteerseheiningen in der Tropen. *Ann. J. Bot. (Buitenzong)* **35**:125-162.
10. Franco, C. M. (1940). Fotoperiodismo em cafeeiro (*C. arabica* L.). *Inst. Café Estado São Paulo Rev.* **15(164)**:1586-1592.
11. Franco, C. M. (1962). Fisiologia do cafeeiro. In *Curso Internacional de Fisiologia Vegetal* (mimeographed), Piracicaba, Brasil.
12. Hacquart, A. (1941). Periodicité de la floraison et de la fructification du caféier "Robusta" á l'Equateur. *Bull. Agr. Congo Belge* **32(3)**:496-538.
13. Mes, M. G. (1957). Studies on the flowering of *Coffea arabica* L.: I. The influence of temperature on the initiation and growth of coffee flower bud. *Portugal. Acta Biol. (Ser. A)* **4(4)**:328-334.
14. Mes, M. G. (1957). Studies on the flowering of *Coffea arabica* L.: II. Breaking the dormancy of coffee flower buds. *Portugal. Acta Biol. (Ser. A)* **4(4)**:342-354.
15. Mes, M. G. (1958). Studies on the flowering of *Coffea arabica* L.: III. Various phenomena associated with the dormancy of coffee flower buds. *Portugal. Acta Biol. (Ser. A)* **5(1)**:25-44.

16. Morales, J. O., Keeper, W. E., and Gomez, O. F. (1951). Estudio economico de fincas cafetaleras. *Agr. Tropical* **7(3)**:33-38.
17. Newton, O. A. (1952). Preliminary Study of the Growth and Flower Habits of *Coffea arabica* L. Processed, Inter-American Institute of Agricultural Sciences, Turrialba, Costa Rica.
18. Pagaez, E. A. (1959). Quelques considerations sur la floraison du cafeier. *Bull. Agr. Congo Belge* **50(6)**:1531-1540.
19. Piringer, A. A., and Borthwick, H. A. (1955). Photoperiodic responses of coffee. *Turrialba* **5(3)**:72-77.
20. Porteres, R. (1946). Action de l'eau après une période seche sur le déclenchement de la floraison chez *Coffea arabica* L. *Agr. Tropicale* **1(3-4)**:148-158.
21. Rees, A. R. (1964). Some observations on the flowering behaviour of *Coffea rupestris* in Southern Nigeria. *J. Ecol.* **52(1)**:1-7.
22. Went, F. W. (1957). The experimental control of plant growth *Chron. Bot. Co. (Waltham, Mass.)* 343 pp.
23. van der Muelen, A. (1939). Over den bouw en de periodieke ontwikkeling der bloem-knoppen by *Coffea*–sooten Mededeeling No. 60. *Lab. Plant Phys. (Onderzoek, Wageningen)*.
24. van der Veen, R. (1968). Plant hormones and flowering in coffee. *Acta Bot. Neerl.* **17(5)**:373-376.

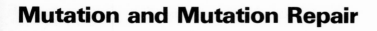

Mutation and Mutation Repair

14

Increasing the Effectiveness, Efficiency, and Specificity of Mutation Induction in Flowering Plants

R. A. Nilan

Department of Agronomy and Soils and Program in Genetics
Washington State University
Pullman, Washington, U.S.A.

Numerous agents are now available for inducing mutations and chromosome aberrations for a variety of investigations in plant genetics, development, and evolution and in plant breeding (mutation breeding). These include the widely used physical mutagens X-rays, γ-rays, neutrons, and β-rays; the potent alkylating compounds ethyl methanesulfonate (EMS), diethyl sulfate (dES), and ethyleneimine (EI); and nitroso compounds, nitroso ethylurethane (NEH), nitroso methylurethane (NMU), ethyl nitrosourea (ENH), and methyl nitrosourea (MNH). Much of the recent research on induced mutation in plants has been reviewed by Auerbach and Kilbey (4). Thus information in this chapter will be largely confined to experiments with flowering plants.

Seeds are most frequently used in experiments where gene and chromosome changes are to be induced. However, meristems of whole plants, pollen, cuttings, tubers, and bulbs have been used. Single diploid and haploid cells are just being introduced in mutation experiments.

As a result of mutagen treatments, a wide variety of changes which affect growth, adaptation, and utilization of flowering plants have been induced. However, of most relevance to this Symposium is that many commercially important traits in agronomic and horticultural plants have been altered in a positive way by the various physical and chemical mutagens, and these so-called beneficial mutations are being utilized in breeding. The broad subject of mutation breeding has been reviewed extensively (11, 25, 31, 67, 73) and was the subject of a symposium of Latin American plant geneticists and breeders held at Buenos Aires in 1970 (e.g., see ref. 11).

Over 100 varieties of cereals, legumes, fruit trees, and ornamentals developed with the aid of induced mutations are or have been in commercial production around the world. An updated list of these varieties is presented in the Proceedings of the Buenos Aires symposium and summarized in Table I. Improvements in these varieties are due to induced mutations of both qualitatively and quantitatively inherited traits such as yield, disease reaction, winter hardiness, maturity, adaptability, flower color, and shape.

Mutations of considerable current interest are those contributing to improvement of quality characters, particularly quantity and quality of protein (21,76). One of the most striking achievements in mutation induction for improved quality has been the recent induction of high-lysine mutants in barley. From among 6000 lines derived from ethyleneimine treatment, Ingversen *et al.* (33) selected six high-lysine lines. One of these mutants exhibits a 45–50% increase of lysine content with only a 10% reduction in yield. It was induced in the best Danish variety and is free of the shriveled endosperm characteristic. This success with induced mutations can be contrasted to the selection of one high-lysine line with a 15% increase from over 1000 entries of the World Barley Collection. This

Table I. Released Varieties Developed Through Induced Mutations

Type of crop		Number of released varieties (1971)
Cereals		42
Bread wheat	7	
Durum wheat	4	
Rice	7	
Barley	19	
Oats	5	
Legumes		16
Fruit trees		3
Other crops		7
Total crops		68
Ornamentals		33
Total induced mutant varieties		101
Number of crop species	19	
Number of ornamental species	7	

Summary supplied by Dr. B. Sigurbjörnsson.

line is of Ethiopian origin and has poor yield and other undesirable character-istics. Thus it is becoming apparent that as selection techniques improve, important induced biochemical and physiological mutations can be detected that can contribute to improving, for example, yield, drought resistance, photosyn-thetic efficiency, quality, and disease resistance. Furthermore, induced muta-tions provide genetic variability in crop plants that may be difficult to obtain through interspecific and intergeneric crosses or that may no longer exist because distant or near relatives containing needed genes are no longer available. The various factors that a plant breeder should consider before employing mutation breeding are well described by Brock (11).

In spite of considerable achievements in the induction and utilization of mutations in various genetic, developmental, evolutionary, and breeding investi-gations, it is evident that further progress in these areas demands mutations in greater numbers per locus to provide many new and different alleles and at an increasing number of loci in most plant species. Thus present mutagens must be made more effective (more numerous mutations per dose of mutagen), more efficient (higher frequency of such desirable events as point mutations in relation to such undesirable or unwanted events as sterility and chromosome aberrations), and more specific (higher frequencies of mutations at specific loci).

This chapter will mainly be an account of recent progress toward these goals in plant mutagenesis. It will also attempt to point out some directions that future research may take.

Progress in increasing mutation effectiveness, efficiency, and specificity has been achieved in spite of the fact that the nature of both spontaneous and induced mutations in flowering plants is still very little understood (56,59). Recent investigations and reviews (*cf.* refs. 51 and 69) indicate that we do not yet have the high resolving power of genetic and chemical analyses of mutants to detect the induction of subtle alterations in DNA structure by ionizing radiation or the chemical agents. Rather, the alterations in genetic material that have been detected as contributing to induced and spontaneous mutations in flowering plants have been determined for the most part by genetic and cytological analyses. These analyses indicate that many mutations inherited in normal Mendelian fashion may not be point mutations but rather small changes in chromosome structure. Further progress in understanding the nature of muta-tional events is hampered by the great structural complexity of the chromo-somes and by the complicated biological cycles which permit only an indirect approach to generalizations about the nature of mutations.

Fortunately, understanding of genetic alterations at the DNA level has considerably progressed in lower plants such as yeast and *Neurospora*. Here, the chromosome structure and arrangement of genetic material are similar to those in the flowering plants, but the resolving power of genetic analyses of mutants more closely resembles that for the prokaryotes (12, 19, 45–47). Results with these organisms suggest that the detection of genetic alterations at the DNA level should be possible with flowering plants once the resolving power for mutant analyses has been increased.

Recently developed techniques for producing and mutagen-treating cultures of somatic cells and haploid plants will surely aid in achieving greater control of the induced mutation process in flowering species. These techniques will permit the induction, selection, and analysis of mutations of single haploid or diploid cells. Haploid cells can subsequently be converted with the aid of colchicine into mature diploid plants homozygous for the mutation. Thus the mutation techniques so widely used in microbial genetics are close at hand for the plant geneticist. Smith (72) and Carlson *et al.* (Chapter 8, this volume) have recently summarized the success of such techniques in *Nicotiana.* Large numbers of haploid plants can now be obtained from anther culture in at least six genera (48, 61, 74; Nitsch and Norreel, Chapter 10, this volume) and from species crosses, as demonstrated in barley by Kasha and colleagues (35) and Lange (40). Indeed, mutations from haploid cell cultures of *Nicotiana* have already been induced (61, 72).

EFFECTIVENESS AND EFFICIENCY

During the past several years, extensive research has produced new information and techniques for increasing the effectiveness and efficiency of chemical mutagens and of ionizing radiations (38, 58). Barley seeds have been the most widely used, since they exhibit easily scored chromosome aberrations and numerous well-defined chlorophyll-deficient mutations after mutagen treatment.

Chemical Mutagens

The full potential of the most widely used chemical mutagens has not been realized because of a wide variety of physical, chemical, and biological factors which influence the biological action and hence the effectiveness and efficiency of these mutagens in plant cells. A list of these factors is lengthy, and experiments to control or manipulate them to increase effectiveness and efficiency and to understand how chemical mutagens induce genetic changes in plant cells are numerous. The most studied factors include several properties of the biological system such as genetic composition and physiological state of the organism or system; physical and chemical properties of the mutagens such as solubility, alkylating group, and half-life; concentration of the mutagen; duration of the mutagen treatment; temperature of the treatment solution and organism; several catalytic agents; hydrogen ion concentration of the treatment solution; and treatment at specific stages in chromosome cycle and genotype. Many of the experiments with these factors have been previously described and summarized

(23, 27, 38, 39, 52). Thus results with only two such factors will be described, namely, pH, which has produced some striking increases in effectiveness and efficiency, and stage of cell cycle, which appears to provide one of the most promising avenues for controlling and directing the induced mutation process in plant cells.

My colleagues and I have increased the effectiveness of the potent mutagen ethyleneimine and of a new mutagen, sodium azide, and the efficiency of methyl nitrosourea by adjusting the pH of the treatment solution when applied to barley seeds.

At pH 7, EI is approximately 89% ethyleneimmonium cation and 11% imine form. The latter, however, can penetrate cell membranes with less difficulty than the immonium cation. We (77) were able to show that very slight increases above pH 7 increased considerably the concentration of the imine form and subsequent EI in the cell, which in turn increased both mutations and chromosome aberrations (Table II).

Sodium azide, the well-known respiratory inhibitor, now appears to be a potent mutagen in barley and possibly bacteria (39, 57, 60). However, when azide was first determined to be mutagenic several years ago its full potential was not realized, because all treatment solutions were at pH 7. This was first recognized in experiments by Dr. E. G. Sideris in which azide solutions at different pHs were used. In Table III, it can be seen that azide produces the highest frequency of mutations at pH 3. These mutations were not accompanied by appreciable frequencies of chromosome aberrations. Viable morphological mutations were also detected in high frequencies among M_2 plants. This demonstrated to us that azide was indeed inducing gene changes and that at least most of the observed chlorophyll-deficient mutations were not caused by plastid changes induced by azide. This was of interest because we knew nothing about the mutagenicity or action of azide at the outset of our experiments.

Table II. Comparison of pH, Imine Form Concentration, and Biological Changes Induced in Barley by Treatment with EI[a]

pH	Concentration of imine form EI (mM)	Seedling injury (%)	Number of fragments/cell	M_2 seedling mutation (%)
6.84	0.85	0.6	0.07	1.09
7.20	1.61	8.4	0.32	1.89
7.60	3.08	24.9	0.82	3.25
7.96	4.67	54.6	1.05	3.30

After Wagner *et al.* (77).

[a] Barley was treated with EI for 4 hr at 20°C.

Table III. Frequencies of Chlorophyll-Deficient
Seedling Mutations Obtained in M_2 Seedlings[a]

	Without azide		With azide	
pH	M_1 spikes tested	Mutation frequency	M_1 spikes tested	Mutation frequency
3	934	0.6	799	17.3
7	904	0.6	971	6.9
11	857	1.1	1014	1.4

After Nilan *et al.* (60).

[a] Mutation frequencies are per 100 M_1 spikes. Barley seeds were treated for 3 hr with 10^{-3} M NaN$_3$ solutions buffered at pH 3, 7, and 11 with 0.1 M phosphate buffer. Data are a summary of two replications.

An understanding of the effect of pH on azide-treated seeds is based on the fact that the pK of sodium azide is at pH 4.8; thus at pH 3 the dominant species is hydrogen azide. We have not yet determined if the greater effectiveness at pH 3 is due to the better permeability of the cell membrane to the neutral HN$_3$ molecule or if HN$_3$ is the mutagenic form. Dr. A. Kleinhofs, using mutagen tester strains of *Salmonella,* has determined that azide induces only base substitutions.

Further increases in mutation yield with azide were obtained by treatments at different stages of the cell cycle, as will be described below.

De Kock (18) and Konzak *et al.* (39) have demonstrated that MNH solutions between pH 6 and 6.7 are the most effective and efficient for mutation induction in barley.

A significant opportunity for increasing efficiency and effectiveness and even specificity of chemical mutagen treatments is afforded by seeds, in which it is possible to control more precisely than in roots or other tissues the stage of interphase in the mitotic cell at which the mutagen treatment is given. Early experiments in which seeds were "presoaked" prior to chemical mutagen treatment gave indications of increased effectiveness and even efficiency. The realization that such results may be due to the fact that treatments were being applied before, during, or after DNA synthesis (S) led to slightly more sophisticated experiments in which the time of treatment in relation to S stage was controlled. There are many problems in delivering the mutagenic form or species of a chemical mutagen precisely at G1 or G2, or S, and these as well as some solutions to the problems are well described in the proceedings of a recent conference (22).

In some recent studies, the time of DNA synthesis under rather specific temperature and seed-soaking conditions was determined. Here, it is important to realize that usually the time of DNA synthesis is determined in untreated soaked seeds. This determination does not take into account the effect of the mutagen on the cell cycle, which may result in delayed DNA synthesis. Thus, times of DNA synthesis established in untreated seeds can lead to somewhat unsuitable treatment times and ultimately to reservations about the relation of a particular stage to induced genetic effects.

There is evidence, chiefly from barley seeds, that maximum rates of mutation frequency with least lethal or physiological effects occur when treatments are presumably applied at the onset of DNA synthesis. This is true for treatments with dES, EMS, and MNU (13, 29, 49, 50, 53, 65, 73). Chromosome aberration frequencies, however, were lowest at the S stage of the cell cycle but were highest at early G1 (49).

It would appear from the above experiments and others that it may be possible to control frequencies of chromosome aberrations and mutations by chemical mutagen treatment at different stages. Indeed, it is becoming evident that maximum aberration frequencies are induced in early G1, while maximum chlorophyll-deficient mutations are induced at S. If this can be confirmed, then it is indicative of a different cause of chromosome aberration and mutation and that at least some mutations are not due to chromosome aberrations. Furthermore, future studies along this line could shed some light on chromosome structure.

Table IV. Frequencies of Chlorophyll-Deficient Mutations[a]

Presoak (hr)	M_1 spikes tested	Mutation frequency
Control	905	1.7
0	960	22.5
1	944	23.2
2	950	32.8
3	1008	35.0
4	706	46.3

After Nilan *et al.* (60).

[a] Mutation frequencies are per 100 M_1 spikes. Barley seeds were treated for 2 hr with 10^{-3} M NaN_3 solutions buffered at pH 3 with 0.1 M phosphate buffer. The seeds were soaked for the indicated time intervals in O_2-saturated water prior to the azide treatment. Data are a summary of two replications.

In our laboratory, Dr. C. Sander has shown that presoaking barley seeds from 1 to 4 hr greatly increases the effectiveness of sodium azide. The seeds were presoaked in oxygen-saturated water and then treated with a sodium azide solution of pH 3. Table IV presents data for the chlorophyll-deficient mutations, while Table V summarizes data for viable morphological mutations. These latter include dwarf, male sterile, curly, and *erectoides* plants.

Chromosome aberration frequencies (bridges and fragments in first mitotic division after germination) measured for the same treatments were only slightly above background levels. Thus azide is an efficient mutagen.

The cause of this increase in mutation frequencies with presoaking is not known. Current experiments show that DNA synthesis in azide-treated seeds does not occur until well after 4 hr.

Ionizing Radiations

Among the radiations, γ-rays, X-rays, and fast neutrons are the most widely used for inducing mutations in plants. Compared to the sparsely ionizing X-rays and γ-rays, the densely ionizing fast neutrons are much more effective for inducing several biological effects. In one recent study, Conger (15) reported that unmoderated fission neutrons were 75 times more effective than γ-rays in inducing chlorophyll-deficient mutations in barley.

Numerous factors that alter the sensitivity of cells to the sparsely ionizing radiations X- and γ-rays have been utilized in experiments aimed at understanding how these mutagens induce genetic changes and increasing effectiveness and efficiency of mutation induction. These factors include nuclear volume; tissue structure; genotype; oxygen, temperature, pH, and water content of the cells;

Table V. Frequencies of Viable Morphological Mutations Obtained in the M_2 Generation[a]

Presoak (hr)	Number of M_1 spikes	Mutations	
		Number	Frequency
0	579	132	22.8
1	439	176	40.1
2	357	138	38.7
3	260	132	50.8
3½	159	93	58.5

[a] Mutation frequencies are per 100 M_1 spikes. Barley seeds were treated as described in Table IV. Data are a summary of two replications.

and stage of the cell cycle. Results of experiments with these factors have been frequently summarized (14, 55, 58).

The effectiveness of X- and γ-rays has been altered by 15 times or more by the manipulation of oxygen, water, and temperature in treated barley seeds (14, 15, 17, 37, 58, 70). The marked increase in efficiency as found with chemicals is yet to be demonstrated for physical mutagens. There have been indications that heat shock, pH, and certain sulfur-containing compounds may alter the ratio of mutations to chromosome aberrations, but these results have not been definitive enough for practical application.

Until recently, it was considered that the biological action of neutrons was little influenced by these factors (28). However, in highly controlled experiments (16) it was shown that the effectiveness of neutrons can be increased by oxygen in very dry barley seeds. These and other recent developments of the modification of neutron effects in plants by environmental factors have been reviewed by Smith (70).

Opportunities exist for irradiating cells at G1, S, and G2 during mitosis in seeds, but relatively little detailed work has been conducted. One experiment (49) suggested that the peak of chromosome fragment production in γ-irradiated barley seeds occurred at G2. It should be recalled that in a similar experiment the peak of fragments in EMS-treated barley seeds occurred at G1. Numerous investigations dealing with radiation effects and the cell cycle are described in Ebert and Howard (22).

EFFICACY

Of practical importance is the problem of increasing the effectiveness and efficiency of useful or beneficial mutations in crop plants. Most of the experimental results discussed in this chapter involve M_2 chlorophyll-deficient seedling mutations, which are relatively easy and inexpensive to grow and score. Determining frequencies of beneficial mutations, which are usually scored on a mature plant basis, is more difficult and expensive. Gaul *et al.* (26) have used the term "efficacy" to indicate the ability of a mutagen to produce beneficial mutations. Certainly any estimate of the efficacy of a mutagen is related not only to the mutagenic treatment but also to the selection technique applied.

A recent experiment has demonstrated the superior efficacy of EMS over X-rays for inducing disease-resistant mutants in barley (26). Mildew-resistant mutants were scored in M_2 after treatment of seeds of eight spring barley varieties with X-rays or EMS. From a total of about 1,300,000 treated plants, 91 mildew-resistant barleys were selected. Of these, the number of partially and completely mildew-resistant plants per 100,000 plants was 12.39 for EMS and 5.70 for X-rays, indicating that EMS produced 2.2 times as many resistant plants as X-rays. This can be compared to induction of chlorophyll-deficient mutations in the same experiment, where the EMS produced 4.2 times as many as X-rays.

MUTAGENIC SPECIFICITY

A long desired goal of plant mutagenesis has been to induce mutations at specific loci and alter the mutation spectrum. For mutation breeding, this goal is more restrictive because the desire here is to produce at will mutations that have beneficial value for crop improvement. Most investigations to this end have involved the search for mutagens that react selectively with certain genes. However, the search for locus-specific mutagens is not realistic because of the nature of the DNA, which is a series of triplet sequences comprising combinations of only four nucleotides and thus provides no apparent differential sites for mutagen specificity.

There are a number of experimental results with flowering plants, however, which suggest that following mutagen treatments mutations of a given phenotype may occur preferentially (4, 56, 57, 68, 70). This type of mutagen specificity appears not to be due to direct interactions between specific genes and specific mutagens. Rather, it may be due to the action of a series of "selection sieves," as proposed by Auerbach (2, 3). She maintains that numbers and types of mutations may be controlled by several secondary steps which determine whether a change in DNA will take place and whether once it has taken place it will give rise to an observable mutation. It is at the level of these steps or "sieves" that specificities may be expected.

Sieves preceding the reaction between mutagen and DNA are concerned with chemical changes that a mutagen may undergo before reaching the gene and the accessibility of the gene to the mutagen. They are influenced by genotype, cell type, and metabolic state and probably depend on the degree of coiling of chomosomes and chromosome regions and on the amount and type of chromosomal components other than DNA. The sieves, following the reaction between mutagen and DNA, determine which of the changes in DNA will eventually appear as an observable mutation. They include processes such as repair, transcription, translation, and competitive cell growth. All of these sieves or secondary steps occur in flowering plants, and it is probably here where explanations of already published examples of mutagen specificity reside and where new approaches to control of the induced mutation process appear most fruitful.

Auerbach (2) and Auerbach and Kilbey (4) have presented examples for several eukaryotic organisms of preferential occurrence of mutation brought about by intervention of secondary steps in the mutation process through selection of biological, physiological (such as nutrition), and environmental conditions, selection of a suitable genetic background, variation of the dose of a mutagen, or a combination of the effects of several mutagens. One of the best examples has come from studies with the double auxotroph *ad-inos* strain of *Neurospora crassa* (5–7). X-rays, diepoxybutane (DEB), and two other chemicals induce more adenine than inositol reversions and hence are adenine specific, while ultraviolet light (UV) and two other chemicals are inositol specific.

Furthermore, specificity changed with dose, and this was particularly striking for DEB. In addition, pre- or post-treatment of UV-treated conidia with weak doses of DEB increased the frequency of UV-induced adenine reversions and decreased that of UV-induced inositol reversions. Moreover, using fractionated doses of DEB it was shown that weak doses given before or after a moderately high dose of DEB act as a booster for the production of adenine reversion.

Intralocus specificity among flowering plants has not been reported even for the well-studied "waxy" gene of maize. In *Neurospora,* de Serres *et al.* (20) have recently reported an apparent case of intragenic specificity at the *ad-3B* locus.

Examples of interlocus specificity or preferential production of mutations in flowering plants are increasing. With increasing data, it becomes increasingly evident that some type of interlocus specificity occurs among some of the 26 known *erectoides* (*ert*) loci (62) and of the 44 known *eceriferum* (*cer*) loci (42, 43) of barley. At certain loci, the number of mutants is now large enough for an analysis of interlocus specificity. As seen in Table VI, there are considerable differences among locus *ert a* (32 mutants), locus *ert c* (34 mutants), and locus *ert d* (26 mutants) in responses to physical and chemical mutagens; *ert a* mutates more frequently after treatment with sparsely ionizing radiation (X- and γ-rays) than after densely ionizing radiation treatments (neutrons). On the other hand, locus *ert c* responds more frequently to neutrons. A differential response of these loci to certain chemical mutagens is also becoming evident. In addition, chromosome breaks occur relatively frequently at or near locus *ert c* but not at locus *ert a*. Tests of heterogeneity indicate the differences in mutagen response of the different loci to be significant.

Certain loci of the *eceriferum* group also show differential responses to the chemical and physical mutagens. The alkylating chemical mutagens mutate preferentially at loci *c, q,* and *u* but produce no mutations at locus *i*. Neutrons, on the other hand, act preferentially on locus *i*.

Table VI. Induction of *erectoides* (*ert*)
Mutations by Different Mutagens in
Barley

Mutagen	ert loci		
	ert a	ert c	ert d
X- and γ-rays	14	11	9
Neutrons, protons	1	16	6
Chemicals	17	7	11
	32	34	26

After Persson and Hagberg (62).

In tomato, Jain *et al.* (34) reported several genes to be highly sensitive to hydrazine. These genes, however, were little affected by other chemical mutagens, such as EMS, which were able to induce mutations at other loci.

The genetic basis for this type of mutagen specificity is not known. It may relate to mutagen-specific chromosome breaking properties at or near the loci in question or may be caused by differential lethal effects (sometimes called "diplontic selection") with the different mutagens. Smith (70, 71) has summarized results of several experiments which demonstrate that products of irradiation can be preferentially recovered depending on environmental conditions during growth of irradiated tissue, e.g., seeds.

A striking case of apparent interlocus specificity has been reported in *Aspergillus nidulans* (1). A differential response of gene loci to forward mutation induced by γ-irradiation was determined by the presence of oxygen or nitrogen at the time of irradiation. Differences in the initial lesions and in repair mechanisms in irradiated conidia under the influence of the two gases are offered as explanations.

Another type of preferential occurrence of mutation has been the alteration of the relative proportion of chlorophyll-deficient mutations. Many experiments, using several plant species, have claimed changes in the proportion of different classes of chlorophyll phenotypes, e.g., *albina, xantha,* or *viridis,* or in the ratios of viable to lethal types produced by different mutagens or treatment conditions. The problems and pitfalls of experimenting with these types of mutations and the reservations about the validity of many reports of alteration of mutation spectrum have been described previously (55, 56).

Nevertheless, substantial data on induced chlorophyll-deficient mutations in barley have now demonstrated a significant difference between the spectra induced by some alkylating chemicals and by sparsely ionizing radiation. Alkylating agents such as diethyl sulfate, ethyl methanesulfonate, and ethyleneimine compared to X-rays or γ-rays induce lower proportions of *albina* and higher proportions of *viridis* and *xantha* mutations (57). For example, results from several large experiments with barley in our laboratory have demonstrated that γ-rays and diethyl sulfate induced 48.6 and 30.3% *albina,* 37.7 and 44.8% *viridis,* and 4.5 and 10.2% *xantha* mutations, respectively. These figures are based on large numbers of mutations and are significant at the 99% confidence interval. Similar data for other alkylating compounds have been reported in barley (24, 30, 57) as well as in rice (64).

Whether this type of group mutability can be attributed to different relative frequencies of induced chromosome aberrations and/or sterility induced by the chemical mutagen compared to X-rays is not known. Alkylating agents induce few chromosome aberrations but do induce appreciable amounts of sterility. From a very careful analysis of the relation of sterility to mutation spectrum, Gustafsson (30) reported that the differences in mutation spectra between the chemical mutagens and radiation in barley occurred at several levels of fertility. Westergaard (78) suggested that the alkylating chemicals, because of their apparent slight effect on chromosomes, may induce a higher proportion of less drastic mutations, such as *viridis,* to extreme mutations, such as *albina,* than produced by radiation.

Mutagen treatments at different stages of the cell cycle not only can alter the frequencies of mutations as described earlier in this chapter but also appear to alter the proportion of mutations. Swaminathan and Sarma (75) and Swaminathan (73) found that using pulse treatments of EMS and NMU during different stages of the S phase in barley seeds resulted in differential induction of chlorophyll-deficient characters, especially those induced by single genes. Explanations for these results may be found in the differential effect of certain mutagens on active *vs.* nonactive genes, in that DNA replication along the chromosome is asynchronous and in that maximum mutation frequencies of some genes occur at the time of their replication (9, 10).

With increased understanding of the genetic control that occurs in plants through cytoplasmic DNA residing in the mitochondria and the chloroplasts, the possibility of differential induction of mutations in the cytoplasm *vs.* the nucleus becomes intriguing and important. In a pilot experiment, Schwaier *et al.* (66) examined the effect of mutagens on genes affecting respiration in the mitochondria and in the nucleus of yeast. In this system, respiratory-deficient mutants are caused by damage in the nuclear DNA or in the mitochondrial DNA. A distinct difference in cytoplasmic *vs.* nuclear mutagen specificity was observed between nitrous acid (NA) and *N*-nitroso-*N*-methylurethane (NMU). Nitrous acid was unable to induce cytoplasmic respiratory-deficient mutants but proved to be highly efficient in the induction of nuclear mutants.

A high degree of specificity or direction of mutation exists with the so-called controlling elements and mutable loci (44, 63) and with the paramutation phenomenon (8) in maize and other species. Furthermore, there is now some indication that these controlling elements may be altered by mutagens (54), and in this way phenotypes of specific structural genes would be altered. As indicated by McClintock and others, it is possible by removing the controlling element to stabilize the changed action of the structural gene to any desired state or level.

Producing desired genetic changes in flowering plants now appears to be a possibility through transformation. The most elegant and detailed work on this problem has been that of Ledoux and his colleagues in Belgium (41). They have conclusively demonstrated the uptake and incorporation of bacterial DNA into cells of barley and *Arabidopsis.* Furthermore, it appears that such exogenous bacterial DNA can "cure" genetic defects in *Arabidopsis* at specific loci. Equally remarkable results have been obtained with flower color genes in *Petunia* by Hess (32). Here, apparent transformation of anthocyaninless alleles to anthocyanin-producing alleles was induced by treatment with DNA from an anthocyanin-producing line.

Before concluding, an important aspect of mutagen specificity should be mentioned. Plant geneticists must recognize that increasing the efficiency and specificity of mutagens for inducing mutations is not the only important goal for plant mutagenesis and mutation breeding. There must also be concern for increasing the efficiency and specificity of the mutagens for inducing chromosomal breaks and aberrations. This is because new karyotypes and hence phenotypes, some of which may not be obtainable through induced mutation and plant hybridization techniques, may be produced through various kinds of gross chromosome aberrations. Ways in which these different chromosome aberrations can contribute to "chromosome engineering" and be utilized, and possibilities for increasing efficiency and specificity of induced chromosome breaks, have been reviewed (25, 36).

ACKNOWLEDGMENT

Scientific Paper No. 4031. College of Agriculture Research Center, Washington State University, Pullman, Project 1068. Some of the results obtained on a grant from the U.S. Atomic Energy Commission Contract AT(45-1)-2221. AEC Paper RLO-2221-T2-16.

REFERENCES

1. Alderson, T., and Scott, B. R. (1971). Induction of mutation by γ-irradiation in the presence of oxygen or nitrogen. *Nature New Biol.* **230**:45-48.
2. Auerbach, C. (1966). The role of mutagen specificity in mutation breeding. *Genetika* **1**:3-11.
3. Auerbach, C. (1967). The chemical production of mutations. *Science* **158**:1141-1147.
4. Auerbach, C., and Kilbey, B. J. (1971). Mutation in eucaryotes. *Ann. Rev. Genet.* **5**:163-218.
5. Auerbach, C., and Ramsay, D. (1968). The influence of treatment conditions on the selective mutagenic action of diepoxybutane in *Neurospora. Japan. J. Genet.* **43**:1-8.
6. Auerbach, C., and Ramsay, D. (1970). Analysis of a case of mutagen specificity in *Neurospora crassa.* II. Interaction between treatments with diepoxybutane (DEB) and ultraviolet light. *Mol. Gen. Genet.* **109**:1-17.
7. Auerbach, C., and Ramsay, D. (1970). Analysis of a case of mutagen specificity in *Neurospora crassa.* III. Fractionated treatment with diepoxybutane (DEB). *Mol. Gen. Genet.* **109**:285-291.
8. Brink, R. A., Styles, E. D., and Axtell, J. D. (1968). Paramutation: Directed genetic change. *Science* **159**:161-170.
9. Brock, R. D. (1969). Increasing the specificity of mutation. In *Induced Mutations in Plants,* STI/PUB/231, International Atomic Energy Agency, Vienna, pp. 93-100.
10. Brock, R. D. (1971). Differential mutation of the β-galactosidase gene of *Escherichia coli. Mutation Res.* **11**:181-186.

11. Brock, R. D. (1972). The role of induced mutations in plant improvement. In *Induced Mutations and Plant Improvement,* STI/PUB/297, International Atomic Energy Agency, Vienna, pp. 513-521.

12. Brockman, H. E., de Serres, F. J., and Barnett, W. E. (1969). Analysis of *ad-3* mutants induced by nitrous acid in a heterokaryon of *Neurospora crassa. Mutation Res.* 7:307-314.

13. Brunner, H., and Mikaelsen, K. (1971). Beeinflussende Faktoren in der mutagenen Wirkung von Äthylmethansulfonat auf Gerste. *Z. Pflanzenzüchtg.* 66:9-36.

14. Conger, B. V. (1972). Contributions of seed meristems to radiobiology. In Miller, M. W., and Kuehnert, C. (eds.), *The Dynamics of Meristem Cell Populations,* Plenum Press, New York.

15. Conger, B. V. (1972). Control and modification of seed radiosensitivity. *Trans. ASAE* 15:780-784.

16. Conger, B. V., and Constantin, M. J. (1970). Oxygen effect following neutron irradiation of dry barley seeds. *Radiat. Bot.* 10:95-97.

17. Conger, B. V., Constantin, M. J., and Carabia, J. V. (1972). Seed radiosensitivity: Wide range in oxygen-enhancement ratio after gamma-irradiation of eight species. *Internat. J. Radiat. Biol.* 22:225-235.

18. de Kock, M. J. (1972). The actions of gamma irradiation and *N*-methyl-*N*-nitrosourea in plants. Ph.D. dissertation, Washington State University, Pullman.

19. de Serres, F. J., Brockman, H. E., Barnett, W. E., and Kölmark, H. G. (1967). Allelic complementation among nitrous acid-induced *ad-3B* mutants of *Neurospora crassa. Mutation Res.* 4:415-424.

20. de Serres, F. J., Brockman, H. E., Barnett, W. E., and Kölmark, H. G. (1971). Mutagen specificity in *Neurospora crassa. Mutation Res.* 12:129-142.

21. Doll, H. (1972). Variation in protein quantity and quality induced in barley by EMS treatment. In *Induced Mutations and Plant Improvement,* STI/PUB/297, International Atomic Energy Agency, Vienna, pp. 331-342.

22. Ebert, M., and Howard, A. (eds.) (1972). Radiation effects and the mitotic cycle. In *Current Topics in Radiation Research Quarterly,* North-Holland, Amsterdam, pp. 244-391.

23. Ehrenberg, L. (1971). Higher plants. In Hollaender, A. (ed.), *Chemical Mutagens: Principles and Methods for Their Detection,* Plenum Press, New York, pp. 365-386.

24. Ehrenberg, L., Gustafsson, Å., and Lundqvist, U. (1961). Viable mutants induced in barley by ionizing radiations and chemical mutagens. *Hereditas* 47:243-282.

25. Gaul, H. (1965). Induced mutations in plant breeding. In Geerts, S. J. (ed.), *Genetics Today,* Vol. 3, Pergamon Press, New York, pp. 689-709.

26. Gaul, H., Frimmel, G., Gichner, T., and Ulonska, E. (1972). Efficiency of mutagenesis. In *Induced Mutations and Plant Improvement,* STI/PUB/297, International Atomic Energy Agency, Vienna, pp. 121-139.

27. Gichner, T., Velemínský, J., Pokorný, V., and Svachulová, J. (1972). Influence of post-treatment washing on the mutagenic effects in propyl methanesulfonate- and isopropyl methanesulfonate-treated barley seeds. *Radiat. Bot.* 12:221-227.

28. Gopal-Ayengar, A. R., and Swaminathan, M. S. (1964). Use of neutron irradiation in agriculture and applied genetics. In *Biological Effects of Neutron and Proton Irradiations,* Vol. 1, STI/PUB/80, International Atomic Energy Agency, Vienna, pp. 409-432.

29. Grant, C. J., Heslot, H., and Ferrary, R. (1969). The effects of chemical mutagens in relation to the chromosome cycle. In Darlington, C. D., and Lewis, K. R. (eds.), *Chromosomes Today,* Vol. 2, Plenum Press, New York, pp. 75-78.

30. Gustafsson, Å. (1963). Productive mutations induced in barley by ionizing radiations and chemical mutagens. *Hereditas* **50:**211-263.
31. Gustafsson, Å., Hagberg, A., Persson, G., and Wiklund, K. (1971). Induced mutations and barley improvement. *Theoret. Appl. Genet.* **41:**239-248.
32. Hess, D. (1970). Versuche zur Transformation an höheren Pflanzen: Genetische Charakterisierung einiger mutmablich transformierter Pflanzen. *Z. Pflanzenphysiol.* **63:**31-43.
33. Ingversen, J., Andersen, A. J., Doll, H., and Köie, B. (1973). Selection and properties of high lysine barley. In *Nuclear Techniques for Seed Protein Improvement.* STI/PUB/320 International Atomic Energy Agency, Vienna, pp. 193-198.
34. Jain, H. K., Raut, R. N., and Khamankar, Y. G. (1968). Base specific chemicals and mutation analysis in *Lycopersicon. Heredity* **23:**247-256.
35. Kasha, K. J., and Kao, K. N. (1970). High frequency haploid production in barley. *Nature* **225:**874-876.
36. Kihlman, B. A. (1966). *Actions of Chemicals on Dividing Cells,* Prentice-Hall, Englewood Cliffs, N.J.
37. Klein, R. M., and Klein, D. T. (1971). Post-irradiation modulation of ionizing radiation damage to plants. *Bot. Rev.* **37:**397-436.
38. Konzak, C. F., Nilan, R. A., Wagner, J., and Foster, R. J. (1965). Efficient chemical mutagenesis. In The Use of Induced Mutations in Plant Breeding. *Radiat. Bot. (Suppl.)* **5:**49-70.
39. Konzak, C. F., Wickham, I. M., and de Kock, M. J. (1972). Advances in methods of mutagen treatment. In *Induced Mutations and Plant Improvement,* STI/PUB/297, International Atomic Energy Agency, Vienna, pp. 95-119.
40. Lange, W. (1971). Crosses between *Hordeum vulgare* L. and *H. bulbosum* L. I. Production, morphology and meiosis of hybrids, haploids and dihaploids. *Euphytica* **20:**14-29.
41. Ledoux, L., Huart, R., and Jacobs, M. (1972). Fate and biological effects of exogenous DNA in *Arabidopsis thaliana.* In Lupton, F. G. H., Jenkins, G., and Johnson, R. (eds.), *The Way Ahead in Plant Breeding,* Cambridge University Press, New York, pp. 165-184.
42. Lundqvist, U., and von Wettstein, D. (1962). Induction of *eceriferum* mutants in barley by ionizing radiations and chemical mutagens. *Hereditas* **48:**342-362.
43. Lundqvist, U., von Wettstein-Knowles, P., and von Wettstein, D. (1968). Induction of *eceriferum* mutants in barley by ionizing radiations and chemical mutagens. II. *Hereditas* **59:**473-504.
44. McClintock, B. (1967). II. The role of the nucleus. Genetic systems regulating gene expression during development. *Develop. Biol. (Suppl.)* **1:**84-112.
45. Malling, H. V. (1971). Hydroxylamine-induced purple mutants (*ad-3*) in *Neurospora crassa. Hereditas* **68:**219-234.
46. Malling, H. V., and de Serres, F. J. (1967). Relation between complementation patterns and genetic alterations in nitrous acid-induced *ad-3B* mutants of *Neurospora crassa. Mutation Res.* **4:**425-440.
47. Malling, H. V., and de Serres, F. J. (1968). Identification of genetic alterations induced by ethyl methanesulfonate in *Neurospora crassa. Mutation Res.* **6:**181-193.
48. Melchers, G. (1972). Haploid higher plants for plant breeding. *Z. Pflanzenzüchtg.* **67:**19-32.
49. Mikaelsen, K. (1968). Comparisons between chromosome aberrations induced by ionizing radiations and alkylating agents at different stages of mitotis in barley seeds. In *Mutations in Plant Breeding II,* STI/PUB/182, International Atomic Energy Agency, Vienna, pp. 287-290.

50. Mikaelsen, K., Brunner, H., and Li, W. C. (1971). Influence of postwash time on the mutagenic effects of ethylmethanesulphonate (EMS) in barley seeds. *Hereditas* **69**:15-18.
51. Mottinger, J. P. (1970). The effects of X-rays on the bronze and shrunken loci in maize. *Genetics* **64**:259-271.
52. Narayanan, K. R., and Konzak, C. F. (1969). Influence of chemical post-treatments on the mutagenic efficiency of alkylating agents. In *Induced Mutations in Plants*, STI/PUB/231, International Atomic Energy Agency, Vienna, pp. 281-304.
53. Natarajan, A. T., and Shivasankar, G. (1965). Studies on modification of mutation response of barley seeds to ethyl methanesulfonate. *Z. Verebungsl.* **96**:13-21.
54. Neuffer, M. G. (1966). Stability of the suppressor element in two mutator systems at the A_1 locus in maize. *Genetics* **53**:541-549.
55. Nilan, R. A. (1964). *The Cytology and Genetics of Barley, 1951-1962*, Washington State University Press, Pullman.
56. Nilan, R. A. (1967). Nature of induced mutations in higher plants. In *Induced Mutations and Their Utilization (Erwin-Bauer Memorial Lectures IV)*, Akademie-Verlag, Berlin, pp. 5-20.
57. Nilan, R. A. (1972). Mutagenic specificity in flowering plants: Facts and prospects. In *Induced Mutations and Plant Improvement*, STI/PUB/297, International Atomic Energy Agency, Vienna, pp. 141-151.
58. Nilan, R. A., Konzak, C. F., Wagner, J., and Legault, R. R. (1965). Effectiveness and efficiency of radiations for inducing genetic and cytogenetic changes. In The Use of Induced Mutations in Plant Breeding. *Radiat. Bot. (Suppl.)* **5**:71-89.
59. Nilan, R. A., Kleinhofs, A., and Sideris, E. G. (1969). Structural and biochemical concepts of mutations in flowering plants. In *Induced Mutations in Plants*, STI/PUB/231, International Atomic Energy Agency, Vienna, pp. 35-49.
60. Nilan, R. A., Sideris, E. G., Kleinhofs, A., Sander, C., and Konzak, C. F. (1973). Azide—A potent mutagen. *Mutation Res.* **17**:142-144.
61. Nitsch, J. P. (1972). Haploid plants from pollen. *Z. Pflanzenzüchtg.* **67**:3-18.
62. Persson, G., and Hagberg, A. (1969). Induced variation in a quantitative character in barley. Morphology and cytogenetics of *erectoides* mutants. *Hereditas* **61**:115-178.
63. Peterson, P. A. (1970). Controlling elements and mutable loci in maize: Their relationship to bacterial episomes. *Genetica* **41**:33-56.
64. Rao, N. S., and Gopal-Ayengar, A. R. (1964). Combined effects of thermal neutrons and diethyl sulphate on mutation frequency and spectrum in rice. In *Biological Effects of Neutron and Proton Irradiations*, Vol. 1, STI/PUB/80, International Atomic Energy Agency, Vienna, pp. 383-391.
65. Savin, V. N., Swaminathan, M. S., and Sharma, B. (1968). Enhancement of chemically-induced mutation frequency in barley through alteration in the duration of pre-soaking of seeds. *Mutation Res.* **6**:101-107.
66. Schwaier, R., Nashed, N., and Zimmermann, F. K. (1968). Mutagen specificity in the induction of karyotic versus cytoplasmic respiratory deficient mutants in yeast by nitrous acid and alkylating nitrosamides. *Mol. Gen. Genet.* **102**:290-300.
67. Sigurbjörnsson, B. (1971). Induced mutations in plants. *Sci. Am.* **224**:86-95.
68. Smith, H. H. (1961). Mutagenic specificity and directed mutation. In *Mutation and Plant Breeding*, Publ. No. 891, NAS-NRC, Washington, D.C., pp. 413-436.
69. Smith, H. H. (1971). Broadening the base of genetic variability in plants. *J. Hered.* **62**:265-276.
70. Smith, H. H. (1972). Environmental modulation of plant response to neutron irradiation. *Radiat. Bot.* **12**:229-237.
71. Smith, H. H. (1972). Comparative genetic effects of different physical mutagens in

higher plants. In *Induced Mutations and Plant Improvement,* STI/PUB/297, International Atomic Energy Agency, Vienna, pp. 75-93.

72. Smith, H. H. (1973). Model genetic systems for studying mutation, differentiation, and somatic cell hybridization in plants. Presented at FAO/IAEA/EUCARPIA Conference on Mutation and Polyploidy, Oct. 2-8, 1972, Bari, Italy (in press).

73. Swaminathan, M. S. (1969). Mutation breeding. In Oshima, C. (ed.), *Proceedings of the XIIth International Congress of Genetics,* Vol. 3, The Science Council of Japan, Tokyo, pp. 327-347.

74. Swaminathan, M. S. (1972). Mutational reconstruction of crop ideotypes. In *Induced Mutations and Plant Improvement,* STI/PUB/297, International Atomic Energy Agency, Vienna, pp. 155-171.

75. Swaminathan, M. S., and Sarma, N. P. (1968). Alteration of the mutation spectrum in barley through treatments at different periods in the S phase of DNA synthesis. *Current Sci.* 37:685-686.

76. Swaminathan, M. S., Austin, A., Kaul, A. K., and Naik, M. S. (1969). Genetic and agronomic enrichment of the quantity and quality of proteins in cereals and pulses. In *New Approaches to Breeding for Improved Plant Protein,* STI/PUB/80, International Atomic Energy Agency, Vienna, pp. 71-86.

77. Wagner, J. H., Nawar, M. M., Konzak, C. F., and Nilan, R. A. (1968). The influence of pH on the biological changes induced by ethyleneimine in barley. *Mutation Res.* 5:57-64.

78. Westergaard, M. (1960). A discussion of mutagenic specificity. 1. Specificity on the "geographical" level. In *Chemische Mutagenese (Erwin-Baur-Gedächtnisvorlesungen I),* Akademie-Verlag, Berlin, pp. 116-121.

15

Repair of Radiation and Chemical Damage to DNA in Human Cells

Steven N. Buhl

*The University of Tennessee - Oak Ridge Graduate School of Biomedical Sciences
and
Biology Division, Oak Ridge National Laboratory
Oak Ridge, Tennessee, U.S.A.*

DNA is susceptible to damage from extracellular sources. Repair of damaged DNA can be divided into (a) prereplication repair, observed in DNA that is present when the insult is given, and (b) postreplication repair, observed in the daughter strands synthesized after the insult. Recovery and repair in human cells have been measured in a number of ways: (a) by a decrease in reproductive death with dose fractionation (1), (b) by unscheduled DNA synthesis (2), (c) by repair replication (3), (d) by sedimentation-velocity studies (4), (e) by a combination of repair replication and sedimentation-velocity studies with photolysis of BrdUrd-sensitized DNA (5), and (f) by excision of chemical products or photoproducts from DNA (6,7).

Recovery of human cells from radiation damage was first described by Lockart *et al.* (1), who noted that fractionated doses resulted in a lower level of reproductive death than did the same amounts of radiation given in single doses. Possible repair of radiation damage to DNA was first detected when unscheduled DNA synthesis was observed after ultraviolet (2) and ionizing (3) irradiation. The types of damage and modes of repair were soon examined and are described in the following paragraphs.

PREREPLICATION REPAIR

Repair of Damage from Ultraviolet Irradiation

Repair of ultraviolet (*UV*) damage involves four steps: (a) incision of the DNA near the dimer, (b) DNA degradation, (c) DNA synthesis (repair replication), and (d) joining of the newly synthesized DNA to the old strand (ligase action).

The presumed repair of DNA after UV irradiation of human cells was first detected by Rasmussen and Painter (2), using autoradiography to detect unscheduled (non-S-phase) DNA synthesis after irradiation. The same authors (3) confirmed their results by showing that after UV irradiation exogenous nucleotides are inserted into the parental DNA (repair replication). Regan *et al.* (7) demonstrated the presence of pyrmidine dimers in UV-irradiated human DNA and their subsequent removal during postirradiation incubation. Cleaver (8) found that in cells derived from individuals with xeroderma pigmentosum (XP) repair replication was reduced or absent. Such individuals are sensitive to sunlight, as indicated by the appearance of skin cancer at an early age. Studies on cells from these individuals were expanded by Setlow *et al.* (9), who showed that XP cells do not excise pyrimidine dimers and do not make the initial incision in the DNA containing the dimer.

The kinetics and mechanisms of repair were examined in more detail by Evans and Norman (10), who studied unscheduled DNA synthesis, and by Regan and Setlow (11), who studied the sedimentation velocities of photolyzed, BrdUrd-containing DNA from UV-irradiated human cells. After UV irradiation,

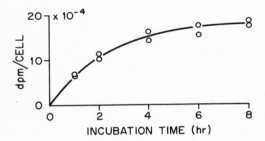

Fig. 1. Kinetics of ^3H-thymidine incorporation (unscheduled DNA synthesis) in human lymphocytes incubated at $37^\circ C$ after UV irradiation with 25 ergs/mm^2. The kinetics describe a single-component repair system that completes its repair within 3–4 hr after irradiation. Data obtained from Evans and Norman (10).

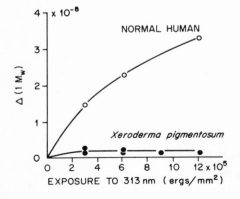

Fig. 2. Kinetics of photolysis, indicating repair of DNA in BrdUrd after 200 ergs/mm^2 of 254-nm radiation. $\Delta(1/M_W) = [(1/M_W)^{BrdUrd} - (1/M_W)^{dThd}]$ represents the presence of photosensitive BrdUrd-containing regions in DNA. Normal human cells repair extensively and contain many photosensitive regions, but XP cells repair minimally and contain few photosensitive regions. Data obtained from Regan and Setlow (11).

unscheduled DNA synthesis is essentially complete after 3–4 hr (Fig. 1). The size and number of repaired regions were investigated by Regan *et al.* (5), using the photolysis technique, by which the length and number of repaired regions can be determined. They found 0.33–0.50 repaired regions per pyrimidine dimer and approximately 100 replaced nucleotides per repaired region. The pattern of photolysis of repaired UV damage was curvilinear (Fig. 2), indicating that saturation had been achieved at higher doses of 313-nm radiation, as expected.

Repair of Damage from Ionizing Radiation

Possible repair of damage from ionizing radiation was first observed as unscheduled DNA synthesis by Rasmussen and Painter (3). The production of breaks in human DNA by ionizing radiation and their subsequent rejoining (repair) was first reported by Lohman (4), using sedimentation-velocity analysis of DNA from X-irradiated human cells. And recently Zhustyanikov *et al.* (12) described a human mutation that causes a lack of repair of damage from ionizing radiation. The kinetics of unscheduled DNA synthesis were studied in detail by Spiegler and Norman (13), who observed that this repair system could be divided into a rapid component, which operates within the first hour after irradiation, and a slower component, which continues through 22 hr (Fig. 3). Regan and Setlow (11), using the technique of photolysis after repair replication, studied the mechanics and kinetics of repair and photolysis of γ-irradiated human DNA and found that three or four nucleotides are replaced per repaired region. Figure

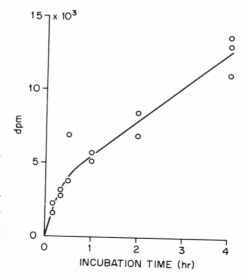

Fig. 3. Kinetics of ^{3}H-thymidine incorporation (unscheduled DNA synthesis) into γ-irradiated (5 krad) human lymphocytes. The data describe a two-component repair system—a rapid system, which is complete within the first hour, and a slow system, which continues through 22 hr. Data obtained from Clarkson and Evans (14).

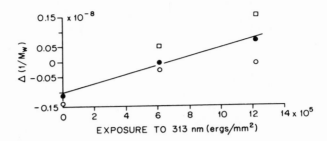

Fig. 4. *Kinetics of photolysis of γ-irradiated (10 krad) human DNA repaired in BrdUrd.* Increasing $\Delta(1/M_W)$ represents the presence of photosensitive BrdUrd-containing regions of DNA. The slowly rising linear line represents small substituted regions with three or four nucleotides per substituted (repaired) region. Data obtained from Regan and Setlow (11).

4 shows the kinetics of photolysis of the repair-replicated regions. The curve is a slowly rising linear line and can be contrasted with the curvilinear line obtained in studies of the repair of UV damage (Fig. 2). The data from studies of unscheduled synthesis after ionizing and UV irradiation (Figs. 1 and 3) should also be contrasted.

To summarize the above observations, there are at least two prereplication repair systems: one (UV-type repair) is examplified by the repair of damage from UV radiation, operates slowly (up to 4 hr), and replaces large amounts of DNA (approximately 100 nucleotides per repaired region); the other (ionizing-type repair) is exemplified by repair of damage from ionizing radiation and consists of two components—rapid repair, which is essentially complete in 1 hr, and a slower repair, which continues through 22 hr after irradiation—both of which replace three or four nucleotides per initial chain break.

Repair of Chemical Damage

The ability of human cells to recover from chemical damage was first described by Crathorn and Roberts (6), who showed chromatographically that HeLa cells excise the chemical products of ^{35}S-labeled mustard gas from DNA and have survival curves that indicate the presence of repair systems. Workers in the same laboratory (15,16) expanded on these results by demonstrating the presence of repair replication and the recovery of the ability to synthesize DNA at the normal rate after treatment with mustard gas.

Chemicals that damage DNA can be divided into three classes, based on the kinetics and mode of the repair system that acts on their damage. Table I is a compilation of chemicals that have been examined and the types of repair

Table I. Repair of Chemical Damage to DNA

Agent	Repair in xeroderma pigmentosum	Type of repair	Reference
N-Acetoxy-2-acetylaminofluorine	No	UV	Setlow and Regan (17)
4-Nitroquinoline oxide	Partial	UV and ionizing	Stich and San (18) Regan and Setlow (11)
Ethyl methanesulfonate	Not tested	Ionizing	Regan and Setlow (11)
Propane sultone	Not tested	Ionizing	Regan and Setlow (11)
Methyl methanesulfonate	Yes	Ionizing	Cleaver (19) Clarkson and Evans (14) Regan and Setlow (11)
Nitrogen mustard	Reduced	UV	Cleaver (19) Clarkson and Evans (14)
Mitomycin C	Not tested	Ionizing	Regan and Setlow (11)
ICR-170[a]	No	UV	Regan and Setlow (11)

[a] (2-Methoxy-6-chloro-9-[3-(ethyl-2-chloroethyl)-aminopropylaminoacridine dihydrochloride.

system they evoke. There are three types of compounds: those which evoke the rapid (ionizing-type) repair system, with the insertion of only a few nucleotides per repaired region; those which evoke the slower (UV-type) repair system, with the insertion of 80–100 nucleotides per repaired region; and those which evoke a combination of the two repair systems. From the data in Table I, it is apparent

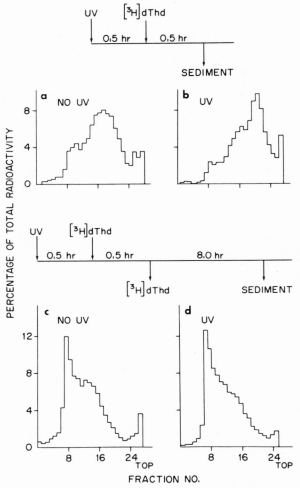

Fig. 5. Alkaline sucrose gradient sedimentation profiles of DNA from normal human fibroblasts (a) nonirradiated or (b) UV-irradiated with 75 ergs/mm², pulse-labeled with ³H-thymidine, and harvested immediately. (c,d) Profiles for (a) and (b), respectively, after incubation for 8 hr. Data obtained from Buhl et al. (20).

that the enzyme that is defective in XP is not specific for UV damage but must recognize damage from a broad spectrum of insults. The common parameter of all the agents not repaired by XP is that they produce only a few single-strand breaks but distort the DNA structure. One can hypothesize that the human mutant lacking repair of ionizing radiation damage (12) would also be deficient in repair of damage from compounds that evoke the ionizing-type repair system.

POSTREPLICATION REPAIR

Ultraviolet Radiation

DNA synthesized by human cells after UV irradiation is synthesized in smaller ($8–10 \times 10^6$ daltons) than normal segments (approximately 40×10^6 daltons), as assayed on alkaline sucrose gradients after pulse-labeling with ^{3}H-thymidine (Fig. 5a,b). When UV-irradiated, pulse-labeled cells are incubated, the short segments are elongated to form high molecular weight DNA (more than 10^8 daltons) (Fig. 5c,d). Table II shows that the size of the DNA segments synthesized after a given dose of UV radiation is comparable to the average distance between pyrmidine dimers produced at the same dose (20,21). As a further investigation of the effect of dimers on the production of short segments of DNA after UV irradiation, the following experiment was done. Normal (excision-plus) and XP (excision-minus) human cells were incubated in medium containing hydroxyurea for 2 hr to stop normal DNA synthesis, after which they were UV-irradiated and incubated in hydroxyurea for various times. The medi-

Table II. Measured Size of DNA and Distance Between Dimers[a]

Dose of UV radiation (ergs/mm²)	Measured dimers[b] (%)	Calculated distance between dimers[c] (10^6 daltons)	Measured size of DNA[d] (10^6 daltons)
200	0.08	2.1	2.1
100	0.04	4.2	3.6–4.5
75	0.03	6.0	4.6–5.2
50	0.02	8.4	6.6–10.3
25	0.01	16.8	15.4

[a] See refs. 20 and 21.

[b] Measurements provided by W. L. Carrier.

[c] From Setlow et al. (9).

[d] Number-average molecular weight of the peak, not corrected for the number-average molecular weight resulting from pulse-labeling of unirradiated cells.

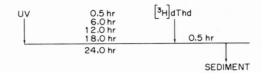

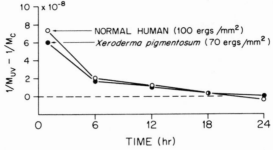

Fig. 6. *Differences in the reciprocals of M_W for nonirradiated and UV-irradiated human cells pulse-labeled for 30 min at various times after irradiation.* Decreasing $\Delta(1/M_W)$ represents recovery of ability to synthesize DNA in normal-size segments. Data obtained from Buhl *et al.* (21).

um was then changed before pulse-labeling and sedimentation. Figure 6 shows results from these experiments. It is apparent that human cells slowly recover the ability to synthesize DNA in segments of normal size and that the presence or absence of dimers does not affect the size of the DNA units synthesized long after irradiation.

We also examined the elongation and joining process that operates on the shorter DNA segments synthesized after UV irradiation and on the intermediate segments synthesized by untreated cells (22). Using the photolysis technique (Fig. 7), we showed that the intermediate segments synthesized by untreated cells are elongated by insertion of large amounts of exogenous nucleotides (normal semiconservative DNA replication) and that the shorter segments synthesized after UV irradiation are elongated and joined by insertion of small amounts (approximately 10^3 nucleotides, which are photolyzed at higher 313-nm doses) in addition to the large amounts of exogenous nucleotides (photolyzed at lower 313-nm doses) observed in the untreated cells. Figure 8 shows a model of DNA chain elongation and joining of the short segments synthesized in human cells shortly after UV irradiation.

Ionizing Radiation

Our results indicate that irradiation with 10 krad from a ^{60}Co source under oxic conditions does not reduce the size of the DNA segments synthesized by

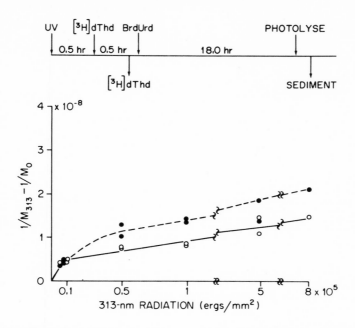

Fig. 7. The effect of various fluxes of 313-nm radiation on the DNA of nonirradiated and UV-irradiated normal human fibroblasts incubated for 8 hr in 0.1 mM BrdUrd. Cells were irradiated with 0 (○) or 100 (●) ergs/mm², pulse-labeled with ³H-thymidine, and incubated in BrdUrd. $1/M_{313}$, reciprocal of the weight-average molecular weight after photolysis with 313 nm and sedimentation; $1/M_0$, reciprocal of the weight-average molecular weight after sedimentation of DNA from cells incubated in BrdUrd. Increasing $\Delta(1/M_w)$ represents additional photosensitive BrdUrd-containing DNA. This additional sensitivity is observed at 0.5×10^5 ergs/mm² of 313-nm radiation, which is equivalent to approximately 10^3 nucleotides of fully substituted BrdUrd-containing DNA (17). Data obtained from Buhl *et al.* (22).

human cells during the first 4 hr after irradiation (S. N. Buhl and J. D. Regan, unpublished results).

N-Acetoxy-2-acetylaminofluorene

Treatment with either 70 or 7 μM *N*-acetoxy-2-acetylaminofluorene for 1 hr does not affect the size of the DNA segments synthesized in human cells during the first 6 hr after treatment, nor is the process of DNA chain elongation and joining severely affected (S.N. Buhl and J. D. Regan, unpublished results). The damage induced by this compound is repaired by UV-type prereplication repair (Table I).

a   UV IRRADIATED DNA

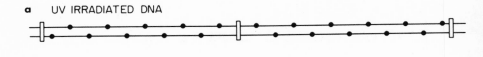

b   DNA OBSERVED AFTER PULSE-LABELED

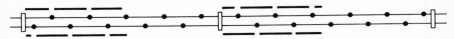

c   COMPLETED DNA SYNTHESIS

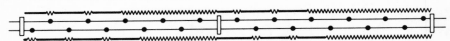

Fig. 8. Model describing elongation of DNA chains and joining of the short segments synthesized within the first hour after UV irradiation of human cells. ▯, beginning or end of replicating unit; •, pyrimidine dimer; ▬, short segment of DNA observed after pulse-labeling for 30 min; ∿, newly synthesized DNA, elongating and joining of the short segments. The size of the regions was determined by the photolysis technique (22).

Methyl Methanesulfonate

Treatment of human cells with methyl methanesulfonate (MMS) reduces the rate of DNA synthesis for several hours; however, the amount of DNA synthesis returns to normal within 4 hr after a 1-hr treatment (Fig. 9). [A similar observation was made in HeLa cells treated with mustard gas (16).] MMS also has a differential effect on the size of the DNA segments synthesized. Figure 10 shows the differences between the reciprocals of the weight-average molecular weights of DNA from untreated and treated cells pulse-labeled at various times after a 1-hr treatment with MMS. The important observation is the reduction in the size of the units synthesized 2.5 hr after treatment and the recovery of the ability to synthesize DNA in normal lengths within 4 hr after treatment (23). As a test of whether the cells could elongate and join the DNA after MMS treatment, they were incubated for 12 hr after pulse-labeling at various times after MMS treatment. Figure 11 shows that the shorter segments (approximately 20×10^6 daltons) synthesized at 2.5 hr are elongated and joined to form high molecular weight DNA (more than 10^8 daltons), as are the intermediate segments (more than $35-40 \times 10^6$ daltons) synthesized by nontreated cells and by treated cells pulse-labeled at 0.5 and 4.0 hr after MMS treatment.

To summarize the postreplication repair systems briefly, there are two general types, one exemplified by the elongation and joining of the short

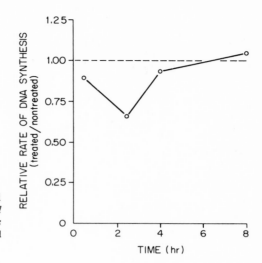

Fig. 9. Relative amounts of DNA synthesized by human cells treated with 1 mM MMS for 1 hr at various times after treatment. Data obtained from Buhl and Regan (23).

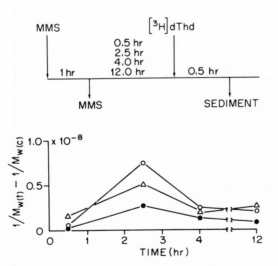

Fig. 10. Differences between the reciprocals of the weight-average molecular weights $(1/M_W)$ obtained from DNA profiles from alkaline sucrose gradients of untreated (c) and MMS-treated (t) normal human fibroblasts. Untreated cells were pulse-labeled for 20 min. Treated cells were exposed to 10^{-5} (●), 10^{-4} (△), or 10^{-3} (○) M MMA for 1 hr before pulse-labeling at 0.5, 2.5, 4.0, or 12 hr for 25, 30, 25, or 25 min, respectively. Data obtained from Buhl and Regan (23).

234 Steven N. Buhl

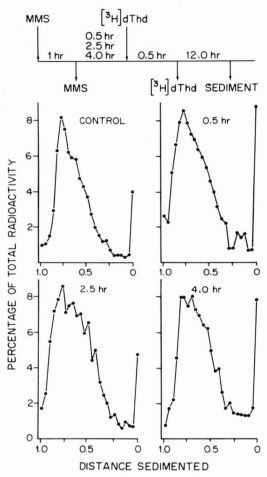

Fig. 11. DNA profiles from alkaline sucrose gradients of normal human fibroblasts treated for 1 hr with 10⁻⁴ M MMS, pulse-labeled for 30 min at various times after treatment, as indicated, and then incubated for 18 hr before sedimentation. Sedimentation was for 75 min at 40,000 rpm. Data obtained from Buhl and Regan (23).

segments synthesized after the insult and the other by the recovery of the ability to synthesize DNA in segments of normal size rather than continuing to synthesize the shorter segments observed immediately after the insult. Recovery of the ability to synthesize DNA in normal segments is faster after MMS treatment than after UV irradiation. Perhaps this difference represents a difference in repair systems. Similarly, the process of chain elongation and joining after MMS treatment needs to be examined to determine whether it differs from the elongation and joining process observed after UV irradiation.

CONCLUSION

There is little correlation of the observations made in studies of prereplication and postreplication repair. In the case of damage from UV radiation, the size of the DNA segments synthesized shortly after UV irradiation is equal to the distance between pyrimidine dimers. However, this correlation does not hold for DNA synthesized at long times after UV irradiation. The data summarized here indicate that the dimer is not the lesion that determines the size of the DNA segments synthesized on UV-irradiated templates, but these data are not conclusive. Another example of the lack of correlation between results from studies of prereplication and postreplication repair is the data from cells incubated in N-acetoxy-2-acetylaminofluorine. This agent causes DNA damage that is recognized by the same prereplication repair system that recognizes UV damage, but it has no effect on the size of the DNA segments observed in studies of postreplication repair.

Equally puzzling are the findings for ionizing irradiation and MMS treatment. Although damage from these agents seems to be recognized by the same prereplication repair system, damage from ionizing radiation has no effect on the size of the DNA synthesized after treatment, whereas damage from MMS has a tremendous effect.

ACKNOWLEDGMENTS

I wish to acknowledge the contributions of Drs. R. B. Setlow and James D. Regan in preparing the manuscript.

This research was sponsored by the U.S. Atomic Energy Commission under contract with the Union Carbide Corporation. The author is a predoctoral trainee supported by Grant GM1974 from the National Institute of General Medical Sciences.

REFERENCES

1. Lockart, R. Z., Elkind, M. M., and Moses, W. B. (1961). *J. Natl. Cancer Inst.* **27**:1393.
2. Rasmussen, R. E., and Painter, R. B. (1964). *Nature* **203**:1360.
3. Rasmussen, R. E., and Painter, R. B. (1966). *J. Cell Biol.* **29**:11.
4. Lohman, P. H. M. (1968). *Mutation Res.* **6**:449.
5. Regan, J. D., Setlow, R. B., and Ley, R. D. (1971). *Proc. Natl. Acad. Sci. (USA)* **68**:708.
6. Crathorn, A. R., and Roberts, J. J. (1966). *Nature* **211**:150.
7. Regan, J. D., Trosko, J. E., and Carrier, W. L. (1968). *Biophys. J.* **8**:319.
8. Cleaver, J. E. (1968). *Nature* **218**:652.
9. Setlow, R. B., Regan, J. D., German, J., and Carrier, W. L. (1969). *Proc. Natl. Acad. Sci. (USA)* **64**:1065.
10. Evans, R. G., and Norman, A. (1968). *Radiat. Res.* **36**:287.
11. Regan, J. D., and Setlow, R. B. (1973). In Hollaender, A. (ed.), *Chemical Mutagens— Principles and Methods for Their Detection,* Plenum Press, New York.

12. Zhustyanikov, V. D., Mikhelson, V. M., Krupnova, G. F., Aikazyan, A. V., Seitkhodzhaev, A. I., Semenova, E. G., Logunova, G. M., and Genter, E. I. (1972). *Abst. IV Internat. Congr. Biophys.*, No. 1, p. 206.
13. Spiegler, P., and Norman, A. (1969). *Radiat. Res.* **39:**400.
14. Clarkson, J. M., and Evans, H. J. (1972). *Mutation Res.* **14:**413.
15. Roberts, J. J., Crathorn, A. R., and Brent, T. P. (1968). *Nature* **218:**970.
16. Roberts, J. J., Brent, T. P., and Crathorn, A. R. (1968). In Campbell, P. N. (ed.), *Biological Council Symposium on the Interaction of Drugs and Subcellular Components in Animals,* Churchill, London, p. 5.
17. Setlow, R. B., and Regan, J. D. (1972). *Biochem. Biophys. Res. Commun.* **46:**1019.
18. Stich, H. F., and San, R. H. C. (1971). *Mutation Res.* **13:**279.
19. Cleaver, J. E. (1971). *Mutation Res.* **12:**453.
20. Buhl, S. N., Stillman, R. M., Setlow, R. B., and Regan, J. D. (1972). *Biophys. J.* **12:**1183.
21. Buhl, S. N., Setlow, R. B., and Regan, J. D. (1973). *Biophys. J.* (in press).
22. Buhl, S. N., Setlow, R. B., and Regan, J. D. (1972). *Internat. J. Radiat. Biol.* **22:**417.
23. Buhl, S. N., and Regan, J. D. (1973). *Mutation Res.* **18:**191.

Evolution and Distribution
of Economically Important Species

16

Geographical Distribution of Cultivated Cottons Relative to Probable Centers of Domestication in the New World

S. G. Stephens

Genetics Department
North Carolina State University
Raleigh, North Carolina, U.S.A.

Most cotton geneticists would agree that the cottons cultivated in the New World separate clearly into two well-defined species, *Gossypium hirsutum* L. and *G. barbadense* L. If modern annual forms are excluded from consideration, most forms of *G. hirsutum* occur in Central America and southern Mexico and most forms of *G. barbadense* in tropical and subtropical South America. The two species are widely sympatric in the Caribbean area, from northern coastal Colombia through Venezuela and extending through the Lesser and Greater Antilles.

Hutchinson (1,2) recognized seven races of *G. hirsutum* and three varieties of *G. barbadense:*

Hirsutum	Barbadense
morrilli	*barbadense* (type)
richmondi	var. *brasiliense*
palmeri	var. *darwinii*
punctatum	
latifolium	
yucatanense	
marie-galante	

Of the *hirsutum* races listed above, the first three are essentially local forms of dooryard or semiferal cottons occurring in the Pacific coastal valley systems of southern Mexico and Guatemala. Race *yucatanense* is a wild form, apparently restricted to the north Yucatan coast. Two races, *punctatum* and *latifolium,* are far more widely distributed and are broadly overlapping in southern Mexico and Guatemala. All the six races so far mentioned are perennial shrubs, and their main distinguishing features are differences in general habit of growth. Although growth habit is not the type of character which lends itself to "classical" taxonomic analysis, it may nevertheless reflect taxonomic differences. The seventh race, *marie-galante,* is well differentiated from the other *hirsutum* races in several aspects. First, it is a well-defined *geographical* race, allopatric with all the other *hirsutum* races over practically its entire range. There is minimal overlap in the upper Motagua valley of Guatemala, and along the Guatemala/El Salvador border, and—at the other end of its range—in the Greater Antilles. Over most of the coastal Caribbean region, it is the only form of *hirsutum* found. Second, *marie-galante* is unique among the *hirsutum* races in its tree form of growth, with pronounced apical dominance. It lacks the shrubby, much-branched habit common to the other races. A third distinguishing feature is its delayed anthesis. In most species of *Gossypium,* pollen shedding begins as the flowers open. In *marie-galante,* pollen shedding may be delayed as long as 2 hr after the flowers are open. Fourth, the bracteoles of *marie-galante,* though more variable in both size and shape than those of other *hirsutum* races, have one consistent distinguishing feature: the bracteole teeth tend to be restricted to the apical half of the bracteole. Finally, two generally rare genes—ck^X (corky complementary) and $R_2{}^V$ (red vein)—are common in *marie-galante* and unkown in other races of *hirsutum.*

Of the three varieties of *G. barbadense* recognized by Hutchinson, var. *darwinii* is a wild form endemic to the Galápagos Islands. Apart from a few cultivated forms of *barbadense,* introduced by settlers on Charles and Chatham Islands, var. *darwinii* is a geographical isolate. *G. barbadense,* excluding var. *darwinii,* exists as a wild form only in the Guayas region of northern Peru and southern Ecuador. Its cultivated forms are widely distributed from the Peruvian coast, across northern South America, and into the Antilles. *G. barbadense* var. *brasiliense* is the commonest form in the Amazon basin and is broadly sympatric with *barbadense* proper in northern and northeastern South America and the Antilles. An apparently secondary center of distribution for var. *brasiliense* occurs in British Honduras, extending from there northwest into the Peten and southern Mexico and, as a rather rare form, southward as far as Costa Rica. I have suggested elsewhere (3) that var. *brasiliense* may have reached British Honduras as a Carib introduction no earlier than the eighteenth century.

The racial differentiation of a cultivated plant clearly implies some form of isolation. In the absence of cytological, genetic, or ethological barriers, this

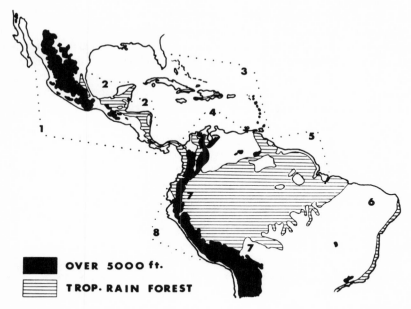

Fig. 1. Map of the American tropics and subtropics showing areas available for the establishment of primitive cottons. Most cottons are found in the more arid, low-lying regions (unshaded) and are confined to riverine settlements in the more humid regions (crosshatched). The numbers indicate eight available subregions partially isolated from one another. From Stephens and Phillips (5).

could take the form of geographical, ecological, or "cultural" isolation. By the term "cultural" I mean to imply the combined effects of human selection, migration, and diffusion. Since all three forms of isolation should be strongly influenced by the topography and accompanying climatic conditions of the area under consideration, it is instructive to consider the distribution of the two cultivated species of *Gossypium* in relation to the physical conditions encountered in the tropical and subtropical Americas. Figure 1 presents a generalized picture of these regions with respect to topography and rainfall. Since few cottons are found at altitudes above 5000 ft, it is clear that the Andes, in particular, and the Mexican cordillera, to a lesser extent, provide barriers to diffusion. The situation is not likely to be affected materially by the fact that cottons could be carried as seeds by human transport from one side of the Andes to the other. It is not likely, for instance, that cottons established in the cool, dry valleys of coastal Peru could easily be transplanted to the upper Amazon basin. All wild forms of *G. hirsutum* and *G. barbadense,* and all cultivated forms of *G. hirsutum,* are restricted actually and potentially to the arid regions on the map. On the other hand, *G. barbadense* var. *brasiliense* is well established throughout the Amazon and Orinoco basins and is, presumably, well adapted to humid tropical conditions. Our field collections indicate that it is not found west of the Andes, with the exception of one form grown by the Cuna Indians in the Darien region of northwestern Colombia. In Central America, it occurs most commonly in the humid Carib settlements of British Honduras and in the equally humid regions of the Peten and lower Motagua valley. The perennial habit combined with nontolerance to frost restricts both species to relatively low latitudes. Until the development through human selection of annual, day-neutral types, primitive cottons could only survive in frost-free areas.

With these considerations in mind, I have indicated (rather arbitrarily) by numbers those subregions on the map in Fig. 1 which should be partially isolated from one another. In Central America, region 1 (Pacific coast) and region 2 (Gulf coast) have relatively unrestricted communication through the Isthmus of Tehuantepec and probably, too, through the Usamacinta and Motagua valley systems. Three of Hutchinson's races of *hirsutum* (*morrilli, richmondi,* and *palmeri*) are included in region 1; one (*yucatanense*) is confined to region 2. Two other races (*latifolium* and *punctatum*) extend beyond both regions. Regions 1 and 4 are connected through the Isthmus of Panama, with no major breaks in an arid coastal habitat. The gap between region 4 (Caribbean coast of South America) and region 3 (Antilles) has been crossed at least twice by the Arawak and Carib (4), who both used cotton. The southern portion of region 1, southward from El Salvador, and regions 4 and 3 include most of the geographical range of race *marie-galante*. An outlying concentration of this race is found in region 6 (the arid "serido" area of northeast Brazil). The origin of these "Moco" cottons is obscure: they may have been introduced by early European colonists (5), and there is good evidence that they have been modified by interracial and interspecific hybridization (6).

Regions 5 and 7, though widely separated geographically, are virtually continuous through the interconnected Amazon and Orinoco river systems. The center of this vast area is little known from the point of view of cotton collection, but on the periphery, in regions 5 and 7, *G. barbadense* var. *brasiliense* predominates. This shows no clear-cut regional differentiation, and seems to be unique among the cultivated cottons in being adapted to growth in the *humid* tropics.

Region 8 (the dry Pacific coast from Ecuador south) is occupied by forms of *barbadense* which are obviously tolerant of extremely arid conditions. Their diffusion to the east is blocked by the almost unbroken Andean chain, to the north by the coastal swamps and jungles of northern Ecuador and Colombia, and to the south by winter temperatures. It is here, surely, that one would expect strong racial differentiation to have developed, but it is not indicated in Hutchinson's classification.

Based on the patterns of racial differentiation in the two cultivated species, it is usually supposed that there are two "centers of origin" (perhaps, more correctly, "centers of domestication"). According to this hypothesis, the center for *G. hirsutum* lies somewhere in southern Mexico and Guatemala, from which region its three major races have diverged geographically and become differentiated (to the north and east *latifolium* and *punctatum,* to the south *mariegalante*). The center for *G. barbadense* is supposedly somewhere in the Peru-Ecuadorean region, west of the Andes. From this center, the cultivated forms would have diffused across the Andes (or around their northern extremity) and into the Amazon basin. It is by no means clear, from this interpretation, what factors were involved in the differentiation of the variety *brasiliense* from *barbadense* since both forms occur sympatrically through much of northern South America and the Antilles.

Since over 90% of the cottons which have been studied in determining patterns of raciation are commensal or dooryard forms, it is reasonable to suppose that human migrations and trading patterns have played a major role in their distribution. Ideally, it should be possible to relate the diffusion and raciation patterns of the cottons to the cultural histories of the peoples who domesticated and used them. But, not surprisingly, the archeological record with respect to cotton remains and associated artifacts is rather meager, and almost certainly biased from the point of view of representative sampling. The oldest cotton remains have been found in those areas (southern Mexico and Peru) where conditions for preservation are remarkably good. It may be a matter of chance that these two regions roughly coincide with the presumptive centers of domestication of *G. hirsutum* and *G. barbadense.*

The oldest cotton remains which have been found so far in the Americas were discovered in the Tehuacán valley of Mexico (7). The earliest reliable date is approximately 3500 B.C., and the cottons were apparently "fully domesticated" (8). These cottons were almost certainly early forms of *hirsutum,* though comparisons made between the archeological samples and samples from living primitive forms of this species have not been published. In Peru, the earliest cotton remains from several sites on the central and north coasts (9–12) are approximately 1000 years later than the Tehuacán valley material. Samples of cotton bolls, seeds, and fibers, recovered from preceramic sites in the Ancon area of central coastal Peru, and dating back to 2500 B.C., have recently been compared with samples of living wild and dooryard forms of *barbadense* from Ecuador and Peru (13). These comparisons suggest that the archeological cottons were primitive forms of *barbadense,* intermediate between present-day wild and cultivated forms of this species. In Colombia, as far as I am aware, no cotton remains of comparable age have been found, and the earliest records of cotton use are provided by the spindle whorls associated with other ceramic artifacts. These first appear at the Momil site in the Sinú valley around 500 B.C. (14). But this apparently late date for cotton in Colombia may be misleading. On the Peruvian coast, cotton was used to make fishing lines and twined fabrics long before ceramics and, in fact, long before corn and several other cultivated crops were used.

The facts that one form of cotton (presumably *hirsutum*) had been domesticated by 3500 B.C. in Mexico and that another (probably *barbadense*) had only reached an *early* stage of domestication 1000 years *later* in Peru indicate rather strongly that the two species were differentiated from each other in the wild state and that their subsequent domestications were initiated independently. If this possibility is accepted, a question which is very pertinent for interpreting the raciation and diffusion of the two species immediately comes to mind. Are *two* centers of domestication, one for *hirsutum* and one for *barbadense,* sufficient to explain the raciation patterns of the two species? Or should we consider the possibility of multiple domestications, i.e., several for each species?

A primary requirement for the initiation of plant domestication is that the wild ancestor should be available in or near an area suitable for agricultural settlement. (The regular use of a wild plant by nomadic food or fiber gatherers would not constitute domestication.) Thus, in theory, an attempt to discover the most probable centers of cotton domestication might focus profitably on archeological evidence for early settled cultures which has been obtained from areas where wild forms of cotton are still extant. In practice, the possibilities of such studies are limited. We cannot assume that the areas now occupied by wild forms have remained constant in size over the past 5000 years. The living forms may well be relics of originally extensive populations. Nor do the best archeological records necessarily coincide with areas likely to have been occupied by wild cottons. On the other hand, any interpretation of raciation patterns which conflicts with the archeological record, or with independent anthropological evidence, stands in need of reconsideration and possible revision.

Over the past 10 years, wild forms and primitive cultivars of *hirsutum* and *barbadense* have been collected extensively in Latin America and studied in culture in a tropical garden, Jamaica, W.I. The maps in Figs. 2 and 3 show the sites of such collections in the presumptive centers of domestication, i.e., in Central America and northwestern South America, respectively. Sites from which samples of *hirsutum* were collected and studied in culture are indicated by dots. Large dots represent *marie-galante;* the small dots represent races *latifolium* and *punctatum,* which are not distinguished from each other in Fig. 2. Sites of *barbadense* collections are indicated by triangles; the distinction between closed and open triangles in Fig. 3 will be explained later. Sites of wild populations are shown by enclosing the appropriate dot or triangle in a circle.

Figure 2 shows that *barbadense* accessions tend to be clustered in British Honduras and the neighboring Motagua and Usamacinta valleys. This is a region of high rainfall, and the cottons are mostly kidney-seeded forms (*G. barbadense*

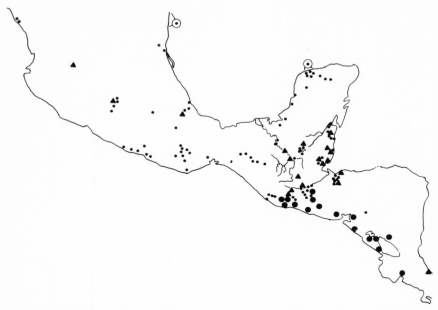

Fig. 2. Collection sites of New World cottons (dooryard and wild) in Central America and southern Mexico. For explanation of symbols, see text.

var. *brasiliense*). They tend to have very long, narrow bolls, and their flowers often have spotless cream petals. In these and other morphological characteristics, they are very similar to the types of *brasiliense* found in the Antilles—as expected if they are relatively recent introductions from those islands (3). They are also found rarely, and at widely scattered locations, northward in southern Mexico and southward as far as Costa Rica. We have found no *brasiliense* so far in Panama.

The *hirsutum* accessions separate geographically into two rather clear groups, with only slight overlap on the Guatemala/El Salvador border. From here, southward along the Pacific coast, the only form of *hirsutum* found is *marie-galante*. So far, wild forms of *hirsutum* have only been found at two widely separated coastal sites; on the northern Yucatan coast (*yucatanense*) and, recently, by Lukefahr (unpublished) in Tamaulipas. None has been found on the Pacific coast, though a wild form is known from Socorro in the Revillagigedos Island, and there may be a similar form near Todos Santos, Baja California (Lukefahr, personal communication). Since wild forms of *hirsutum* often occur as extremely small and localized populations, it is entirely possible that a careful search among salt marshes and along sea cliffs—on both the Gulf and Pacific

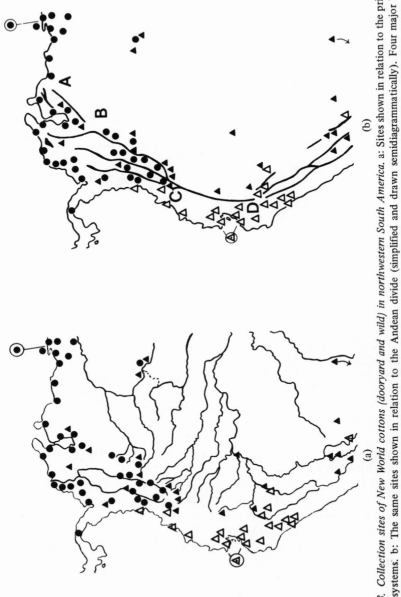

Fig. 3. Collection sites of New World cottons (dooryard and wild) in northwestern South America. a: Sites shown in relation to the principal river systems. b: The same sites shown in relation to the Andean divide (simplified and drawn semidiagrammatically). Four major breaks through which cottons have apparently diffused are indicated by letters as follows: (A) Coastal gap north of Sierra de Perija (*marie-galante*). (B) Rio Apure gap between Cordillera Oriente and Cordillera de Merida (Amazonian-type *barbadense*). (C) Rio Patia/Upper Cauca gap (Ecuadorean-type *barbadense*). (D) Rio Chamaya/Upper Marañon gap (Ecuadorean-type *barbadense*).

coasts—will discover more of them. From the information presented in Fig. 2, the Gulf coast in the Tehuantepec region would seem to be a likely center for the initiation of cotton domestication in Mesoamerica. This conclusion, though speculative, is consistent with current thinking in archeological circles concerning the origin of settled agriculture in Mesoamerica. Coe and Flannery (15) have suggested that easy access to a diversification of microenvironments (with a concomitant diversification of food resources) would be a prime necessity in determining the locations of the earliest settlements. They have suggested that some of the earliest permanently occupied villages in Mesoamerica, near Ocos on the Pacific coast just east of Tehuantepec, are particularly well located with respect to these requirements and that similar conditions "are found all along the Pacific coast of Guatemala and along the Gulf coast of southern Veracruz and Tabasco." Similar conclusions have been reached by Puleston and Puleston (16).

The diffusion of *marie-galante* southward along the Pacific coast from El Salvador to Colombia would surely be accompanied by other, independent evidences of cultural migration. Reichel-Dolmatoff (14) finds such evidence in the rather abrupt appearance, in about 500 B.C., of stone "metates" for corn grinding and pottery styles showing Mesoamerican influence at Momil and other contemporary sites. Thus the earliest hard evidence for corn usage (metates) and that for cotton spinning (spindle whorls) seem to coincide. But Reichel-Dolmatoff believes that the Mesoamerican influences arrived in a series of waves by sea-going transport, rather than by land through the Isthmus of Panama, and were introduced through the west coast of southern Colombia. The map in Fig. 2 suggests that cotton followed the land route.

I am going to suggest an alternative hypothesis for the origin of *marie-galante,* namely, that its initial domestication may have occurred separately from that of the other races of *hirsutum,* and in Colombia rather than Mesoamerica. There are two reasons for considering an alternative hypothesis: first, the apparent absence of a transition zone between *marie-galante* and the other *hirsutum* races in Central America, and, second, the relative morphological uniformity of *marie-galante* along the Pacific coast of Central America as compared with its diversity in northern Colombia. If *marie-galante* had been differentiated southward from a common center in Mesoamerica, one might expect that forms located near to the center (in Guatemala and El Salvador) would be more variable, and with racial characteristics less pronounced, than forms more distant from the center (in Nicaragua and Colombia). Our collections indicate the opposite situation. Accessions from Guatemala and Nicaragua are very similar and uniform with respect to certain racial characteristics (in particular, narrow bracteoles with apical teeth restricted to three or less). It is in Colombia that morphological and genetic variability seems to be associated with geographical and topographical diversity. The maps in Fig. 3 show how our collections of *marie-galante* are distributed in relation to the major topographical features of northern Colombia. In the northwest corner of the maps, i.e., in a triangular area roughly bounded by Barranquila in the north, the Isthmus of Darien to the west, and Monteria to the south, forms of *marie-galante* with small bracteoles and very small seeds are common in dooryards. Perhaps 50% of the plants carry a red-vein gene (R_2V), which is uncommon elsewhere in *marie-galante* and unknown in other *hirsutum* races. Branching out from this area, the distribution of *marie-galante* can be traced in four different directions, all isolated from one another by topographical features. One route leads to the east along the Caribbean coast, through the Guajira peninsula, around Lake Maracaibo, and so into Venezuela and the Antilles. Along this route, the bracteoles become bigger and broader, small round bolls become replaced by larger more oval bolls, and red-veined types occur only sporadically. To the northeast through Panama and into Central America, the bracteoles become larger and relatively narrower, bolls remain round, but the red-vein gene is missing. To the south, *marie-galante* follows two routes, along the Cauca and Magdalena valleys, which are isolated from each other by the Cordillera Centrale. Red-veined types occur infrequently along the Cauca valley but seem to be absent entirely from the upper Magdalena valley. In both valleys, the bracteoles tend to become larger and broader, and in the Magdalena valley there is an increase in the number of bracteole teeth (approximately seven as compared to three or four in the Monteria area).

Some of the earliest sites of coastal settlements in the Americas have been discovered in northwestern Colombia. The oldest, Puerto Hormiga, dates back to at least 3000 B.C. (14,17). The artifacts preserved at these sites indicate that shellfish, and to a less extent bony fish, contributed a substantial part of the food resources available. Stone grinding implements suggest that seeds were also used as food, but apparently no plant remains were preserved. Similar resources were exploited in early Peruvian coastal settlements (11,12), but there plant materials were preserved which indicate that cotton was used in the construction of fishing lines and nets. Most wild forms of *hirsutum* and *barbadense* which exist today occur as coastal ecotypes, and it seems possible that wild forms of *hirsutum* may have been available to the early settlers in northwestern Colombia. However, no wild populations have so far been found anywhere along the Caribbean coastline of Colombia, from Darien to Lake Maracaibo, although several apparently suitable habitats have been explored.

In Fig. 4, I have shown diagrammatically an interpretation based on separate domestications of (a) the Central American races of *G. hirsutum* and (b) *marie-galante*. In both maps, the broken lines indicate possible *recent* routes of migration which may have no bearing on the distribution of cottons in pre-Columbian times. For example, in Fig. 4a, one of the Central American races

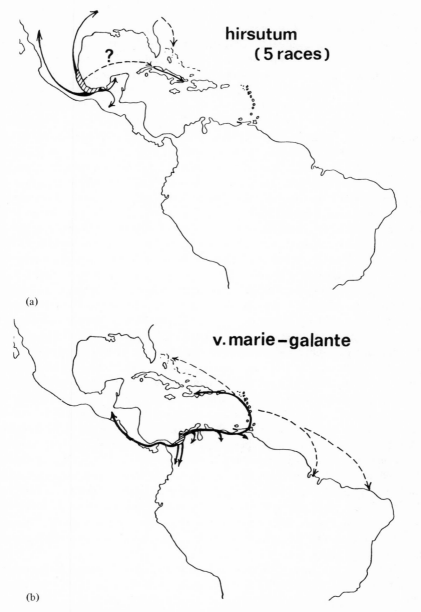

Fig. 4. Interpretations of possible centers of domestication and migration. a: Central American races of *G. hirsutum.* b: *G. hirsutum* race *marie-galante.*

(*punctatum*) is found in both Central America and Cuba. There is little archeological evidence for pre-Columbian contacts between these areas (4), but later, in the sixteenth and seventeenth centuries, a main Spanish trade route linked Veracruz and Havana. In Fig. 4b, there is historical evidence for an eighteenth-century introduction of *marie-galante* from the Virgin Islands into the Bahamas and of contacts between European colonists in the West Indies and northeast Brazil, which *may* account for the presence of *marie-galante* in the latter area.

Before considering the distribution of *barbadense* west and east of the Andes, which is shown in Fig. 3, it is necessary to explain the symbols (closed *vs.* open triangles) which are used to indicate this species. I have mentioned earlier that Hutchinson's classification (1) of the cultivated forms (*barbadense* and its variety *brasiliense*) does not correlate clearly with the major break in the distribution, namely, the Andean divide. In 1966, collections made in the Guayas region of Ecuador and Peru suggested that the cottons found there differed sharply in several characteristics from cottons collected east of the Andes. For convenience, I will call the contrasted forms "Ecuadorean type" and "Amazonian type," respectively. Their contrasting features are summarized in Table I. Subsequently, further collections were made in coastal Peru, in the intra-Andean valleys of the upper Marañon and Utcubamba rivers, and along the northwestern edge of the Amazon basin in eastern Colombia. These collections were supplemented by others made by Dr. C. M. Rick in the Urubamba valley and in eastern Ecuador, and by Dr. D. L. Timothy and Dr. J. Giles S. in northeastern Colombia and eastern Peru, respectively. On the maps in Fig. 3, all collection sites in which "Ecuadorean" features predominate are indicated by open triangles, those in which "Amazonian" features predominate by closed triangles. The maps show that the Ecuadorean types tend to be restricted to the western side of the divide and the Amazonian types to the eastern side of the divide. There are four major breaks in the divide, indicated in Fig. 3b by letters (A through D). It is through these gaps that cottons have apparently diffused from one side of the Andes to the other. The Amazonian type has apparently diffused along the Apure river (B). Ecuadorean-type *barbadense* penetrates into the head of the Cauca valley along a northern branch of the Patia river (C). There, mixed plantings of *barbadense* and *marie-galante* are found. Farther south, in Peru, the Ecuadorean type has apparently diffused via the Chamaya valley (D) into the valleys of the eastward-flowing Marañon, Huallaga, and Ucayali rivers.

In general, the patterns of distribution shown in Fig. 3 agree with the current hypothesis that the center of domestication for *barbadense* lies to the west of the Andes, in or near coastal Peru. As shown in Table I, the cultivated Ecuadorean types have several features in common with wild forms of *barbadense* which are not shared with Amazonian types. Excluding var. *darwinii* in the Galápagos Islands, wild forms of *barbadense* have been found only in the Guayas

Table I. Characters Distinguishing Ecuadorean and Amazonian
Types of *Barbadense*

	Ecuadorean	Amazonian
Leaves	Broader, often pubescent[a]	Narrower, nearly glabrous
Bolls	Smaller, rounded, with 3-4 locules	Larger and longer, usually 3 locules
Seeds	Often fuzzy,[a] never conjoined	Rarely fuzzy, often conjoined
Bracteoles	Smaller, finely toothed[a]	Larger, coarsely toothed
Staminal column	Shorter[a]	Longer
Floral nectary	Fringe hairs often present[a]	Fringe hairs absent
Genetic characters		
a. Corky complementary	ck^Y or ck^{0a}	ck^Y
b. Anthocyanin	Always R_2 (petal spot)[a]	R_2 or R_2V (red vein)

[a] Characters common to Ecuadorean cultivated forms and wild forms of
barbadense.

region near the Ecuador/Peruvian border. The earliest archeological records of
cotton domestication in South America have been obtained at several sites on
the northern and central coasts of Peru. Cotton remains, including bolls, seeds,
and fibers, obtained from sites near Ancon on the central coast have recently
been studied in detail (13). Within the limits of the materials preserved, these
studies indicate that the archeological cottons were intermediate between present-day wild and cultivated forms of *barbadense*. Thus it might be supposed that
early domesticated forms of Ecuadorean-type *barbadense* were eventually transported—probably through the Chamaya/Marañon gap—and became adapted to
the very different ecological conditions prevailing in the Amazon basin. From
this interpretation, the cottons now found in the Marañon, Huallaga, and
Ucayali river systems should represent transitional forms between Ecuadorean
and Amazonian types of *barbadense*.

Unfortunately, the foregoing hypothesis, which requires the derivation of
Amazonian types in the east from ancestral Ecuadorean types in the west, does
not agree at all well with other anthropological evidence. Although the climatic
conditions prevailing in the Amazon basin are not suitable for the preservation
of plant remains and perishable artifacts, Lathrap (18) has recently assembled an
impressive body of evidence which suggests that this region, rather than the

Andean highlands or the Pacific coast, may represent the primary "hearth" from which South American cultures ultimately derive. His evidence is based on similar diffusion patterns shown by (a) linguistic differentiation, (b) styles of pottery construction and decoration, and (c) the development of agricultural techniques, particularly the use of ridged fields and terracing. According to his interpretation, the diffusion patterns moved upstream along the interconnected Amazon and Orinoco waterways, and the plant resources were based on root-crop culture primarily, with cotton being the outstanding exception. A major barrier to westward diffusion was the Andean divide. This general pattern of a diffusion *from the east* does not appear to conflict with the fact that most of the crop plants, together with pottery, make their first appearance on the Peruvian coast about 1000 years later than the first evidence for cotton usage. Further, prior to the use of pottery on the north and central coasts of Peru, the cotton fabrics were constructed by a *twining* technique (19), while true *woven* textiles were found later, at the Hacha site near Acari on the southern coast, in a deposit containing pottery "and abundant plant remains, including squash, beans, peanuts, guava, capsicum, gourds and cotton (plant parts) but no maize" (20). The Hacha site dates back to about 1900 B.C., i.e., almost 800 years later than the preceramic sites on the northern and central coasts.

Is it possible that the cottons east of the Andes were domesticated independently of those on the Pacific coast? Is it possible, further, that the art of weaving was discovered on the eastern side of the Andes and that the *art,* rather than the cottons themselves, was transferred to the Pacific coast where weaving was previously unknown? The late appearance of weaving, pottery, and the use of crops more typical of the Amazon region would seem to suggest that these may all have been introduced to the coast from across the Andes. With these possibilities in mind, it is clear that the patterns of cotton distribution shown in Fig. 3 *could* be interpreted as the bringing together of two historically independent races, instead of the progressive differentiation of one race from the other. Clearly, further collections are needed from the upper Marañon and neighboring river systems in order to obtain more critical information on these questions.

Without exception, all wild species of cotton, and all wild forms of the cultivated species *hirsutum* and *barbadense,* have only been found in extremely arid habitats. Thus, in seeking for a possible wild ancestor of the Amazonian types, there is a rather limited choice of localities which would provide suitable ecological conditions. A possible clue which should be actively explored is the fact that cottons having the smallest bolls and seeds yet found in the Amazon basin occur in Bolivia between the eastern slopes of the Andes and the Mamoré river (a tributary of the Amazon). Very close to this region, and overlapping the borders of Bolivia and Paraguay, is an extensive area of dry thorn-scrub which, as far as I am aware, is one of the few extensive and ecologically suitable habitats in South America which has not yet been searched for wild cottons.

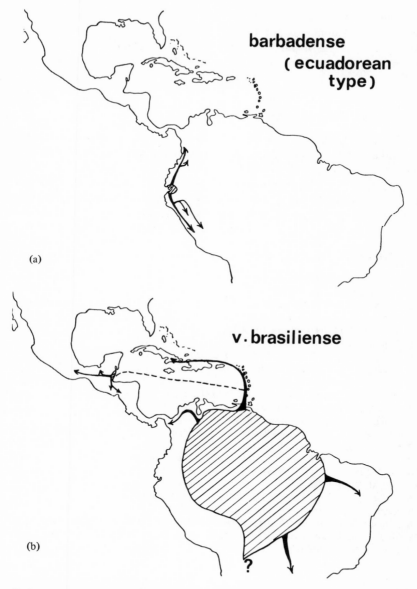

Fig. 5. Interpretations of possible centers of domestication and migration. a: Ecuadorean-type *barbadense.* b: Amazonian-type *barbadense.*

Figure 5 presents an admittedly speculative interpretation of two independent centers of domestication for *barbadense* in South America. The interpretations offered in Figs. 4 and 5 may or may not prove valuable in bringing together viewpoints hitherto derived independently from botanical and archeological research.

ACKNOWLEDGMENTS

The collections on which this study was based were made possible by grants from the John Simon Guggenheim Memorial Foundation and the National Science Foundation (GB 7769). I am also indebted to the following individual collectors for pertinent information and gifts of seeds: I. M. Bowman, H. Brücher, J. Giles, S. M. J. Lukefahr, C. R. Parks, L. L. Phillips, G. Reichel-Dolmatoff, T. R. Richmond, C. M. Rick, Karl Schwerin, and D. L. Timothy.

REFERENCES

1. Hutchinson, J. B. (1947). In *The Evolution of Gossypium,* Oxford University Press, New York, Chap. 3.
2. Hutchinson, J. B. (1951). *Heredity* **5**:161.
3. Stephens, S. G. (1967). *Ciencia e Cultura* **19**:118.
4. Rouse, I. M. (1964). *Science* **144**:499.
5. Stephens, S. G., and Phillips, L. L. (1972). *Biotropica* **4**:49.
6. Boulanger, J., and Pinheiro, D. (1971). *Coton et Fibres Tropicales* **26**:319.
7. Smith, C. E., Jr. (1967). In *The Prehistory of the Tehuacán Valley,* Vol. I: *Environment and Subsistence,* Texas University Press, Austin.
8. Smith, C. E., Jr., and Stephens, S. G. (1971). *Econ. Bot.* **25**:160.
9. Bird, J. B. (1948). *Nat. Hist.* **57**:296.
10. Engel, F. (1963). *Trans. Am. Phil. Soc.* **53**:1.
11. Lanning, E. P. (1967). *Peru Before the Incas,* Prentice-Hall, Englewood Cliffs, N.J.
12. Moseley, M. E., (1968). Ph.D. thesis, Harvard University.
13. Stephens, S. G., and Moseley, M. E. (1973). *Am. Antiq.* (in press).
14. Reichel-Dolmatoff, G. (1965). *Colombia,* Praeger, New York.
15. Coe, M. D., and Flannery, K. V. (1964). *Science* **143**:650.
16. Puleston, D. E., and Puleston, O. S. (1971). *Archaeology* **24**:330.
17. Reichel-Dolmatoff, G. (1971). *Archaeology* **24**:338.
18. Lathrap, D. W. (1970). *The Upper Amazon,* Thames and Hudson, New York.
19. Moseley, M. E., and Barrett, L. K. (1969). *Amer. Antiq.* **34**:162.
20. Gayton, A. H. (1967). *Nawpa Pacha* **5**:1.

17

Potential Genetic Resources
in Tomato Species:
Clues from Observations in Native Habitats

Charles M. Rick

Department of Vegetable Crops
University of California
Davis, California, U.S.A.

Interspecific hybridization is playing an increasingly important role in the breeding of improved cultivars of higher plants. *Lycopersicon* is a good example of a genus in which the cultivated species (*L. esculentum* Mill.) is being improved in this fashion. The advantages offered by the tomato species for this purpose are:

a. All species can be readily grown for experimental purposes, and *L. esculentum* is widely cultivated under a wide range of environmental conditions.

b. Excellent sources of germ plasm now exist in the wild species as well as in modern and primitive cultivars of *L. esculentum.*

c. All of the wild species can be hybridized with *L. esculentum,* albeit requiring special aids in certain combinations; fertility and viability of the hybrid generations permit the intended gene transfers. All species have 12 pairs of chromosomes, which are essentially homologous.

d. The cultivated species is well known genetically; its chromosomes have been mapped cytologically and genetically; it behaves as a basic diploid (27, 28).

Heretofore, interspecific hybridization has been exploited to a great extent in breeding improved tomato cultivars. To mention only the category of disease resistance, successful control of the following pathogens has been achieved in this fashion: *Cladosporium* (18), *Fusarium* (3), root-knot nematodes (13), *Septoria* (2), *Stemphyllium* (15), tobacco mosaic virus (1), and *Verticillium* (31) (this bibliography is not intended to be complete; only one pertinent reference is cited per disease). Many cultivars in which such resistance is combined with desirable horticultural type have been introduced to the trade and are widely cultivated. Cultivars have been bred, furthermore, with combined resistance to three or more of these diseases.

The foregoing research was conducted largely without benefit of information concerning the ecological relations of the tomato species or the range of genetic variation. It is the thesis of this chapter that a survey of the species in their native habitats can shed light on the extent of genetic variability and furnish clues as to their potential as sources of agriculturally valuable genes. Certainly not all of the useful germ plasm can be detected in this way; many traits may require precise testing for their detection; others may not even be observed until hybridization and considerable introgression have been completed, as in the case of the so-called novel variations (30). It can be safely assumed that the capacity of a species or one of its biotypes to survive in a particular environment implies the evolution of a genotype that determines that capacity. Appropriate breeding experiments can reveal the nature of genetic determination and the feasibility of exploiting the character for improvement of the cultivated species.

The substance of this chapter is partly derived from observations made in the field during several extended trips to the areas of natural distribution of the tomato species. The features of their autecology were observed concomitantly with recording phenotypic variation and collecting seeds, herbarium specimens, and other pertinent material. Field observations are correlated with résumés of known pertinent published and unpublished tests.

The time available in the Symposium limits the extent of this chapter. An attempt is made to survey the known findings without presenting any aspects in detail. Consequently, because it is so highly polymorphic both within and between populations (26), the very useful species *L. peruvianum* must be omitted. I have chosen to delimit consideration to certain biotypes of certain species as examples of useful characters that are observed, principally under conditions of environmental stress.

Space limitations also preclude presentation of a complete account of the autecology of the tomato species; instead, only the features pertinent to the present considerations will be mentioned. The natural distribution of the genus is limited to western South America, extending from northern Chile to southern Colombia, the western limits being the Pacific shore (embracing the Galápagos Islands), and the eastern boundary, although not precisely known, probably lying in the lower foothills of the Andes. With the exception of var. *cerasiforme* (Dun.) A. Gray of *L. esculentum,* the species occupy well-defined distributions, which will not be described in detail; but mentioned only in respect to ecological considerations. In many areas, the specific ranges overlap. Yet, despite such sympatry, convincing evidence for natural introgression has been provided only between *L. esculentum* and *L. pimpinellifolium* (Jusl.) Mill. (25).

TOMATO SPECIES

L. esculentum **var.** *cerasiforme*

The wild form of the cultivated tomato is highly diverse morphologically. It is consequently difficult to set any limits that clearly distinguish it from *L. pimpinellifolium* or from the other diverse forms of *L. esculentum*. Intergrades of many sorts exist, not only for fruit size, but also for fruit shape, leaf shape, and pubescence. As arbitrarily treated here, var. *cerasiforme* includes those forms that have fruit diameters between 1.5 and 3.0 cm. Within these limits, no other subspecific form of *L. esculentum* needs recognition; such entities as var. *pyriforme* Bailey and *L. humboldtii* Willd. defy definition and probably have little or no biological significance.

Some biotypes of *cerasiforme* are so successful as weeds that they have spread throughout all of tropical America as far north as southern Texas and Florida and to most of the tropical regions of the world. In this enormous range, the wild form tolerates a wide range of environmental conditions varying to a great extent in amounts of available moisture. Certain biotypes survive the droughts of the western deserts of Perú; others successfully withstand wetter conditions than any other tomato species. Figure 1 illustrates the conditions of its habitat in the tropical rainforests of the eastern slopes of the Andes in Ecuador, where up to 4–5 m of rainfall is received annually. Here a major share of the land surface may be covered by water, and elsewhere the water table is close to the ground surface. In tolerating such conditions, *cerasiforme* is a blatant exception to the general preference of tomato species for dry climates and well-drained soils. Such adaptation implies resistance to wilt and root-rotting fungi that are usually prevalent under such conditions. The concomitant high humidity of this habitat is also highly favorable for the activity of leaf-spotting fungi.

It has been possible to verify this moisture tolerance in at least 20 different localities of collection in eastern Ecuador and Perú. In every instance, observations made by us agree with those of local agriculturists and naturalists regarding this capacity of *cerasiforme*. Large-fruited cultivars of *L. esculentum*, which are frequently tested under the same conditions, seldom survive conditions of the rainy season. We have observed plantings of the latter to succumb completely to *Cladosporium* and other fungi within the first 2 weeks of the advent of the rainy season, while *cerasiforme* continues to grow and fruit throughout the year. Although this taxon has been tested for resistance to certain fungi (32), the resources of its many variants have scarcely been tapped in this respect.

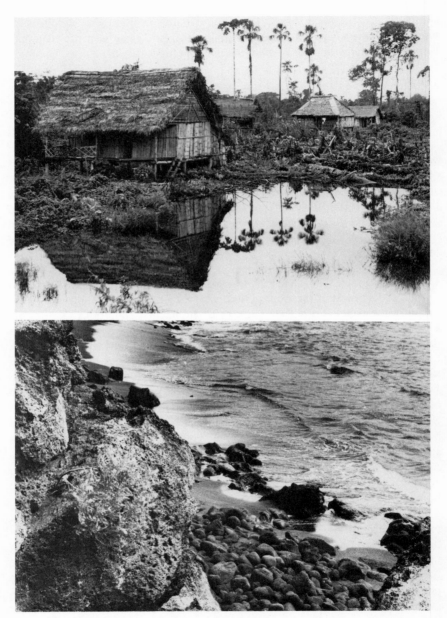

Figs. 1 and 2. Illustrations of the habitats of tomato species. Fig. 1 (top). Typical scene at Lago Agrio in northeastern Ecuador. Plants of *L. esculentum* var. *cerasiforme* were found growing in the dooryards of this settlement. *Fig. 2 (bottom).* Littoral zone on western shore of Isla Isabela, Galápagos, approximately 4 km north of Punta Tortuga. Plant of *L. cheesmanii* var. *minor* is growing in sand and basalt in the left foreground.

L. minutum

The rather poorly understood array of wild tomatoes that bear the unofficial label of "*L. minutum*" (4, 6) occupy a restricted area in the interandean region of central Perú. Two distinct subspecific forms exist: the more widespread entity has diminutive plant parts and extremely reduced flower size, the other is somewhat more robust. Within the limited extent of our field observations, both forms maintain their morphological integrity despite occasional intermingling of branches. The habitats of both are generally rather moist, although always in well-drained, rocky situations. No unusual features have been noted in their autecology, save the scarcity of ripe fruits in the more robust form of the complex. This apparent deficiency of ripe fruit does not reflect unfruitfulness; to the contrary, both have always been observed to set heavy loads of fruit, presumably by self-pollination. The scarcity of ripe fruit suggests animal predation, which, in turn, implies attractivity of the fruit to predators. On ripening, the fruits undergo a slight change in color from green to greenish white and they soften somewhat. A characteristic odor is also developed. But of particular interest to us is the remarkably high content of sugars that are measured in the ripe fruit. Mean values that we have measured by refractometer readings over several seasons under summer field conditions at Davis vary from 10 to 11% soluble solids.

Since soluble solids content is a vital factor in quality of tomato fruits, particularly for processing purposes, we have been transferring this character by hybridization and selection to horticultural tomatoes. The more robust subspecific form was chosen as the wild parent because it lacks the extreme wilt susceptibility and semilethal defoliator (*Df*) gene (5) present in the diminutive type. Following four and five backcrosses to VF-145, the principal canning cultivar in California, followed by pedigree selection, it has been possible to attain and maintain mean readings of 7.5% and higher in breeding lines that have satisfactory fruit size and color. In contrast, the recurrent parent has values of 5.5% or less. The details of this program, for which space does not permit elaboration here, will be the subject of a forthcoming publication.

L. cheesmanii

L. cheesmanii Riley (*sensu* Wiggins and Porter, 1971) is endemic to, and widely distributed throughout, the Galápagos archipelago. Several subspecific taxa can be distinguished, and, to a certain degree, ecological preferences can be discerned among them. The physiological nature of site preferences for the various races is not well understood; however, the following features in the autecology of ssp. *minor* (Hook.) C. H. Mull. are so apparent that they deserve mention.

Subspecies *minor* is rather widespread in the islands, but prefers the lower elevations, where the climate is less overcast, dryer, and warmer. It is often the only form of the species that inhabits such areas. As illustrated in Fig. 2, its range actually extends into the littoral zone, where it is subject to such marine influences as salt spray and salt accumulation in the soil. In certain situations, as depicted in Fig. 2, ssp. *minor* grows scarcely 2 m above, and 5 m total distance from, the high-tide line, where it associates with such halophytes as *Cacabus miersii* (Hook. f.), *Ipomoea pes-caprae* (L.) R. Br., and *Nolana galapagensis* (Christoph.) Johnston. Although its growth there is not maximal, revealing that environmental conditions are not optimal, it does survive well, and the size of the stem of some specimens attested that the plants must have been growing there for periods of 2–3 years.

Tests on salt tolerance of tomato species have been made by Tal (36). Although several tested biotypes of ssp. *minor* did not withstand the high levels of NaCl applied, progeny of uncontrolled hybridization between *minor* and presumably *L. esculentum* showed significantly higher gains in dry weight than the *esculentum* controls. Although the interpretation of these results is subject to an element of conjecture, it seems likely, as Tal concludes, that, although the *minor* parent did not itself perform well under this stress, it did contribute genes which interacted with those of the other parent to lend salt tolerance. It should also be noted that biotypes surviving such exposure to marine influence as that illustrated in Fig. 2 were not tested.

L. hirsutum

The species *L. hirsutum* H. and B. inhabits a zone extending from central Perú to northern Ecuador at elevations from 500 to 3300 m—the latter being the highest known elevation for any tomato species. It generally prefers fairly moist areas, often on stream banks, although generally in well-drained situations. Its altitudinal preferences might suggest cold or frost tolerance, yet it is doubtful whether *hirsutum* is subject to such temperature extremes, even at its highest haunts, which are within the zones of cultivation of such frost-tender cultigens as maize and potatoes. Also, according to repeated observations in cultivation at Davis and elsewhere in temperate zones, *hirsutum* accessions are observed to be no less sensitive to frost than other tomato species.

In our experience, the most notable feature in the autecology of *L. hirsutum* is its freedom from insect predation. From inspecting populations in more than 50 localities throughout its range, I have detected little or no insect damage to leaves, fruits, or other parts (Fig. 5). The presence of virus disease symptoms in two populations in the Andes of southern Ecuador provides the only evidence in *hirsutum* autecology of either disease susceptibility or visits of insects that presumably act as the vectors of the virus disease.

Other wild tomato species, although generally more resistant to insect species than *L. esculentum,* are subject to a substantial attack by a wide variety of predators. The same freedom from insect attack is observed when *L. hirsutum* is grown in cultivation and thereby exposed to the same or different pests than those of the native region.

The behavior of *L. hirsutum* under conditions of natural infestation correlates with experiments on controlled exposure to specific predatory insects. Recent systematic tests have revealed resistance to more species of noxious insects in *L. hirsutum* than any other tested tomato species. Resistance of this tomato species has been demonstrated against two species of spider mite (12,33, 34), leaf miner (37), tobacco flea beetle (10), greenhouse whitefly (11), and Colorado potato beetle (A. K. Stoner and H. G. Mason, unpublished). Only in the case of potato aphid did *L. hirsutum* exhibit lower resistance than other tested tomato species (9,35). Of particular interest among these investigations is the discovery that removal of the glandular exudate from *L. hirsutum* rendered it more susceptible to attack by flea beetles (10) and by whiteflies (11). The strong odor of the exudate in this species, generally considered obnoxious by humans, might thereby be implicated in its resistance. For its offensive pungency, *L. hirsutum* has earned a reputation among natives in several areas for being a poisonous species and is known by such derogatory names as *monte gallinazo*.

S. pennellii

The most striking feature in the autecology of *S. pennellii* Corr. (a species that according to all experimental criteria behaves like a *Lycopersicon* yet has the taxonomic key characters of *Solanum*) is its ability to withstand drought. Its native territory consists of the exceedingly dry, lower, west slopes of the Andes in central Perú. Here it occupies a narrow band of about 500–1500 m elevation, extending from Atico in the south to Ascope in the north. In the lowest places, it may intermingle with *L. peruvianum* and *L. pimpinellifolium,* but in the higher, more arid extensions of its habitat, it associates only with species of cactus and bromeliads (Fig. 3).

The research of Yu (39) has elucidated considerably the nature of water relations in this species. Astonishingly, its root system is so poorly developed that it amounts to less than 5% of the proportional weight in *L. esculentum.* Its leaves, however, exhibit a remarkable ability to retain water, requiring longer dehydration to induce wilting symptoms than those of other species. They are unique also in respect to the much higher proportion of stomata located on the upper leaf surface.

In recent experiments (Rick, unpublished), I have attempted to supply water to plants of this species by applying mists to the upper leaf surface. In this way, it is feasible to keep plants in turgid condition for several days, while under the same regime plants of *L. esculentum* will quickly and severely wilt. The same response can be evoked in detached leaves (Table I), the *pennellii* leaves sometimes actually gaining weight during the period of detachment. My tests agree

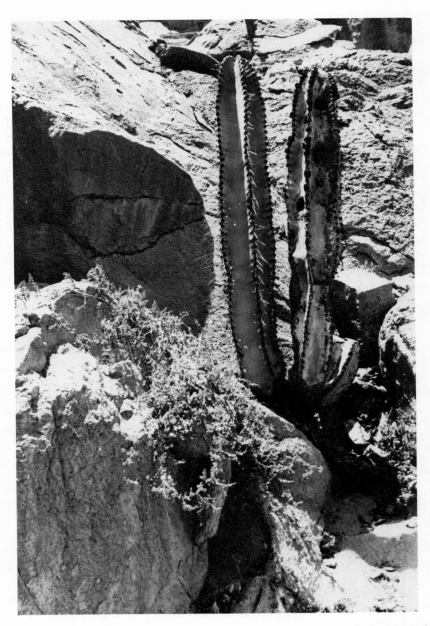

Fig. 3. *Steep quebrada slopes near Pisaquera in west central Perú, elevation approximately 1000 m.* Mature plant of *S. pennellii* in center is associating with the columnar cactus, *Cereus macrostibus* (K. Schum.) Berg.

Table I. Response of Detached Mature Leaves to Moisture Applied on Upper Surface[a]

| | L. esculentum | | F₁ hybrid | | S. pennellii | |
	Untreated	Hydrated	Untreated	Hydrated	Untreated	Hydrated
First test[b]						
Original wt.	34.50	28.90	29.25	26.30	14.90	15.00
Final wt.	29.50	26.50	26.80	26.45	14.00	16.00
% change	−14.5	− 8.3	− 8.4	+ 0.57	− 6.0	+ 6.7
Second test[c]						
Original wt.	37.05	33.95	37.05	34.85	17.60	17.65
Final wt.	33.35	32.60	35.20	36.15	16.90	18.60
% change	− 9.4	− 4.0	− 5.0	+ 3.7	− 3.4	+ 5.4

[a] Six leaves per sample, 2 hr dehydration, water applied as mist to keep upper surface continuously moist.

[b] Leaves exposed to average greenhouse conditions: 30°C, high sunlight intensity, 55% rh.

[c] Leaves exposed in artificial dehydrator: 37°C, no light, very low rh.

with those of Yu in showing a much smaller water loss in the untreated leaves of *pennellii* (3–6%) than in those of *esculentum* (9–14%) under the same conditions. The F_1 hybrids behaved in a fashion similar to the *pennellii* parent.

It is noteworthy in respect to these peculiar features of the anatomy and physiology of *pennellii* that its territory is subject to heavy dews and periodic fogs, although not nearly so intense as those of the Peruvian *lomas*. Our experiments therefore suggest that, like the sympatric bromeliads *Puya* and *Tillandsia, pennellii* may resist drought by evolving a high capacity to absorb and retain atmospheric moisture in its leaves. Also, through lack of selection pressure, its root system might be suffering evolutionary degeneration. The nature of adaptation of *pennellii* to the native xeric conditions is thereby suggested.

Despite the resemblance between *pennellii* and certain bromeliad species in respect to its water economy, the stomatal opening regulation system and other features of the former rule out its having the crassulacean acid metabolism (CAM) (23) characteristic of the latter. Neither does it have the anatomical features peculiar to species with C-4 carbon fixation metabolism (8). Thus, in respect to various aspects of its water economy, *pennellii* is a unique xerophyte.

Dr. Yu's experiments included the measurement of water retention by leaves of the F_2 generation and backcross of the F_1 hybrid to *L. esculentum*. In all tests of these segregating generations, the distributions spread to and beyond the extreme of the *pennellii* parent (Fig. 6). This transgressive variation not only implies interaction between the genotypes of the parental species, but also augurs well for the exploitation of this character in tomato breeding programs.

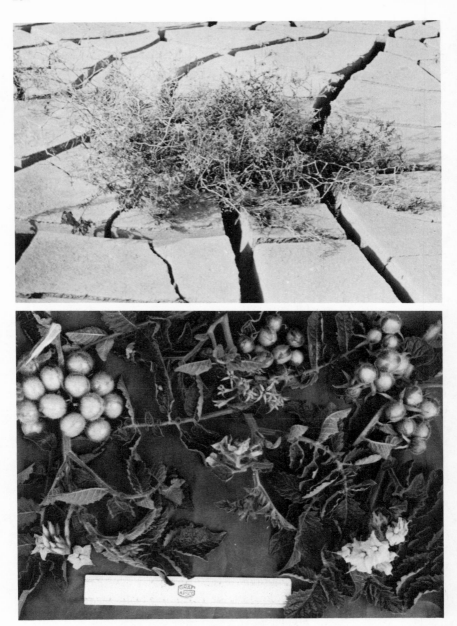

Figs. 4 and 5. Illustrations of tomato species. Fig. 4 (top). Mature plant of *L. chilense* bearing flowers and fruit and growing in bottomland near Sama Grande (Depto. Tacna) in southern Perú. *Fig. 5 (bottom).* Typical assortment of leaves, flowers, and fruit of *L. hirsutum* from eastern outskirts of Loja (Prov. Loja), south-central Ecuador. All parts exhibit typical freedom from insect damage.

L. chilense

One aspect usually observed in the autecology of *L. chilense* Dun., as well as certain other green-fruited species, is the intense activity of its pollinating insects (ref. 24 and Rick, unpublished). Not surprisingly, this feature is correlated with the self-incompatibility that controls the mating system in all tested biotypes of *L. chilense* (29), *L. hirsutum* f. *typicum* (20), and, with one reported exception (16), *L. peruvianum* (26), and in most tested races of *S. pennellii* (14).

Another manifestation of self-incompatibility is the low fruit set usually observed on single plants distantly isolated from other individuals (Fig. 4). Since this character is inherited in dominant fashion in crosses with the self-compatible *L. esculentum,* it markedly affects breeding operations in the F_1 and immediately segregating generations.

It has often been proposed that such self-incompatibility might be utilized to convert closely related autogamous species into cross-fertilizers as a means of expediting large-scale production of F_1 hybrid varieties. Martin (19, 21) explored this proposal by backcrossing self-incompatibility from *chilense* and *hirsutum* into *esculentum.* He discovered that the reaction was controlled by two independent major genes and polygenic modifiers. Although certain *S* alleles could be identified during the backcrossing, their effect became weakened, presumably by dilution of the nonrecurrent parent polygenes, and, anomalously, derivatives having different alleles failed to intermate. Similar diminution of the reaction was reported by Mather (22) for *S* alleles bred from *Petunia violacea* to *P. axillaris.*

Despite such discouraging experiences, Denna (7) has recently revived this proposal for producing cross-fertilizing lines of certain vegetable crops. The rewards for achieving such a goal would certainly justify intensive research efforts. Denna justifiably points out the related problems of improving systems of pollen transfer and restoring self-compatibility in F_1 hybrids of fruit or seed cultigens.

Another fascinating aspect of the autecology of *L. chilense* is its inhabiting the bottoms and slopes of *quebradas* in coastal southern Perú and northern Chile—one of the most arid of the world's temperate deserts. Whereas the more northerly habitat of *pennellii* receives sporadic moisture through movements of ground water, this desert is even dryer. Figure 4 illustrates that, although the *quebradas* may occasionally be flooded, *chilense* will live long afterward as the only surviving herbaceous plant species. As in the case of *pennellii,* we attempted to obtain measurements of native soil moisture but were completely thwarted by the very rocky nature of most habitats. It proved impossible to obtain soil samples at depths that *chilense* roots reach.

Although the nature of water relations in this species has not been properly investigated, we know that its drought resistance must be vested in different anatomical-physiological characters than those of *S. pennellii. L. chilense* actual-

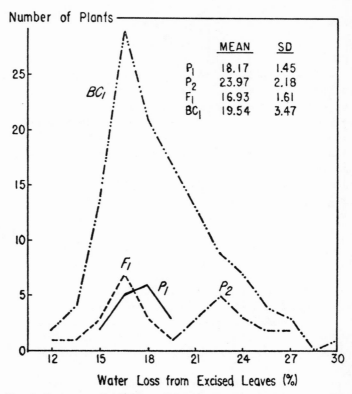

Fig. 6. Frequency distribution of the percent water loss from excised leaves of S. pennellii (P₁), L esculentum cv. VF-36 (P₂), F₁, and first backcross generation to P₂. Plants were grown in containers in the greenhouse. Proportion of water loss during 2-hr period is given. From Yu (39).

ly ranks far below *pennellii* and about the same as the other tomato species in the ability of either detached leaves or whole plants growing in containers to withstand desiccation. Its root system, furthermore, is well developed. It seems likely, accordingly, that the adaptation of *L. chilense* to the temperate deserts depends on the foraging ability of its root system. If this assumption is correct, the problem of assaying the drought tolerance in this species must be approached in a different fashion, possibly by measuring its reaction to high temperatures, as for *Zea* (17). To the best of my knowledge, the inheritance of various characters that affect water usage of *L. chilense* has not yet been studied.

Thus germ plasm with another, probably different, system of water economy is available for the plant breeder. In these days of increasing awareness of diminishing natural resources available for agriculture, it certainly behooves us to assay the potentialities of all such genetic reserves that might be exploited for better conservation of resources.

CONCLUSIONS

The wild species of tomato afford a potential source of many kinds of useful germ plasm. It is possible by casual study of their natural ecological relations to deduce certain genetic potentialities. Particularly in respect to their responses to the dramatic stresses extant in the western Andes, it has been possible to detect, among other characteristics, resistance to drought, excessive moisture and humidity, salinity, and predatory insects. Studies have been initiated on the measurement and genetic determination of these characteristics under cultural conditions. For the most part, their potential value for improvement of tomato cultivars remains to be determined, but the prospects for certain traits appear to be promising. Such genetic resources clearly deserve more intensive investigation than they are currently receiving.

ACKNOWLEDGMENTS

Support for part of the investigations by grants from the National Science Foundation and The Rockefeller Foundation is gratefully acknowledged. Progress in no small measure hinged on the devotion, intuition, and sharp eyes of my wife, Martha, who, despite frequent adversities, accompanied me on most of the travels incident to these studies. The list of other colleagues, whose aid was indispensable in myriad ways, is too long to be presented here; this regrettable circumstance in no way reflects the extent of my gratitude for their assistance.

REFERENCES

1. Alexander, L. J. (1963). Transfer of a dominant type of resistance to the four known Ohio pathogenic strains of TMV from *Lycopersicon peruvianum* to *L. esculentum*. *Phytopathology* **53**:869.
2. Andrus, C. F., and Reynard, G. B. (1945). Resistance to *Septoria* leaf spot and its inheritance in tomatoes. *Phytopathology* **35**:16-24.
3. Bohn, G. W., and Tucker, C. M. (1940). Studies on *Fusarium* wilt of the tomato. I. Immunity in *Lycopersicon pimpinellifolium* Mill. and its inheritance in hybrids. *Mis. Agr. Expt. Sta. Res. Bull.* **311**:1-82.
4. Chmielewski, T. (1962). Cytological and taxonomical studies on a new tomato form. I. *Genet. Polon.* **3**:253-264.
5. Chmielewski, T. (1968). New dominant factor with recessive lethal effect in tomato. *Genet. Polon.* **9**:39-48.
6. Chimielewski, T. (1968). Cytogenetical and taxonomical studies on a new tomato form. II. *Genet. Polon.* **9**:97-124.

7. Denna, D. W. (1971). The potential use of self-incompatibility for breeding F_1 hybrids of naturally self-pollinating vegetable crops. *Euphytica* **20**:542-548.
8. Downton, W. J. S. (1971). Adaptive and evolutionary aspects of C_4 photosynthesis. In Hatch, M. D., Osmond, G. B., and Slatyer, R. A. (eds.), *Photosynthesis and Photorespiration,* Symposium Proceedings, Interscience, New York, pp. 3-17.
9. Gentile, A. G., and Stoner, A. K. (1968). Resistance in *Lycopersicon* and *Solanum* species to the potato aphid. *J. Econ. Entomol.* **61**:1152-1154.
10. Gentile, A. G., and Stoner, A. K. (1968). Resistance in *Lycopersicon* spp. to the tobacco flea beetle. *J. Econ. Entomol.* **61**:1347-1349.
11. Gentile, A. G., Webb, R. E., and Stoner, A. K. (1968). Resistance in *Lycopersicon* and *Solanum* to greenhouse whiteflies. *J. Econ. Entomol.* **61**:1355-1357.
12. Gentile, A. G., Webb, R. E., and Stoner, A. K. (1969). *Lycopersicon* and *Solanum* spp. resistant to the carmine and two-spotted spider mite. *J. Econ. Entomol.* **62**:834-836.
13. Gilbert, J. C., and McGuire, D. C. (1956). Inheritance of resistance to severe root-knot from *Meloidogyne incognita* in commercial-type tomatoes. *Proc. Am. Soc. Hort. Sci.* **68**:437-442.
14. Hardon, J. J. (1967). Unilateral incompatibility between *Solanum pennellii* and *Lycopersicon esculentum. Genetics* **57**:795-808.
15. Hendrix, J. W., and Frazier, W. A. (1949). Studies on the inheritance of *Stemphyllium* resistance in tomatoes. *Hawaii Agr. Expt. Sta. Bull.* **8**:1-24.
16. Hogenboom, N. G. (1968). Self-compatibility in *Lycopersicum peruvianum* (L.) Mill. *Euphytica* **17**:220-223.
17. Hunter, J. W., Laude, H. H., and Brunson, A. M. (1936). A method for studying resistance to drought injury in inbred lines of maize. *J. Am. Soc. Agron.* **20**:694-698.
18. Kerr, E. A., and Bailey, D. L. (1964). Resistance to *Cladosporium fulvum* Cke. obtained from wild species of tomato. *Can. J. Bot.* **42**:1541-1554.
19. Martin, F. W. (1961). The inheritance of self-incompatibility in hybrids of *Lycopersicon esculentum* Mill. $\times$ *L. chilense* Dun. *Genetics* **46**:1443-1454.
20. Martin, F. W. (1963). Distribution and interrelationships of incompatibility barriers in the *Lycopersicon hirsutum* Humb. and Bonpl. complex. *Evolution* **17**:519-528.
21. Martin, F. W. (1968). The behavior of *Lycopersicon* incompatibility alleles in an alien genetic milieu. *Genetics* **60**:101-109.
22. Mather, K. (1943). Specific differences in *Petunia.* I. Incompatibility. *J. Genet.* **45**:215-235.
23. Ranson, S. L., and Thomas, M. (1960). Crassulacean acid metabolism. *Ann. Rev. Plant Phys.* **11**:81-110.
24. Rick, C. M. (1950). Pollination relations of *Lycopersicon esculentum* in native and foreign regions. *Evolution* **4**:110-122.
25. Rick, C. M. (1958). The role of natural hybridization in the derivation of cultivated tomatoes in western South America. *Econ. Bot.* **12**:346-367.
26. Rick, C. M. (1963). Barriers to interbreeding in *Lycopersicon peruvianum. Evolution* **17**:216-232.
27. Rick, C. M. (1971). Some cytogenetic features of the genome in diploid plant species. *Stadler Symp.* **2**:153-174.
28. Rick, C. M., and Khush, G. S. (1969). Cytogenetic explorations in the tomato genome. *Genet. Lect.* **1**:45-68.
29. Rick, C. M., and Lamm, R. (1955). Biosystematic studies on the status of *Lycopersicon chilense. Am. J. Bot.* **42**:663-675.
30. Rick, C. M., and Smith, P. G. (1952). Novel variations in tomato species hybrids. *Am. Naturalist* **87**:359-373.

31. Schaible, L., Cannon, O. S., and Waddoups, V. (1951). Inheritance of resistance to *Verticillium* wilt in a tomato cross. *Phytopathology* **41**:986-990.
32. Skrdla, W. H., Alexander, L. J., Oakes, G., and Dodge, A. F. (1968). Horticultural characters and reaction to two diseases of the world collection of the genus *Lycopersicon. Ohio Agr. Res. Sta. Res. Bull.* **1009**:1-110.
33. Stoner, A. K., and Gentile, A. G. (1968). Resistance of *Lycopersicon* species to the carmine spider mite, U.S.D.A. A.R.S. Prod. Res. Rept. No. 102, pp. 1-9.
34. Stoner, A. K., and Stringfellow, T. (1967). Resistance of tomato varieties to spider mites. *Proc. Am. Soc. Hort. Sci.* **90**:324-329.
35. Stoner, A. K., Webb, R. E., and Gentile, A. G. (1968). Reaction of tomato varieties and breeding lines to aphids. *HortScience* **3**:77.
36. Tal, M. (1971). Salt tolerance in the wild relatives of the cultivated tomato: responses of *Lycopersicon esculentum, L. peruvianum* and *L. esculentum minor* to sodium chloride solution. *Austral. J. Agr. Res.* **22**:631-638.
37. Webb, R. E., Stoner, A. K., and Gentile, A. G. (1971). Resistance to leaf miners in *Lycopersicon* accessions. *J. Am. Soc. Hort. Sci.* **96**:65-67.
38. Wiggins, I. L., and Porter, D. M. (1971). *Flora of the Galápagos Islands,* Stanford University Press, Stanford, Calif., 998 pp.
39. Yu, A. T. T. (1972). The genetics and physiology of water usage in *Solanum pennellii* Corr. and its hybrids with *Lycopersicon esculentum* Mill. Ph.D. thesis, University of California, Davis.

18

Chromosome Knob Patterns in Latin American Maize

Almiro Blumenschein

Instituto de Genética
E.S.A. "Luiz de Queiroz"
Universidade de São Paulo
Piracicaba, SP, Brazil

Although much has been written about the history of maize, important unanswered questions still remain. Some highly speculative studies have motivated new and intensive research, which has developed important information. Most of such studies are based on archeology, botany, genetics, geography, and history. Nevertheless, cytological data have been used, mainly those referring to the chromosome knobs.

The chromosome knobs are well-defined heterochromatic masses formed in the chromosomes of several species of grasses and other plant families. In maize, they can be formed in 21 different positions of the chromosomes; some plants are knobless and others can carry different numbers of knobs. The maximum so far reported was 18 knobs in one plant. The knobs vary in size from plant to plant but maintain their characteristics through the reproductive cycle of the plant and are normally inherited. In maize, the knob-forming positions may be interstitial or terminal.

Teosinte and *Tripsacum*, plants closely related to maize, also have chromosome knobs which vary in size. Teosinte, however, has more knob-forming positions than maize, and in *Tripsacum* the positions are mainly terminal.

According to the "tripartite theory" developed by Mangelsdorf and Reeves (5), the knobs from maize and teosinte originated from *Tripsacum* through crosses between *Tripsacum* and wild maize. Since *Tripsacum* has mainly terminal knobs and maize has several interstitial knobs, structural changes in the maize chromosomes would be expected according to this theory. Extensive work done

271

by Cooper and Brink (3) and Rhoades and Dempsey (9), however, did not show such changes.

Randolph (8) was uncertain about the value of the knob chromosomes as indicators of the importance of maize, teosinte, and *Tripsacum* hybridization for the development of the modern maize varieties. The *Tripsacum* diploid species do not occur in Central America, where the hybridizations were supposed to have happened.

Chromosome knob characteristics, mainly number, were used by several authors for the description of maize races in an extensive program supported by the National Academy of Sciences of the United States of America. McClintock's methodology (6, 7) in her maize chromosome knob studies offers more details and new concepts. She examined pachytene chromosomes from several plants collected in South, Central, and North America and determined the presence or absence of knobs in each of the several knob-forming positions. When the knob was present, it was classified by size, and whether the knob was formed in one or both of the homologous chromosome pairs was determined. The data thus obtained were plotted on a geographical map in such a way that the distribution of individual knobs and the pattern of variation of the several knobs in different regions could be observed.

McClintock was able to show clearly the influence of several germ plasms, characterized by the knob constitutions, on the origin of the races analyzed. She concluded that the geographical distribution of the knobs strongly suggests the derivation of the modern maize from several different centers.

THE KNOB COMPLEXES IN NORTH AND CENTRAL AMERICA

Using McClintock's methodology, T. A. Kato from CIMMYT, Mexico, and I developed studies on maize from the American continent. The work was advised by Dr. McClintock and supported by the Rockefeller Foundation and the CIMMYT. The publication of this work is expected in the near future. Here I will give a summary of the results obtained.

In this work, we tried to cover the largest possible geographical area. As much as feasible, we included samples from all the races collected in a same locality. In general, two to five plants from each sample were examined.

The data showed fundamental groups of knobs which are most frequent at their distribution center and show characteristic distribution patterns. These fundamental groups constitute the Chromosome Knob Complexes, and each characterizes a particular maize germ plasm.

The results obtained by Kato for the United States, Mexico, the Caribbean Islands, and Central America indicated the existence in these areas of seven knob complexes.

A group of knobs is distributed along the Pacific coast of Mexico and concentrated mainly in the race Zapalote Chico and to a lesser extent in the races Zapalote Grande and Bolita from the Oaxaca-Chiapas region. This group of knobs characterizes the Zapalote Chico Complex and is absent in almost all the rest of Mexico. It is found, however, in samples from the south Guatemala lowlands and in the northern countries of Central America. In South America, this germ plasm was introduced into Venezuela. Kato found the Zapalote Chico Complex very diluted in the eastern and western United States.

The Palomero Toluqueno Complex is concentrated in the race Palomero Toluqueno from the Central Mesa of Mexico. It spread to the neighboring regions, mainly toward the north, and was introduced into the United States, migrating toward the southwest of that country. It is also found in Guatemala, other countries from the upper part of Central America, in Venezuela, Colombia, and the Lesser Antilles.

The Pepitilla Complex is concentrated in Balsas basin, Mexico. It is relatively rare along the Pacific coast in northern Mexico but is found in the United States in Arizona, New Mexico, Oklahoma, and Texas and in Venezuela.

The South Guatemala Complex is concentrated in the lowlands of Guatemala and found in maize from the Yucatan peninsula, Chiapas, Oaxaca, Guerrero, the eastern coast of Mexico, the southeastern and southwestern United States, and northern Central America up to Costa Rica. It is also found in the Large Antilles, where it was probably introduced from northern Costa Rica.

A group of medium-sized knobs evolved on the eastern coast of Mexico and spread north, reaching the southern United States and south, reaching the Yucatan peninsula and northern Central America as far as the north of Costa Rica. From western Mexico, it was introduced into eastern Mexico spreading north along the coast. From Costa Rica, it was introduced into the Caribbean Islands and the region around Lake Maracaibo in Venezuela. This group of knobs is concentrated in the Tuxpeno race, and for this reason is called Tuxpeno Complex.

The Small Knob Complex evolved in the highlands of Guatemala and was introduced into the Mexican central mesa, spreading from there to the neighboring regions. From Guatemala, it was distributed south to the highlands of Panama. From Costa Rica, it was introduced into the Large Antilles and western Venezuela. From the Large Antilles, it spread through the islands toward the continent.

The Knobless Complex evolved in the Central Mesa in Mexico. It spread to the neighboring region and northern Mexico and was introduced into the eastern United States, where it spread west. It was also introduced into the highlands of Guatemala and Costa Rica, the Large Antilles, and western Venezuela. From the Large Antilles, it was distributed along the islands toward the continent.

THE KNOB COMPLEXES IN SOUTH AMERICA

Our results for South America show a completely different picture from that of North and Central America.

The Andean highlands is the center for the Andean Complex, characterized by a small knob in the long arm of chromosome 7 and a small knob in the third position of the long arm of chromosome 6. This complex spread into the South American lowlands in all directions, covering almost all the continent. In several places, however, it is "diluted" by other complexes centered in Venezuela and North and Central America.

The Venezuelan Complex is concentrated in central Venezuela and spread to Colombia, Panama, south Costa Rica, the Lesser Antilles, and the Guianas. It was introduced into southeastern Mexico, migrating from there north along the Pacific and Atlantic coasts and reaching the southeastern and southwestern United States. It also spread south to the lowlands of south Guatemala. The Venezuelan Complex seems to have been introduced directly into the Large Antilles from Venezuela. This complex was also introduced in a small area in eastern Brazil and in eastern Argentina, spreading from there north toward Uruguay. It is found in Equador and Bolivia, but the lack of data from southern Colombia and Peru makes it difficult to conclude whether this occurrence is a consequence of a migratory route from northern Colombia or Panama or of direct introduction. Nevertheless, the distribution of this complex, following an apparent line from northwest to southeast, suggests that the migratory route is more probable.

Palomero Toluqueno and Zapalote Chico Knob Complexes are found in one sample or a few samples of maize in Uruguay, Equador, and southeastern Bolivia. Probably they are isolated or accidental introductions.

The South Guatemala Complex was introduced in eastern Brazil, mainly in Pernambuco and Paraiba; it spread north and south along the São Francisco river and reached the north of Minas Gerais. It was also introduced in south Minas Gerais and the north of São Paulo in Brazil, spreading southwest to Paraguay. It was introduced into Rio Grande do Sul, Brazil, spreading north and south, and was also introduced in Uruguay, spreading toward Argentina.

The knobs of the Venezuelan and South Guatemala Complexes are almost all in common. As a matter of fact, their distribution can be distinguished only because of differences found in the distribution pattern of the small knob formed at the short arm of chromosome 1 (characteristic of the South Guatemala Complex) and the large knob formed at the long arm of chromosome 7 (characteristic of the Venezuelan Complex). In eastern South America, some of these common knobs follow the Venezuelan Complex and others the South Guatemala Complex, indicating that both complexes were introduced separately into this region.

The Tuxpeno and Small Knob Complexes follow similar distribution patterns in eastern South America. Both are found around the Amazon river mouth. In northeastern and eastern Brazil, they follow the same pattern described above for the South Guatemala Complex. They are, however, much more frequent than the South Guatemala Complex both in the number of samples and in the number of plants within the samples. Yet the Small Knob Complex is more frequent than the Tuxpeno Complex. The differences in frequency became more clear in the regions far from the coast. The South Guatemala Complex is mainly found in samples from flint maize (mainly *cateto* type), and the Tuxpeno and Small Knob Complexes are found in flint and floury maize (*caingang* and *avati moroti* races, which are local native races). Differently from the South Guatemala Complex, the Tuxpeno and Small Knob Complexes spread in southern Paraguay and were distributed north, reaching eastern Bolivia, northeast and northwest Mato Grosso, and the Rondônia and Acre regions in western Brazil. They are also found in the western Parana and the Small Knob Complex in the western Rio Grande do Sul.

Both complexes are found in eastern Argentina and are distributed north, reaching the border with Bolivia, and east, reaching Uruguay and Rio Grande do Sul in Brazil. In western South America, both complexes are found in Equador and Bolivia, following the migration route or the introduction pattern mentioned for the other complexes.

The presence of the Knobless Complex in South America is not clear, since the Andean Complex is mainly knobless. One possibility is to study the knobless condition in long arm of chromosome 7, since in the Andean Complex a small knob is always expected at this position. The Knobless Complex follows more or less the distribution pattern described for the Tuxpeno and Small Knob Complexes in the same area.

In Roraima, located in the north of Brazil, almost all the knob complexes are present. The kinds of knobs and their frequencies are very similar to those found in western Venezuela. The Roraima situation will certainly be clarified when more data are obtained for the Amazonia region. It seems reasonable to infer, however, that the Andean Complex is concentrated in this region, because the dominant races in this area belong to the interlocked group (2) which is pure Andean Complex. Whether other complexes were introduced into the area is still not known.

Chile is another complex area in South America. In the northern regions, the Andean Complex can be found almost pure; in the south, however, almost all complexes are present in a confused mixture.

THE ORIGIN OF MAIZE FROM EASTERN SOUTH AMERICA

There are some arguments about the origin of the yellow flint maize known as *cateto* which is found in the Caribbean Islands and on the Atlantic coast of South America. Around 1949, several authors believed that Brazilian or Argentinean *cateto* came from Italy. Brieger (1), however, argued against this idea. Although a tropical flint maize was introduced into Europe from Central America, it seems more logical that it was introduced into South America from the Antilles by the Arawak and Carib Indians during their migrations from the north along the eastern coast.

Hatheway (4) suggested a polyphyletic origin for the *cateto,* one origin in the Antilles and another in South America. Brieger *et al.* (2) observed that the *cateto* group reached its maximum development in southeastern Brazil, Uruguay, and Argentina, and the purest types are found in these locations. Based on these observations, they concluded that *cateto* originated in South America.

It is clear, however, from chromosome knob data that *cateto* is formed by the combinations of at least three germ plasms (Tuxpeno, South Guatemala, and Small Knob Complexes) which were introduced into eastern South America. The three germ plasms are also found in the Antilles in the tropical yellow flint. It seems reasonable to consider the Antilles as the original center for *cateto,* from which they were introduced into South America.

THE ORIGIN OF MAIZE

Based on what we have so far discussed, the modern races of maize seem to be derived directly from the nine knob complexes or from combinations of these complexes. Most of the complexes' centers are concentrated around southern Mexico, a fact which points to this region as the main center of origin for modern maize varieties. The Venezuelan Knob Complex could well be the result of a secondary evolutionary process. Historical, geographical, and morphological data provide some indication that the Andean Complex could have been derived from the Small Knob Complex of the highlands of Guatemala or Mexico.

Literature data indicate that different knob complexes can also be detected in teosinte and *Tripsacum.* The data obtained by Kato in Mexico suggest some relation between the origin of maize and origin of teosinte. More studies, mainly with teosinte, must be done, however, before definite conclusions can be made.

REFERENCES

1. Brieger, F. G. (1949). Origem e centro de domesticacao do milho II. Centros de domesticacao. Melhoramento. *Ciencia e Cultura* 1:191-201.
2. Brieger, F. G., Gurgel, J. T. A., Paterniani, E., Blumenschein, A., and Alleoni, M. R. B. (1958). Races of Maize in Brazil and Other Eastern South American Countries, Publication 593, National Academy of Sciences, National Research Council, Washington, D.C.
3. Cooper, D. C., and Brink, R. A. (1931). Cytological evidence for segmental interchange between non-homologous chromosomes in maize. *Proc. Natl. Acad. Sci.* 17:334-338.

4. Hatheway, W. H. (1957). Races of Maize in Cuba, Publication 453, National Academy of Sciences, National Research Council, Washington, D.C.
5. Mangelsdorf, P., and Reeves, R. G. (1939). The origin of Indian corn and relatives. *Texas Agr. Exp. Sta. Bull.* **574**:1-315.
6. McClintock, B. (1959). Genetic and cytological studies of maize. *Carnegie Inst. Wash. Yearbook* **58**:452-456.
7. McClintock, B. (1960). Chromosome constitution of Mexican and Guatemalan races of maize. *Carnegie Inst. Wash. Yearbook* **59**:461-472.
8. Randolph, L. F. (1955). Cytogenetic aspects of the origin and evolutionary history of corn. In Sprague, G. F. (ed.), *Corn and Corn Improvement,* Academic Press, New York, pp. 16-61.
9. Rhoades, M. M., and Dempsey, E. (1953). Cytogenetic effects of deficient duplicate chromosomes derived from inversion heterozygotes in maize. *Am. J. Bot.* **40**:405-424.

Population Genetics

19

Population Genetics in the American Tropics. IX. Rhythmic Genetic Changes That Prove the Adaptive Nature of the Detrimental Load in *Drosophila melanogaster* from Caracolisito, Colombia

H. F. Hoenigsberg, L.E. Castro, L.A. Granobles, and A. Saez

Instituto de Genética
Universidad de los Andes
Bogotá, D. E. Colombia

Our comparative genetic study with the second chromosome of *Drosophila melanogaster* from Hungary and Colombia (25) produced a quantitative appraisal of the detrimental, normal, subvital, and supervital loads. Results such as these lend support to the theory that the genetic characteristics of a gene pool reflect the ecological situation of the population. The most prominent and significant data in this direction were reported for populations of *D. pseudoobscura* on Mount San Jacinto in California (6,9,16), and of *D. pseudoobscura* and *D. persimilis* in Yosemite Park, California (7,8). These pioneering works and our present one detected changes in time. However, while Dobzhansky's shifts were described in terms of the relative frequencies of various karyotypes for which they were found to be polymorphic, our present report deals with genetic modifications in viability similar to those found in Fusagasugá (26). The profound changes in the organization of the genetic architecture found in Fusagasugá were caused by recurrent cycles of rainfall-bound seasons in the area. Our analysis revealed surprising shifts in the mean viability of homozygotes. Furthermore, a suggestive correlation appeared between rain cycles and the genetic load observed. If maximum and minimum temperatures had been used to describe the climatogical situation, as was done in the past, we would not have detected anything consistent with the cyclic shifts in lethals and semilethals. Other work (27) revealed that even within 7 months significant shifts in the sterility content in the second chromosome of *D. melanogaster* from Fusagasugá could be effected by the cyclic rainfall-bound seasons. Testing for heterogeneity among homozygotes of the different temporal populations showed the coexistence of a high- and a low-sterility group. Further partitioning of χ^2 in contingency tables revealed that through female sterility in the dry season and male sterility in the wet season the local demographic unit is altered. Still other works (21,22) have shown how even reforestation can produce profound genetic changes within a single area.

Moreover, results such as Wallace's (42–45), Dobzhansky's (ref. 10 and references therein), and ours (23,26) force us to regard the "load" in its possible adaptive role whenever analysis of the cumulative effects of the advantageous detrimentals is carried out. Only then will we uncover their relative importance to heterozygote fitness. On the other hand, in this chapter we endeavor to show new evidence of the ecological and genetic mutual dependency which is basic in understanding the adaptive role of many detrimental loci in natural populations.

MATERIALS AND METHODS

Since 1962, individual males of *D. melanogaster* collected in Caracolisito (Table I) have been brought to the laboratory and mated singly with CyL/Pm females (e.g., ref. 23). The F_1 heterozygous males are crossed again to six CyL/Pm females to use the resultant $CyL/+$ and $Pm/+$ heterozygous for the same wild chromosome in the F_2. The F_2 was made with five pairs of $CyL/+$ and

Table I. *D. melanogaster* Collections in Caracolisito[a]

Populations	Ecological conditions	Date
IIIb	Woods	Nov. 1, 1962
IVb	Woods	March 8, 1963
Vb	Wood cutting	May 11, 1963
VIb	Cotton plantation, pesticides	Nov. 16, 1963
VIII,IX	Cotton picking	March 6, 1966 and 1967
X	Cotton plantation, pesticides	June 6, 1967
XI	Cotton picking	May 6, 1968
XII	Cotton plantation, pesticides	Oct. 6, 1968
XIV	Cotton picking	June 10, 1969
XIII, XV	Cotton plantation, pesticides	April 4, 1969, and Sept. 22, 1969

[a] All collections were done during the dry season.

Table II. Detrimental and Quasi-Normal Chromosomes in the Homozygous Condition[a]

Caracolisito	N	Detrimentals					Quasi-normals								
		0	10	20	30	40	50	60	70	80	90	100	110	120	>120
IIIb	78	19	3	1	7	3	5	3	3	6	7	8	4	6	3
IVb	168	36	8	6	7	12	12	13	6	19	18	14	11	2	4
Vb	78	14	7	0	3	4	4	2	5	6	5	12	4	6	6
VIb	154	9	8	16	10	7	6	7	15	11	22	20	12	5	6
VIII	351	122	14	5	5	7	5	15	33	34	30	30	28	10	13
IX	281	106	1	2	5	9	9	20	13	20	20	26	17	12	21
X	295	52	40	27	24	26	27	21	10	14	20	8	11	9	6
XI	455	122	15	12	15	14	24	24	28	41	42	41	27	26	24
XII	437	104	2	7	8	12	22	37	50	63	50	27	21	16	18
XIII	369	175	1	2	8	10	14	18	26	20	31	20	16	15	13
XIV	347	147	1	3	5	1	8	13	13	32	46	33	25	12	8
XV	307	150	1	5	5	10	16	18	22	28	22	13	11	4	2
Totals	3320	1057	100	86	102	115	152	191	224	294	313	252	187	123	124

a The numbers from 0 to 120 in the head of the table represent the percent viability of the homozygous chromosomes in relation to the mean viability of the random combinations (heterozygotes) of the chromosomes from the same locality. N stands for the number of chromosomes tested each time.

Pm/+ in either experimental cultures (homozygotes) or controls (heterozygotes). The experimental cultures were those resulting from sib matings in the F_2, while the control ones resulted from crossing the F_2 males to unrelated females coming from different F_1 cultures. The resulting F_3 is made up of equal proportions of +/+, *CyL*/+, *Pm*/+, and *CyL*/*Pm* if the wild chromosome does not contain genes which decrease the viability of the homozygotes. The other kind of cross between unrelated *CyL*/+ and *Pm*/+ from different cultures produces the same genotypes, where one wild type $(+_x)$ is different from its homolog $(+_y)$. Three replicate cultures were made for the control and experimental crosses. Oviposition in each bottle continued for 48 hr. The cultures were maintained in incubators at 24°C, and three counts were made every 3 days after the first imagoes appeared.

Following Haldane's suggestion (18), the viability of *CyL*/*Pm* serves as control since these flies lack the wild chromosome. As shown in Table II, every viability class can be recognized in the homozygous and in the heterozygous condition. Therefore, combinations of detrimentals with normals in wild-type heterozygotes can be distinguished from the detrimental/detrimental and from the normal/normal combinations. Of course, each chromosome has to be marked beforehand. Moreover, as our crosses yield four distinct genotypes, we are in a position to identify the outcome of mutant combinations (*CyL*/+ or *Pm*/+) carrying a particular drastic (detrimental) or a particular normal homolog. For instance, the cross $CyL/+_i$ by $Pm/+_m$ can give $+_i/+_m$, $CyL/+_m$, $Pm/+_i$, and *CyL*/*Pm*. If $+_i$ is a normal (quasi-normal) and $+_m$ is a drastic, we can compare *CyL*/*D* and *Pm*/*N* which coexist in the same culture. We get the viability class which corresponds to each chromosome from the outcome of the experimental cultures. Then quasi-normals (*N*) and detrimentals (*D*, for lethals and semilethals together) can be accurately classified. Occasionally, heterozygous combinations (controls) may include two drastics which are lethals or semilethals. Such chromosomes are considered alleles and are removed from these data.

The chromosomes classified as lethals are those with 10% or less of the normal viability (38). The normal viability is by definition that observed in the control experiments. Semilethals are those chromosomes which in the homozygous condition produce from 10 to 50% of the normal viability. Subvitals are those chromosomes which in the homozygous state fall below 2 standard deviations of the mean viability of the heterozygotes. Supervitals are the chromosomes which in the homozygous condition stand above 2 standard deviations of the same mean heterozygote viability. Moreover, the normal chromosomes are those whose viability occupies the area between two limits as defined by the 2 standard deviations below and above the average viability. With these definitions, we calculate the estimated frequencies of subvital and of supervital chromosomes (*cf.* ref. 23).

The chromosomes which are neither lethals nor semilethals in the homozygous condition are called "quasi-normals." The viability of the homozygotes for quasi-normals includes chromosomes which are below the average normal viability of heterozygotes; therefore, some of the quasi-normals are subvitals while others may be normals and even supervitals (*cf.* refs. 11,12,47). The method is essentially a comparison of the total observed variances of the viabilities among the homozygotes in the quasi-normal class and the variances found among the heterozygotes. The sampling variance is that portion of the total variance which results from using different numbers of individuals in different cultures. The environmental variance, on the other hand, is the part of the total variance attributed to the fluctuations in viability found among the three replicate cultures. The difference between the total and the sum of the environmental and the sampling variances gives the real variance ascribed to genetic differences. With the standard deviation of the genetic variance, we estimate the frequencies of the different classes of quasi-normal chromosomes.

Caracolisito is a lowland and hot valley environment with about three rainy seasons per year. While collections III, IV, and V took place when some of the original wood was present, after the IV collection a great change occurred in the area because the jungle was cut and the area was used to grow cotton. Concomitant with the environmental change brought about by removing the original wood in the area, the rainy seasons changed to different dates and became less uniform. Before the cutting took place, the strong rains lasted for 2 hr at a time and the seasons recurred every 3–4 months: thus there were three rainy seasons per year. After the cutting was completed (October 1963), the rains lasted for 4–5 hr and their intensity became unpredictable. After 1964, we could count as many as four rainy seasons per year and as few as one real and complete rainy season. Furthermore, under such chaotic conditions some traps (Nos. VIII and IX) were totally wiped out by unexpected strong tropical rains during a normally dry period. New traps were placed, and a good dry season collection was picked within the dry season sampling. Before our XIVth collection (May 1969), strong rains flooded our collecting area (a small patch 10 by 10 m in diameter) and we had to wait for the next month's dry season to set in (June 1969). All our collections were done during the dry season in order to balance the rainy variable already studied in Fusagasugá (26). Our intention is to concentrate on the floral changes brought about by the new cotton growth produced in the valley. Our traps are always made up of *Musea sapientum* (bananas), *Carica papaya* (papayas), *Citrus sinensis* (oranges), and *Mangifera indica* (mangoes). They are put in the same area about 1 month before the collection begins and at weekly intervals for a full month to attract all the possible representatives of the area. The collecting site is under the shade of fruiting trees (mangoes), and therefore it is always a good *Drosophila* breeding ground.

RESULTS

The frequency distributions of the two most important viability classes are assembled in Table II. In a frequency *vs.* viability graph, a typical bimodal curve results, with one peak at the lethal level and another peak at the quasi-normal level. This is true both for the first environment (the original woods) and for the

Table III. Percentages of Lethals and Drastics in the Second Chromosomes of *D. melanogaster* from Caracolisito[a]

Populations	N	Percent lethals	Percent drastics
IIIb	78	28.20 ± 5.095	48.72 ± 5.518
IVb	168	26.19 ± 3.394	48.21 ± 3.855
Vb	78	26.92 ± 5.022	41.02 ± 5.569
VIb	154	11.04 ± 2.525	36.36 ± 3.876
VIII	351	38.75 ± 2.601	45.01 ± 2.655
IX	281	38.08 ± 2.896	46.97 ± 2.977
X	295	31.19 ± 2.697	66.44 ± 2.749
XI	455	30.11 ± 2.151	44.40 ± 2.329
XII	437	24.26 ± 2.050	35.47 ± 2.289
XIII	369	47.70 ± 2.600	56.91 ± 2.576
XIV	347	42.65 ± 2.655	47.55 ± 2.681
XV	307	49.19 ± 2.853	60.91 ± 2.784
Unweighted means	3320	34.85 ± 0.2615	48.55 ± 0.2743

[a] N stands for the number of chromosomes tested. The standard deviation is multiplied by 10^{-2}.

Table IV. Percent of Semilethal and Quasi-normal Chromosomes in Samples of *D. melanogaster* at Different Times but in the Same Site in Caracolisito over a 7-year span[a]

Populations	N	Percent semilethals	N	Percent quasi-normals
IIIb	38	20.52	40	51.28
IVb	81	22.02	87	51.79
Vb	32	14.10	46	58.98
VI	56	25.32	98	63.64
VIII	158	6.27	193	54.99
IX	132	8.89	149	53.03
X	196	35.25	99	33.56
XI	202	14.29	253	55.60
XII	155	11.21	282	64.53
XIII	210	9.21	159	43.09
XIV	165	4.90	182	52.45
XV	187	11.72	120	39.09
Unweighted means	1608	13.70	1712	51.57

[a] N stands for the number of chromosomes sampled each time.

second environment (the cotton plantation). But important differences must be considered: while populations from the first environment (III, IV, and V) produced from 26 to 28% lethals, the other populations (apart from VI, which felt the first impact) disclosed from 31 to 50% (approximately). Population XII produced lethals which are below the mark for both groups (*cf.* Table III). Table III indicates the percentage of lethals and drastics for each population under observation. One item is interesting: while populations coming from the first environment (natural woods) have a relatively uniform percentage of lethals, the populations from the second environment (artificial) produce large fluctuations both in lethals and in total drastics. Table IV presents the percentage of semilethals and quasi-normals in the same site over the years. This table shows similar results and conclusions, namely, uniform percentage for the populations of the first environment and large fluctuations for the second environment. The

Table V. Mean Viability of the Wild-Type Class of Second Chromosomes
of *D. melanogaster* from Caracolisito

Populations	N^a (homo).	Homozygotes	N	Heterozygotes
		With detrimentals		
IIIb	78	15.97 ± 1.3466	93	27.72 ± 0.6125
IVb	168	16.16 ± 0.8676	177	28.92 ± 0.4728
Vb	78	16.74 ± 1.3220	80	26.23 ± 0.5186
VIb	154	19.18 ± 0.8734	164	28.92 ± 0.4352
VIII	351	14.22 ± 0.6282	321	26.50 ± 0.3023
IX	281	13.56 ± 0.6902	259	23.73 ± 0.2972
X	295	11.07 ± 0.5643	224	25.97 ± 0.5419
XI	455	15.47 ± 0.5352	427	25.78 ± 0.2962
XII	437	17.69 ± 0.5181	421	27.42 ± 0.3672
XIII	369	11.57 ± 0.5874	328	25.27 ± 0.3408
XIV	347	12.14 ± 0.5955	315	24.68 ± 0.3349
XV	307	10.46 ± 0.5993	288	27.14 ± 0.3794
		Without detrimentals		
IIIb	40	24.77 ± 0.9344	93	27.72 ± 0.6125
IVb	88	24.18 ± 0.5859	175	28.80 ± 0.4597
Vb	46	24.49 ± 0.7875	80	26.23 ± 0.5186
VIb	98	25.58 ± 0.5703	163	29.05 ± 0.4280
VIII	194	22.72 ± 0.3935	321	26.50 ± 0.3023
IX	149	21.78 ± 0.5550	259	23.73 ± 0.2966
X	99	22.52 ± 0.5936	221	26.05 ± 0.5394
XI	255	23.23 ± 0.3769	427	25.78 ± 0.2962
XII	284	22.72 ± 0.3473	413	26.90 ± 0.3407
XIII	159	22.27 ± 0.4776	323	25.31 ± 0.3336
XIV	182	22.01 ± 0.3307	309	24.59 ± 0.3244
XV	120	21.62 ± 0.4288	287	26.81 ± 0.3772

[a] Number of chromosomes tested.

significant level of the differences among the various populations grouped according to cotton growth and collection is shown in Table XIV and will be discussed later. The mean viability of the wild-type class of second chromosomes of these populations is shown in Table V. As expected from previous tables, the homozygotes (which contain lethals and semilethals) coming from the natural environment remain approximately the same, while the others fluctuate in a rhythmic cycle that can best be shown for detrimentals in χ^2 figures of Table XIV. From Table V, we can appreciate the rhythmic changes: starting with a high mean viability of about 19% in VI, we get 14–13 and 11% approximately by VIII, IX, and X, high again (around 15.5–18%) in XI and XII, low again in XIII–XIV (11.5–12%), and lowest in XV (around 10%).

The lower part of Table V presents the average viability of the wild-type class, after detrimentals are removed. The results are startling. While populations from the natural environments have mean viabilities for homozygotes around 24%, those from the artificial environment have means around 22%. The two groups are significantly different (Table VI).

In Table VII, the observed, environmental, sampling, and real variances are presented. These variances are essential to calculate the percentages of quasi-normal chromosomes. As expected from theory (31), homozygous variances are larger than for the more buffered heterozygous. Since one of the replicates from III, IV, V, and VI was lost due to carelessness, those populations do not have environmental variances. Table VIII presents the frequency distribution of quasi-normals. As expected, subvitals and normal chromosomes are more fre-

Table VI. Significance of Differences of Mean Viabilities Between the Observed Mean and the Expected Mendelian Value for the Second Chromosomes of the Wild-Type Class of *D. melanogaster* [a]

Populations	$\overline{X}$ (obs.)	d	S_d	$n-1$	t	P
IIIb	0.2477	0.0023	0.009344	39	0.2461	0.50
IVb	0.2418	0.0082	0.005859	87	1.3995	0.10–0.20
Vb	0.2449	0.0051	0.007875	45	0.6476	0.50
VIb	0.2558	0.0058	0.005703	97	1.0170	0.30–0.40
VIII	0.2272	0.0228	0.004089	193	5.5759	<0.001
IX	0.2178	0.0322	0.005550	148	5.8018	<0.001
X	0.2252	0.0248	0.005936	98	4.1778	<0.001
XI	0.2323	0.0177	0.003769	254	4.6962	<0.001
XII	0.2272	0.0228	0.003473	283	6.5649	<0.001
XIII	0.2227	0.0273	0.004776	158	5.7160	<0.001
XIV	0.2201	0.0299	0.003307	181	9.0414	<0.001
XV	0.2162	0.0338	0.004288	119	7.8824	<0.001

[a] These results exclude detrimental chromosomes, and the S_d (standard error of the difference) is that of the total variance observed for the various populations.

quent than supervitals. Here again, as in previous tables, normals and subvitals from natural environments are more or less uniform (45–49%), while populations from the unnatural agricultural environment fluctuate considerably: from 48 to 88% among the normals and from 12 to about 50% among the subvital chromosomes. As for the homozygote viabilities, we find even greater cyclic fluctuations for normals on subvitals coming from artificial environments, i.e., from VI to XV (*cf.* Table VIII).

The rate of elimination of "detrimentals" through homozygosis can be calculated by multiplying the frequency of lethals and semilethals in drastic/

Table VII. Total, Environmental, Sampling, and Genetic Variances of the Various Temporal Populations of Caracolisito[a]

Caracolisito	S_T^2	S_e^2	S_s^2	S_g^2
Homozygous				
IIIb	142.19	—	11.81×10^{-8}	142.19
IVb	125.45	—	3.15×10^{-8}	125.45
Vb	136.42	—	14.10×10^{-8}	136.42
VIb	117.60	—	3.65×10^{-8}	117.60
VIII	138.54	0.4121	0.51×10^{-8}	138.13
IX	133.40	0.2289	0.89×10^{-8}	133.18
X	93.61	0.4386	$0.41 \times 10^{'8}$	93.17
XI	130.34	0.1181	0.40×10^{-8}	130.22
XII	117.31	1.6449	0.75×10^{-8}	115.67
XIII	127.31	1.3567	0.75×10^{-8}	125.95
XIV	123.04	2.7635	0.65×10^{-8}	120.28
XV	110.25	0.3359	0.59×10^{-8}	109.92
Heterozygous				
IIIb	34.89	—	12.71×10^{-8}	34.89
IVb	39.57	—	3.35×10^{-8}	39.57
Vb	21.50	—	1.63×10^{-8}	21.50
VIb	31.03	—	3.36×10^{-8}	31.03
VIII	29.34	0.1604	0.78×10^{-8}	29.18
IX	22.79	1.2117	1.31×10^{-8}	21.58
X	65.80	1.5833	1.44×10^{-8}	64.22
XI	37.47	1.9166	0.57×10^{-8}	36.90
XII	56.77	2.3389	0.86×10^{-8}	55.91
XIII	38.09	0.1966	1.57×10^{-8}	36.52
XIV	35.34	1.6700	1.38×10^{-8}	33.96
XV	41.46	4.2540	1.34×10^{-8}	37.21

[a] The numbers should be multiplied by 10^{-4} except the sampling variance. We are including lethal and semilethal chromosomes.

Table VIII. Percentages of "Quasi-normal" Chromosomes in Caracolisito

Caracolisito	Percent normals	Percent subvitals	Percent supervitals
IIIb	47.5	49.6	2.9
IVb	49.2	49.6	1.2
Vb	45.3	49.2	5.5
VIb	84.9	12.3	2.8
VIII	52.7	44.8	2.5
IX	48.5	46.8	4.7
X	88.0	11.9	0.1
XI	54.3	43.3	2.4
XII	67.7	31.2	1.1
XIII	54.5	44.4	1.1
XIV	51.8	46.8	1.4
XV	66.3	33.4	0.3

drastic (D/D) combinations by the frequency of drastics squared in the same populations. In other words, these heterozygous combinations in which both chromosomes are classified as drastics in their homozygous state and which produce lethality are obviously eliminated in such individuals. If we multiply such a number by the square of the frequency which the drastics have in homozygous lines, we get the proportional number eliminated as homozygotes (A. H. Sturtevant, cited in ref. 14). Table IX summarizes those results.

Table X indicates the relative contributions of each combination to the heterozygote viability shown in Table XI for the quasi-normals present in each population. While it is the D/D heterozygous combinations that sometimes produce a higher average viability, at other times it is the D/N or N/N combinations. Others (2,30) have found similar results for natural populations and even for irradiated artificial populations. This latter kind of work (45) revealed an increase in viability for heterozygotes for two detrimental chromosomes, in marked contrast with other but not strictly comparable investigations documented by Crow *et al.* (e.g., ref. 20).

The relative fitness of the mutants heterozygous for $CyL/+$ or Pm against CyL/Pm is shown in Table XII. The heterozygotes have either a "normal" or a detrimental chromosome. As expected, $Pm/+$ individuals are better competitors than $CyL/+$ individuals. In general, the quasi-normal heterozygous mutants prove to have a higher adaptive value than those carrying detrimentals. Nevertheless, in some cases (XII, XIV, and XV) the heterozygotes for drastics scored better adaptive points (see *Discussion*).

Table XIII shows the general test for homogeneity of all our populations. This table, which shows a χ^2 of 11.31 for 11 degrees of freedom, indicates that

Table IX. Combined Elimination of Detrimentals Through
Near-Lethal Combinations

	Rate of elimination of "drastics" through homozygosis[a]		
Populations	D/D	(frequency of D)^2	Rate of elimination
IIIb	0.0206	0.2374	0.0049
IVb	0.0111	0.2268	0.0025
Vb	0.0122	0.1683	0.0021
VIb	0.0060	0.1322	0.0008
VIII	0.0061	0.2000	0.0012
IX	0.0038	0.2206	0.0085
X	0.1107	0.4414	0.0489
XI	0.0115	0.1932	0.0022
XII	0.0047	0.1226	0.0006
XIII	0.0030	0.3251	0.0010
XIV	0.0308	0.2261	0.0070
XV	0.0170	0.3710	0.0063
Grand average	0.0192	0.2345	0.0045

	Rate of elimination of drastic genes through their heterozygote carriers in drastic/normal combinations		
	Frequency of drastics (q)	$q(1-q)$	Frequency of drastics in D/N combination	Rate of elimination
IIIb	0.4872	0.2498	0.0103	0.0026
IVb	0.4762	0.2494	0.0055	0.0014
Vb	0.4102	0.2419	0.0122	0.0030
VIb	0.3636	0.2314	0.0060	0.0014
VIII	0.4501	0.2475	0.0152	0.0038
IX	0.4697	0.2491	0.0114	0.0028
X	0.6644	0.2230	0.0344	0.0077
XI	0.4395	0.2463	0.0023	0.0006
XII	0.3524	0.2282	0.0095	0.0022
XIII	0.5691	0.2452	0.0091	0.0022
XIV	0.4755	0.2494	0.0185	0.0046
XV	0.6091	0.2381	0.0034	0.0008
Grand average	0.4843	0.2498	0.0113	0.0028

[a] D stands for drastics (lethals and semilethals combined).

all our temporal populations result from a single statistical universe. However, when confronted populations are compared for single degrees of freedom according to the cotton growth and picking cycles referred to in Table I, the rhythmic changes in terms of significant comparisons appear to full extent (*cf.*

Table X. Relative Contributions of Each Genotype (*D/D*, *D/N*, and *N/N*) to Each of the Heterozygote Experiments

Population	Quasi-normals			Drastics		
	D/D	*D/N*	*N/N*	*D/D*	*D/N*	Σ(total)
IIIb	0.3299	0.3711	0.2680	0.0206	0.0103	0.9999
IVb	0.2389	0.4555	0.2833	0.0055	0.0111	0.9943
Vb	0.1585	0.3902	0.4268	0.0122	0.0122	0.9999
VIb	0.1145	0.4277	0.4337	0.0060	0.0060	0.9879
VIII	0.1860	0.4543	0.3323	0.0061	0.0152	0.9939
IX	0.2053	0.4715	0.3042	0.0038	0.0114	0.9962
X	0.4046	0.3588	0.0878	0.1107	0.0344	0.9963
XI	0.1778	0.4226	0.3857	0.0115	0.0023	0.9999
XII	0.1214	0.3976	0.4667	0.0095	0.0047	0.9999
XIII	0.2165	0.4817	0.2896	0.0030	0.0091	0.9999
XIV	0.1785	0.5015	0.2708	0.0308	0.0185	0.9999
XV	0.2891	0.5170	0.1701	0.0170	0.0034	0.9976

Table XI. Average Viability Contributed by Each Genotype (*D/D*, *N/D*, and *N/N*) in the Heterozygous Combination Used in These Experiments[a]

Population	*D/D*	*D/N*	*N/N*
IIIb	0.2594 ± 0.0105	0.2817 ± 0.0120	0.2677 ± 0.0123
IVb	0.2996 ± 0.0086	0.2884 ± 0.0070	0.2716 ± 0.0066
Vb	0.2493 ± 0.0095	0.2557 ± 0.0121	0.2630 ± 0.0078
VIb	0.3022 ± 0.0105	0.2929 ± 0.0061	0.2843 ± 0.0340
VIII	0.2530 ± 0.0057	0.2563 ± 0.0053	0.2632 ± 0.0061
IX	0.2454 ± 0.0080	0.2268 ± 0.0042	0.2388 ± 0.0050
X	0.2489 ± 0.0074	0.2525 ± 0.0089	0.2800 ± 0.0222
XI	0.2468 ± 0.0064	0.2591 ± 0.0050	0.2538 ± 0.0045
XII	0.2720 ± 0.0095	0.2636 ± 0.0051	0.2696 ± 0.0052
XIII	0.2557 ± 0.0086	0.2529 ± 0.0049	0.2483 ± 0.0065
XIV	0.2445 ± 0.0066	0.2403 ± 0.0041	0.2470 ± 0.0069
XV	0.2738 ± 0.0066	0.2664 ± 0.0051	0.2633 ± 0.0090
Unweighted means	0.2594 ± 0.0025	0.2576 ± 0.0017	0.2605 ± 0.0020

[a] Only quasi-normal combinations are included.

Table XIV). We have the plantation growing after population V. Samples III and IV originate from the natural environment (the original woods) and score a low χ^2; VI, when the plantation and pesticides begin, produces a high χ^2; VIII and IX are at cotton-picking time and score a low χ^2; X is a population coming from a plantation growth where pesticides are used and produces a high χ^2; XI represents a cotton-picking environment and produces a low χ^2; XII corresponds

Table XII. Competitive Ability of the Mutant Heterozygotes for Lethals, Drastics, and Quasi-Normal Chromosomes[a]

Populations	Lethals		Drastics		Quasi-normals	
	Pm/+	CyL/+	Pm/+	CyL/+	Pm/+	CyL/+
IIIb	1.1477	1.0830	1.2141	1.1621	1.3890	1.2399
IVb	1.2127	1.1016	1.2848	1.1331	1.3541	1.1623
Vb	1.1196	1.3122	1.0685	1.2181	1.4149	1.2214
VIb	1.3905	1.3611	1.2979	1.1164	1.4046	1.1298
VIII	1.0216	1.0460	1.0244	1.0691	1.0302	1.1545
IX	0.9848	0.9661	1.0030	0.9941	1.0549	1.0114
X	1.1253	1.3238	1.1116	1.3296	1.3379	1.6145
XI	1.0364	0.8886	0.9963	0.9156	1.0489	1.0591
XII	1.1581	0.9869	1.1608	1.0638	1.1460	1.1542
XIII	1.0320	0.9926	1.0316	1.0008	1.0382	1.0400
XIV	1.1367	1.1537	1.1314	1.1504	1.0585	1.0593
XV	1.1884	1.1003	1.1870	1.1007	1.1873	1.1449
Unweighted means	1.1295 ± 0.0346	1.1097 ± 0.0139	1.1259 ± 0.0096	1.1045 ± 0.0100	1.2054 ± 0.0148	1.1659 ± 0.0144

[a] Each ⊕ or + is the same for each viability class (Pm or CyL). These data come from the homozygous (experimental) lines where +/+, Pm/+, CyL/+, and CyL/Pm are expected. As CyL/Pm individuals lack the + chromosome, we have used their viability to provide relative fitness of the mutant heterozygotes in the same vial, e.g., Pm/+ individuals divided by CyL/Pm and CyL/+ individuals divided by the same CyL/Pm of that vial.

Table XIII. General χ^2 Table to Test the Homogeneity of the Temporal
Populations present in Caracolisito[a]

Populations	Detrimentals (x_j)	Normals $(n_j - x_j)$	Totals (n_j)	$p_j = x_j/n_j$	$(p_j)(x_j)$
IIIb	38	40	78	0.4871	18.5098
IVb	81	87	168	0.4821	39.0501
Vb	32	46	78	0.4102	13.1264
VIb	56	98	154	0.3636	20.3616
VIII	158	193	351	0.4501	71.1158
IX	132	149	281	0.4697	62.0004
X	196	99	295	0.6644	130.2224
XI	202	253	455	0.4439	89.6678
XII	155	282	437	0.3546	54.9630
XIII	210	159	369	0.5691	119.5110
XIV	165	182	347	0.4755	78.4575
XV	187	120	307	0.6091	113.9017
	1612	1708	3320	5.7794	810.8875

[a] $p = 0.4855$, $q = 0.5145$. $\chi^2 = \dfrac{(\Sigma x_j\, p_j - \hat{p}\, \Sigma x_j)}{(\hat{p}\, \hat{q})} = 11.31$.

Table XIV. Confronted Populations by Partitioning χ^2 in Contingency
Tables According to the Ecological Changes in Caracolisito

Confronted populations	df	χ^2	P
A. III, IV *vs.*			
V, VI, VIII, IX, X, XI, XII, XIII, XIV, XV	1	0.2598	0.50–0.70
B. VI *vs.*			
III, IV, V, VIII, IX, X, XI, XII, XIII, XIV, XV	1	9.4235	0.01
C. VIII, IX *vs.*			
III, IV, V, VI, X, XI, XII, XIII, XIV, XV	1	2.3442	0.10–0.20
D. X *vs.*			
III, IV, V, VI, VIII, IX, XI, XII, XIII, XIV, XV	1	41.1705	0.01
E. XI *vs.*			
III, IV, V, VI, VIII, IX, X, XII, XIII, XIV, XV	1	3.6140	0.05–0.10
F. XII *vs.*			
III, IV, V, VI, VIII, IX, X, XI, XIII, XIV, XV	1	34.2638	0.01
G. XIV *vs.*			
III, IV, V, VI, VIII, IX, X, XI, XII, XIII, XV	1	0.3459	0.50–0.70
H. XV, XIII *vs.*			
III, IV, V, VI, VIII, IX, X, XI, XII, XIV	1	35.1677	0.01
I. Within III, IV	1	0.0016	0.95–0.98
J. Within VIII, IX	1	0.2585	0.50–0.70
K. Within XIII, XV	1	1.2141	0.20–0.30
Totals	11	11.31	0.50–0.30

to plantation growth and use of pesticides and results in a high χ^2; XIV is the result of cotton picking in the area and produces, as expected, a low χ^2; XIII and XV correspond to plantation growth and pesticides and, as expected, produce a high χ^2. In other words, certain characteristics of the agricultural treatment of the surrounding environment result in rhythmic changes in detrimentals that prove their adaptive nature! We do not know, however, which of the ecological variables may be interacting with the local genotypes. Perhaps the periodic use of pesticides changes the effective breeding size to exert the selection-dependent demographic challenge that causes the cyclic changes reported here.

DISCUSSION

The cyclic genetic changes brought about by recurrent man-made ecological modifications in Caracolisito over a 7-year span have been demonstrated in the previous section.

In this part of the chapter, we shall discuss some of the effects produced by the genetic loads on their carriers. The need for brevity forces us to refer to a previous paper (26) for more extensive discussion of this important but confusing topic. Moreover, additional results (Hoenigsberg et al., unpublished) which will appear elsewhere will allow us to discuss more thoroughly the role of the genetic load in natural populations.

Perhaps any work on population genetics today gives a distorted view of the strength of selection acting on alternative alleles. Moreover, the documentation on strongly selected polymorphisms has revealed the wealth of genetic and environmental instruments by which alleles may be balanced in a population. Nevertheless, we still have only hazy ideas about which balancing mechanisms are most prevalent, in part because a great many of these ideas are based either on theoretical models using unrealistic parameters or on experimental set-ups whose conditions are artificial, although highly imaginative (e.g., refs. 35–37).

Despite considerable criticism of Fisher's fundamental theorem of natural selection (e.g., refs. 1,15,32,33,40,41), at least in Drosophila, populations tend toward the maintenance of an average fitness when a single genetic locus is considered to be under constant genotypic selection. In Drosophila, we have all noted that fitness measured as viability, population size, egg productivity, and developmental or genetic homeostasis increases under the action of selection.

In reference to drastic alleles, the relatively high proportion of detrimentality in natural populations has usually been explained in one of two ways: (a) that an appreciable fraction of the deleterious genes or even of deleterious chromosomes is due to their heterotic effect in conditions of balanced polymorphism which allow for high allelic substitution because of high initial and final frequencies and (b) that the genetic load produced by unselected mutations persists until population-size dependent homozygosity eliminates it. When recessives penetrate in heterozygotes, elimination occurs in both homozygotes and heterozygotes (5).

When or if the first condition does not operate to maintain an allele, even if only slightly important to fitness, many individuals will be lost because they do not possess the new allele (19). This is Kimura's (28, 29) "substitutional load." However, when such mutations are beneficial when heterozygous there will result an accumulation of even advantageous detrimentals. Conversely, consistently deleterious alleles will be eventually eliminated (46).

Works by Morton *et al.* (34) and Hiraizumi and Crow (20) have contributed the most to the erroneous assumption that most lethals or even detrimentals formed in natural populations are harmful in heterozygotes (*cf.* ref. 5). Accordingly, those detrimentals are subject to prompt elimination by homozygosis. However, Crow's works have the serious drawback that they were done with artificial laboratory conditions and cultures and therefore with unnatural genetic backgrounds. In fact, their 2.6% reduction (which turns out to be even more) of preadult viability, slower development, and decrease in fecundity and longevity of the heterozygous carriers were scored for individuals with different cinnabar and brown genetic backgrounds. As laboratory cultures have their own long-standing adaptability, it is not surprising that through ecological load (called "environmental misplacement load" by Dobzhansky and Spassky in ref. 13) and even through segregational load they could present a reduced fitness in new environments and crosses. We do not mean that there is no elimination through heterozygosis (Table IX demonstrates its possibility). However, the conclusion that most lethals and semilethals found in natural populations are detrimental in heterozygotes is unwarranted (*cf.* Tables XI and XII).

Many newly arisen mutations are likely to be deleterious in heterozygous combinations. Before such heterozygotes are totally eliminated, the so-called detrimental alleles have time to get into adaptable permutations that may make them fit population-wise, even though singly and in certain combinations they may prove to be inferior mixers. For the preservation of such "deserving" alleles, epistatic modifiers tend to accumulate and modify the previously unfavorable fitness of deserving alleles toward a favorable one that maintains them at least by virtue of their heterotic advantage. The hypothesis implicit in such an interpretation can be verified by scoring the viability values of induced mutations both at the beginning and after several generations. Wallace (45) obtained results that confirm the increasing heterotic values of "early" induced drastics. Furthermore, most such studies have been carried out on the basis of whole chromosomes and not individual gene loci. It is worthwhile to consider the possibility that if such structural heterozygotes were desynthesized the separate parts might turn out to have lesser effects on viability. Such considerations emphasize that particular viabilities may often be conditioned by the appropriate genotypic background or ecological circumstances.

A study of Table XII shows that there are populations (III, IV, VIII, IX, X, XI, and XIII) in which the structural heterozygotes (CyL/+ or Pm/+) for quasi-normals (those wild types within 2 standard deviations above and below the mean, plus the genetic elite that stand more to the right of 2 standard deviations above the mean) have superior fitness to that of the structural heterozygotes (D/+, where + is a drastic, i.e., lethal or semilethal) for drastics. Indeed, such cases are the majority, as expected on the assumption by Crow (3) and Crow and Temin (5) that recessive lethals from nature have deleterious effects as heterozygotes because of their ever-present penetrance.

Moreover, and notwithstanding some recent models (e.g., ref. 35) which claim a 3% reduction in heterozygotes' fitness using Nei's γ-distribution, some populations (V, VI, XII, and XIV) produce structural heterozygotes for drastics (D/+, in which the + chromosome is a lethal or a semilethal) which have a fitness superior to that of those carrying normals and the genetic elite. Why has it been that detrimentals which in homozygotes are lethals do not cripple their carriers in their heterozygous condition? Moreover, if our natural drastics are the result of recurrent mutations which are eventually destined to be wiped out in homozygous combinations, why are they more adaptive in some combinations (e.g., in Table XII see populations V and VI for CyL/+ and populations III and IV for Pm/+) and in some populations? Furthermore, Table XII also demonstrates that even within a single culture (as our methods permit us to observe) certain populations show better fitness belonging to those CyL/+ carrying drastics, rather than to their CyL/+ counterparts carrying quasi-normals (see populations, V, VI, and XIV in that table). These questions can be resolved, as proposed by Dobzhansky (10), by assuming that newly arising mutations range in their heterozygous effects from deleterious, to near neutral, to downright heterotic.

The changes which we have now reported reflect the magnitude of selective forces which appear as responses to environmental fluctuations to which each deme adapts even by using its labile genetic load. We have found that the gene pool is able to place different fitness values in different heterozygous combinations (CyL/+ or Pm/+ as the case may be) to change in the desirable direction. However, the full role of the various genetic loads (mutational or the various balanced loads) is still unclear, and much information is still needed to understand their dynamics in population genetics.

ACKNOWLEDGMENTS

The authors are grateful to COLCIENCIAS (Colombian National Science Foundation) for their partial support of this work.

REFERENCES

1. Arunachalam, B. (1970). Fundamental theorem of natural selection in two loci. *Ann. Hum. Genet. (Lond.)* 34:195-199.
2. Band, H. T., and Ives, P. T. (1962). Correlation between heterozygote and homozygote viabilities and the nature of the genetic load in a natural population of *Drosophila melanogaster. Rec. Genet. Soc. Am.* 31:72.
3. Crow, J. F. (1963). The concept of genetic load: A reply. *Am. J. Hum. Genet.* 15:310-315.
4. Crow, J. F., and Morton, N. E. (1955). Measurement of gene frequency drift in small populations. *Evolution* 9:202-214.
5. Crow, J. F., and Temin, R. G. (1964). Evidence for the partial dominance of recessive lethal genes in natural populations of *Drosophila. Am. Naturalist* 98:21-33.
6. Dobzhansky, T. (1947). A directional change in the genetic constitution of a natural population of *Drosophila pseudoobscura. Heredity* 1:53-64.
7. Dobzhansky, T. (1952). Genetics of natural populations. XVI. *Evolution* 6:234-243.
8. Dobzhansky, T. (1956). Genetics of natural populations. XXV. *Evolution* 10:82-92.
9. Dobzhansky, T. (1958). Genetics of natural populations. XXVII. *Evolution* 12:385-401.
10. Dobzhansky, T. (1964). How do the genetic loads affect the fitness of their carriers in *Drosophila* populations? *Am. Naturalist* 98:151-166.
11. Dobzhansky, T., and Spassky, B. (1953). Genetics of natural populations. XXI. Concealed variability in two sympatric species of *Drosophila. Genetics* 38:471-484.
12. Dobzhansky, T., and Spassky, B. (1954). Genetics of natural populations. XXII. A comparison of the concealed variability in *Drosophila prosaltans* with that of other species. *Genetics* 39:472-487.
13. Dobzhansky, T., and Spassky, B. (1963). Genetics of natural populations. XXXIV. Adaptive norm, genetic load and genetic elite in *Drosophila pseudoobscura. Genetics* 48:1467-1485.
14. Dobzhansky, T., and Wright, S. (1941). Genetics of natural populations. V. Relations between mutational rate and accumulation of lethals in populations of *Drosophila pseudoobscura. Genetics* 26:23-51.
15. Edwards, A. W. F. (1967). Fundamental theorem of natural selection. *Nature* 215:537-538.
16. Epling, C., and Lower, W. R. (1957). Changes in the inversion system during a hundred generations. *Evolution* 11:248-258.
17. Fisher, R. A. (1930). *The Genetical Theory of Natural Selection,* Oxford University Press, London.
18. Haldane, J. B. S. (1956). The estimation of viabilities. *J. Genet.* 54:294-296.
19. Haldane, J. B. S. (1957). The cost of natural selection. *J. Genet.* 55:511-524.
20. Hiraizumi, Y., and Crow, J. F. (1960). Heterozygous effects on viability, fertility, rate of development and longevity of *Drosophila* chromosomes that are lethal when homozygous. *Genetics* 45:1071-1083.
21. Hoenigsberg, H. F. (1968). Rate of elimination of natural lethals. *Am. Naturalist* 102:185-187.
22. Hoenigsberg, H. F. (1968). An ecological situation which produced a change in the proportion of *Drosophila melanogaster* to *Drosophila simulans. Am. Naturalist* 102:389-390.
23. Hoenigsberg, H. F., and de Navas, Y. G. (1965). Population genetics in the American tropics. I. Concealed recessives in different bioclimatic regions. *Evolution* 19:506-513.
24. Hoenigsberg, H. F., Castro, L. E., and Granobles, L. A. (1968). Population genetics in

the American tropics. III. The genetic role of heterozygous individuals in various Colombian populations of *D. melanogaster. Evolution* **22**:66-75.

25. Hoenigsberg, H. F., Castro, L. E., Granobles, L. A., and Idrobo, J. M. (1969). Population genetics in the American tropics. II. The comparative genetics of *Drosophila* in European and neo-tropical environments. *Genetica* **40**:43-60.

26. Hoenigsberg, H. F., Granobles, L. A., and Castro, L. E. (1969). Population genetics in the American tropics. IV. Temporal changes effected in natural populations of *Drosophila melanogaster* from Colombia. *Genetica* **40**:201-215.

27. Hoenigsberg, H. F., Castro, L. E., and Granobles, L. A. (1969). Population genetics in the American tropics. V. The sterility content in the second chromosomes of *Drosophila melanogaster* from Fusagasuagá, Colombia. *Genetica* **40**:543-554.

28. Kimura, M. (1960). Optimum mutation rate and degree of dominance as determined by the principle of minimum genetic load. *J. Genet.* **57**:21-34.

29. Kimura, M. (1961). Natural selection as a process of accumulating genetic information in adaptive evolution. *Genet. Res.* **2**:127-140.

30. Krimbas, C. B. (1959). Comparison of the concealed variability in *Drosophila willistoni* with that in *Drosophila prosaltans. Genetics* **44**:1359-1370.

31. Lerner, I. M. (1954). *Genetic Homeostasis.* John Wiley, New York.

32. Li, C. C. (1967). Fundamental theorem of natural selection. *Nature* **214**:505-506.

33. Mandel, S. P. H. (1968). Fundamental theorem of natural selection. *Nature* **220**: 1251-1252.

34. Morton, N. E., Crow, J. F., and Muller, H. J. (1956). An estimate of the mutational damage in man from data on consanguineous marriages. *Proc. Natl. Acad. Sci. (USA)* **42**:855-863.

35. Murata, M. (1970). Frequency distribution of lethal chromosomes in small populations of *Drosophila melanogaster. Genetics* **64**:559-571.

36. Nei, M. (1968). The frequency distribution of lethal chromosomes in finite populations. *Proc. Natl. Acad. Sci. (USA)* **60**:517-524.

37. Nei, M. (1969). Heterozygous effects and frequency changes of lethal genes in populations. *Genetics* **63**:669-680.

38. Pavan, C., Cordeiro, A. R., Dobzhansky, T., Dobzhansky, N., Malogolowkin, C., Spassky, B., and Wedel, M. (1951). Concealed genetic variability in Brazilian populations of *Drosophila Willistoni. Genetics* **36**:13-30.

39. Simpson, G. G. (1953). *The Major Features of Evolution,* Columbia University Press, New York.

40. Turner, J. R. G. (1967). Fundamental theorem of natural selection. *Nature* **215**:1080.

41. Turner, J. R. G. (1970). Changes in mean fitness under natural selection. In Kojima, K. (ed.), *Mathematical Topics in Population Genetics,* Springer-Verlag, Berlin.

42. Wallace, B. (1956). Studies on irradiated populations of *Drosophila melanogaster. J. Genet.* **54**:280-293.

43. Wallace, B. (1958). The average effect of radiation induced mutations on viability in *Drosophila melanogaster. Evolution* **12**:532-556.

44. Wallace, B. (1959). The role of heterozygosity in *Drosophila* populations. *Proc. Xth Internat. Congr. Genet.* **1**:408-419.

45. Wallace, B. (1962). Temporal change in the roles of lethal and semilethal chromosomes within populations of *Drosophila melanogaster. Am. Naturalist* **96**:247-256.

46. Wallace, B. (1965). The viability of spontaneous mutations in *Drosophila melanogaster. Am. Naturalist* **99**:335-348.

47. Wallace, B., and Madden, C. (1953). The frequencies of sub- and supervitals in experimental populations of *Drosophila melanogaster. Genetics* **38**:456-470.

Applications of Genetics

20

Breeding for Specific Amino Acids

Oliver E. Nelson, Jr.

Laboratory of Genetics
University of Wisconsin
Madison, Wisconsin, U.S.A.

The demonstration that single-gene substitutions can result in marked increases in the content of the limiting essential amino acids for nutrition of humans or monogastric animals has been made for maize (6,12) and barley (9). It is then naturally a question of the extent of our ability to manipulate the amino acid content of economically important plants. Could one enhance the content of any desired amino acid in any plant tissue? The answer to this question clearly is negative, and the reasons for so concluding are the subject of this chapter. They constitute an essential background for any investigator interested in the improvement of plant protein quality. Understanding the severe restrictions on the system allows a reasonable estimation of the probability of success. The restrictions to which I refer take this form: The primary sequence (the order of amino acids) of a polypeptide chain is specified by the structural gene for that polypeptide in the DNA codescript. Decoding takes place through transcription into an RNA intermediate and translation into a polypeptide chain via ribosome-based protein synthesis. Because the sequence is specified, polypeptide chains synthesized on the same RNA message are identical, barring the occurrence of relatively infrequent mistakes in translation.

The majority of the proteins in most tissues have a role to play either catalytically or structurally, and their amino acid sequences have evolved to permit them to carry out this role effectively. Thus it is that proteins such as cytochrome *c,* hemoglobins, or histone IV can be shown either to be identical or to embody relatively minor differences in amino acid sequence in organisms that are quite different. The functional role of proteins is a conservative force with regard to amino acid substituions. Further, such aberrations in the protein-synthesizing system as an amino acid activating enzyme that attached an amino acid to a tRNA species recognizing the messenger RNA code word for another amino acid would almost certainly be lethal. These and additional reasons for concluding that the amino acid content of functional proteins cannot be altered sufficiently to make any significant impact on the nutritional quality of the collective proteins of a plant tissue have been considered at greater length (11).

In contrast to the functional proteins of most plant tissues, the seeds of many plant species contain large quantities of metabolically inert storage proteins that serve as a reservoir of readily available reduced nitrogen for the embryo during germination. Osborne (13) and his collaborators played a key role in the characterization of storage proteins. Osborne divided the seed proteins into the albumin, globulin, prolamine, and glutelin fractions on the basis of solubility. The albumins and globulins, which are the protein fractions soluble in water and dilute salt solution, respectively, contain the enzymatic proteins. In addition, the bulk of the storage proteins in the legumes are found in the globulin fraction. The prolamines, soluble in 70% ethanol, and the glutelins, soluble in dilute alkali, contain only storage protein. These latter two fractions comprise the greater part of the protein synthesized in the endosperm of various cereals. In maize, for example, the prolamine fraction contains approximately 60% of the total protein of the endosperm and the glutelin fraction about 32%. By contrast, the albumin and globulin fractions together contain only about 6% of the total protein (4).

In addition to the investigations of the biochemical properties of the storage proteins, Osborne and his collaborators also demonstrated the poor nutritive quality for monogastric animals of some of these storage protein fractions from cereals. Osborne and Mendel (15,16) found that rats of any age would go into a rapid decline and ultimately die on diets in which protein was solely the alcohol-soluble fraction (zein) of maize seeds. On the other hand, when lysine and tryptophan were added to the diet, rats grew at nearly normal rates. Osborne and Leavenworth (14) had previously shown that zein contains no lysine. This brief example utilizing maize proteins indicates the basis of the nutritive inadequacy for humans or monogastric animals of all the cereals in which the prolamine fraction is large. In maize, more than half of the endosperm protein is this fraction, with a negligible content of two essential amino acids, lysine and tryptophan. Therefore, the proteins of the endosperm collectively are markedly deficient in these two amino acids. The prolamine fractions of other cereals may differ with respect to lysine content, but in none is the content adequate (8).

A former colleague, E. T. Mertz, and I instituted attempts in 1963 to identify mutations that would disqualify the seeds carrying them from producing the prolamine fraction with the hope that other protein fractions of greater nutritive value would be enhanced. My initial choice of experimental material was fortunate since two of the first four mutants investigated, *opaque-2* and *floury-2,* proved to have a lysine content approximately 100% higher than common maize (6,12). The tryptophan content was shown to be increased by the same factor (12). Table I gives the amino acid composition of the total endosperm proteins of normal, *opaque-2,* and *floury-2* maize following hydroly-sis of the proteins. It should be noted that other amino acids are changed in quantity when the mutants are compared to normal. Aspartate, glycine, and arginine also are increased markedly in the mutants, while the contents of glutamate, leucine, and alanine are decreased. Additionally, there is a notable increase in methionine in *floury-2.* The amino acid composition of the embryos in the three genotypes is not altered. It should be mentioned also that recently McWhirter (5) has isolated a third mutation in maize, *opaque-7,* that effects changes in amino acid composition similar to those effected by *opaque-2.*

Jiménez (4) has studied the effect of these mutations on the production of storage proteins, and his results are shown in Table II. Clearly, synthesis of the alcohol-soluble fraction has not been completely blocked, but synthesis is markedly depressed with a concomitant increase in the albumin and globulin fractions. The change in the overall amino acid composition of these mutants

Table I. Amino Acid Content[a]

Amino acid	W64A +	W64A o_2	fl$_2$	W22 o_7,[b]	W22 +[b]
Lysine[c]	1.6	3.7	3.4	3.8	2.3
Tryptophan[c]	0.3	0.7	0.9	0.7	0.4
Arginine	3.4	5.2	4.3	5.2	3.7
Aspartate	7.0	10.8	10.9	9.4	6.7
Glutamate	26.0	19.8	20.6	25.5	27.4
Glycine	3.0	4.7	3.7	5.2	4.0
Alanine	10.1	7.2	8.6	7.9	8.5
Cysteine	1.8	2.0	1.6	1.9	2.4
Methionine[c]	2.0	1.8	3.4	3.2	3.2
Isoleucine[c]	4.5	3.9	4.2	4.3	4.3
Leucine[c]	18.8	11.6	13.9	12.5	15.9
Tyrosine	5.3	3.9	4.7	4.9	5.8
Phenylalanine[c]	6.5	4.9	5.4	5.2	6.7
Percent protein	12.7	11.1	13.6	7.3	8.5

[a] In g/100 g protein. The values are given only for the amino acids where the mutant content differs from normal.

[b] Data from Misra *et al.* (7).

[c] Amino acids essential for human nutrition.

Table II. Solubility Fractions of Endosperm Proteins from Various Maize Genotypes, Together with the Lysine Content of These Fractions[a]

Fraction		+ Per 10 g defatted endosperm[d]	+ Per endosperm	o^2 Per 10 g defatted endosperm	o^2 Per endosperm	fl_2 Per 10 g defatted endosperm	fl_2 Per endosperm	o_7[b] % saline extractable
H_2O (protein)	Mg	46.8 (3.8)[d]	0.81	96.0 (3.7)[d]	1.21	73.6 (3.4)[d]	0.76	
	%[c]	3.3		7.7		5.8		
H_2O (A.A.)	Mg	7.0	0.11	56.5	0.71	49.7	0.50	16.6
	%[c]	0.5	4	4.5		3.9		
5% NaCl	Mg	28.2 (5.0)	0.48	64.3 (5.6)	0.81	92.6 (6.0)	0.95	
	%[c]	2.2		5.7		8.4		
70% ETOH	Mg	775.2 (0.2)	13.34	288.5 (0)	3.6	370.7 (0.1)	3.80	20.3
	%[c]	59.4		25.4		33.4		
0.2% NaOH	Mg	447.6 (3.2)	7.70	629.0 (4.5)	7.9	521.3 (4.4)	5.35	60.3
	%	34.3		55.4		47.0		
Residue	Mg	47.9 (2.7)	0.82	56.6 (2.9)	0.71	182.9 (2.2)	1.88	
	%[c]	3.4		4.5		14.3		
Total protein recovered	Mg	1352.7	23.3	1190.9	15.0	1290.8	13.24	
	%	96.1		94.9		101.2		

[a] From the data of J. Jiménez.

[b] Data from Misra et al. (7).

[c] Percent total N found in this fraction.

[d] Percent lysine of the fractions. For the water-soluble fraction, this is the lysine content of proteins and free amino acids combined.

can be accounted for by the change in the relative proportions of the solubility fractions together with the change in the composition of the *opaque-2* glutelin fractions. Similar results have been reported by Mossé (8). Misra *et al.* (7), in fractionation studies of *opaque-7* endosperm, also reported similar results for that mutant.

The other species in which simply inherited variants enhance the lysine content is barley, *Hordeum vulgare.* Munck *et al.* (10) reported such a mutation in an Ethiopian barley accession, while Doll (2) has isolated several higher lysine mutants following ethyl methanesulfonate mutagenesis. In these instances, it appears that the observed changes are a consequence of shifts in the relative proportions of the storage proteins (3,9). The Risφ mutant 1508, which has a lysine content 50% higher than its parental variety, has an albumin plus globulin content that is 46% of the total nitrogen and a prolamine content that is 9% of total nitrogen. The parental variety had an albumin plus globulin content that was 27% and a prolamine content that was 27% of total protein. The glutelin content was 39% of total nitrogen for both mutant and parental strains (Ingversen, Köie, and Doll, manuscript in preparation).

The amino acid composition of seeds may also be altered by changes in the relative proportions of various tissues that contain quite different species of proteins. For example, the proteins of the embryo in all cereals contain adequate quantities of lysine and tryptophan, and any increase in embryo size relative to the endosperm will result in an increase in lysine and tryptophan content (11). Such shifts can be carried to impractical extremes, as in certain starch-synthesizing mutants of maize (7). These mutants synthesize only a fraction of the starch synthesized in normal seeds. As the amount of starch decreases, so does the amount of the storage proteins, although the mechanism is not understood. The size of the embryo in these mutant seeds, however, is not decreased. Therefore, the more extreme the mutant in loss of starch-synthesizing capabilities, the larger the proportion of the total seed protein that is supplied by the endosperm albumins and globulins and by the embryo proteins and the higher the lysine becomes (stated as a percent of protein or as percent of total dry weight). The total amount of carbohydrate, protein, or lysine per plant, however, is much less for the mutants than for normal.

Other possibilities exist for alterations in the normal proportions of tissues within a seed. Wolf *et al.* (19) have reported in maize a dominant gene that conditions an aleurone layer two to four cells rather than one cell in thickness, as is characteristic of ordinary maize. In addition, the multilayer aleurone may have a higher protein content stated as a percentage of aleurone weight. The lysine content (as a percentage of protein) in endosperms plus aleurones from multilayered seeds was higher (approximately 0.2% units) than in endosperms plus aleurones from single-layered seeds. Our own data with the same gene substantiate the conclusion that a multilayer aleurone is inherited as though conditioned by a single dominant gene. Further, the changes in content of the basic amino acids effected by the gene are in the same direction as those effected by *opaque-2* and further enhance the effect of *opaque-2* (Table III).

Most of the amino acids present in mature seeds are peptide bound. In the mature endosperm of normal maize, for example, between 0.05 and 0.1% of the amino acids are free. The small size of the pool, which consists largely of the simpler amino acids, indicates that synthesis of the amino acids is regulated by their requirement for protein synthesis. In bacterial systems, mutants exist that have lost the ability to respond to the usual signals that repress enzyme synthesis or in which an altered enzyme is not inhibited by the factors that inhibit the normal enzyme. This loss of responsiveness to control mechanisms results in overproduction of the amino acid which is the end product of that particular biosynthetic sequence. Such mutations have rarely been identified in higher plants, although Widholm (18) has reported a 5-methyltryptophan-resistant culture of *Nicotiana tabacum* cells. The basis of this resistance is an altered anthranilate synthetase which is not inhibited by L-tryptophan or 5-methyltryptophan to the extent that the normal enzyme is. Anthranilate synthetase is believed to be a key regulatory enzyme for tryptophan biosynthesis, and it is significant that cells of this mutant line have a pool of free tryptophan ten times that in normal cells. There is no report to date of plants reconstituted from this mutant cell clone. It would be useful to know what the effect of the mutation on the growth of the sporophyte might be.

Mutants of this type, releasing synthesis of a particular amino acid from the usual regulatory restraints, would constitute, if viable and healthy, a possible means of increasing the quantity of a particular amino acid in a plant tissue (11). One laboratory is making a systematic investigation of the possibility of increasing lysine content by such means (1). Since bacteria and higher plants apparently synthesize lysine by similar pathways (from aspartate via dihydrodipicolinic and diaminopimelic acids), the question that has been asked is how many mutations are necessary to produce lines that are resistant to an inhibitory lysine analog, S-(β-aminoethyl)-cysteine, in *Escherichia coli.* This analog was also shown to be inhibitory to the growth of barley seedlings. The results indicate that two separate mutations are required to convert *E. coli* into an overproducer of lysine. One mutation affects the aspartate kinase allozyme that is specifically inhibited by lysine, and the other affects the dihydrodipicolinic acid synthetase. The necessity of obtaining two separate mutations for lysine overproduction is a reflection of the branched pathway for lysine synthesis with feedback inhibition by lysine operating at two separate steps. If the same steps in lysine biosynthesis in higher plants are key regulatory steps, then the necessity for two independent mutations to provide the biochemical background for lysine overproduction would obtain in plants as well.

Assuming the ability to produce and identify these mutants in higher plants,

Table III. Protein and Lysine, Arginine, Leucine, and Glutamate Content of the Endosperms of Segregates from (C12 o_2/o_2 × Mo 316 ae/ae) ⊗

Kernel type		Percent protein	Percent lysine[a]	Percent arginine[a]	Percent leucine[a]	Percent glutamate[a]
3418-1+/+	I[b]	13.8	1.5	2.8	14.3	20.3
+/+	III[c]	13.8	1.5	2.9	14.2	20.4
o_2/o_2	I	11.3	3.3	4.1	10.1	19.6
o_2/o_2	III	11.5	3.5	4.6	10.0	19.2
3418-2+/+	I	11.6	1.7	2.9	14.0	20.5
+/+	III	11.7	1.9	3.3	14.4	21.4
o_2/o_2	I	10.6	3.6	4.4	10.2	18.9
o_2/o_2	III	10.6	3.8	4.6	9.8	18.7
3418-3+/+	I	12.0	1.7	2.9	14.1	20.5
+/+	III	12.1	1.7	2.9	14.3	20.9
o_2/o_2	I	10.2	3.7	4.6	9.8	17.9
o_2/o_2	III	10.3	4.1	5.1	9.6	17.0
3418-1-2, -3	ae/ae I	13.6	2.1	3.2	13.7	20.1
	ae/ae III	13.5	2.3	3.4	13.6	20.2

[a] As a percentage of protein.

[b] One aleurone layer.

[c] Two to three aleurone layers.

it is not yet clear what effect such lysine overproduction would have on the growth of the sporophytic generation or even whether plants carrying such mutations would be viable. If they are healthy, a further point of uncertainty is whether such overproduction by the plant would be reflected in the grain produced by that plant. Sodek and Wilson (17) injected either ^{14}C-lysine or ^{14}C-leucine into the stalks of selfed heterozygous $(+/o_2)$ plants at various time intervals after pollination and then examined the label in the kernels of each phenotype at harvest. When the label was injected at 23 days after pollination and the ears were harvested 24 days later, 97% of the recovered label in both types of kernels after ^{14}C-leucine injection was in the form of leucine. When ^{14}C-lysine was injected, however, 90% of the recovered label was in lysine in opaque kernels but only 53% in normal kernels. The remainder was in the form of proline or glutamate. Since only small quantities of the amino acids were injected, the results suggest that even if a lysine overproducer was detected in one of the cereals the presence of a gene such as *opaque-2*, which conditions greater synthesis of relatively lysine-rich proteins, might be required for realization of maximum potentialities for lysine content of the seeds.

The investigations to date indicate the complexities of attempting to enhance specifically the quantity of a particular amino acid by altering the regulatory processes affecting its synthesis. Feasibility studies such as that of Brock *et al.* (1) are necessary to indicate the potentialities of such an approach and should be encouraged.

Briefly, I have endeavored to show why our knowledge of the genetic control of protein structure requires that marked changes in the overall amino acid composition of a seed arise from shifts in the proportion of the normally synthesized proteins without changes in the primary sequence of these proteins. Such shifts can be genically mediated in the seeds of many plants where large quantities of storage proteins are synthesized. A second and less effective method of affecting amino acid composition is to change the proportion of tissues that contain protein populations which are quite disparate in their amino acid composition. Limitations to the magnitude of changes effected by this approach are obvious. A corollary of this conclusion as to the origin of changes in amino acid composition is that the probability of effecting changes in plant tissues such as leaves, in which most proteins synthesized are functional, is low indeed.

There remains the possibility of enhancing the quantity of a given amino acid by a mutation or mutations rendering inoperative the regulatory mechanisms on its biosynthetic pathway. Studies on such mutants in higher plants are not sufficiently advanced to allow an estimate of probable success.

REFERENCES

1. Brock, R. D., Friederich, E. A., and Langridge, J. (1972). The modification of amino acid composition of higher plants by mutation and selection. In *Proceedings of the FAO/IAEA/GSF Meeting on Nuclear Techniques for Seed Protein Improvement,* Neuherberg, June 26-30, 1972, IAEA, Vienna, pp. 329-338.
2. Doll, H. (1971). Variation in protein quantity and quality induced in barley by EMS treatment. In *Proceedings of the Latin America Meeting on Induced Mutations and Plant Improvement,* IAEA/FAO, Vienna.
3. Ingversen, J., Andersen, A. J., Doll, H., and Köie, B. (1972). Selection and properties of high lysine barleys. In *Proceedings of the FAO/IAEA/GSF Meeting on Nuclear Techniques for Seed Protein Improvement,* Neuherberg, June 26-30, 1972, IAEA, Vienna, pp. 193-198.
4. Jiménez, J. R. (1966). Protein fractionation studies of high lysine corn. In Mertz, E. T., and Nelson, O. E. (eds.), *Proceedings of the High Lysine Corn Conference,* Corn Industries Research Foundation, Washington, D.C., pp. 74-79.
5. McWhirter, K. S. (1971). A floury endosperm, high lysine locus on chromosome 10. *Maize Genet. Coop. News Letter* 45:184.
6. Mertz, E. T., Bates, L. S., and Nelson, O. E. (1964). Mutant gene that changes protein composition and increases lysine content of maize endosperm. *Science* 145:279-280.
7. Misra, P. S., *et al.* (1972). Endosperm protein synthesis in maize with increased lysine content. *Science* 176:1425-1426.
8. Mossé, J. (1966). Alcohol-soluble proteins of cereal grains. *Fed. Proc.* 25:1663-1669.
9. Munck, L. (1972). Barley seed proteins. In *Proceedings of the American Chemical Society Symposium on Seed Proteins,* Los Angeles, March 29, 1971 (in press).
10. Munck, L., Karlsson, K. E., Hagberg, A., and Eggum, B. O. (1970). Gene for improved nutritional value in barley seed protein. *Science* 168:985-987.
11. Nelson, O. E. (1969). Genetic modification of protein quality in plants. *Advan. Agron.* 21:171-194.
12. Nelson, O. E., Mertz, E. T., and Bates, L. S. (1965). Second mutant gene affecting the amino acid pattern of maize endosperm proteins. *Science* 150:1469-1470.
13. Osborne, T. B. (1924). *The Vegetable Proteins,* 2nd ed., Longmans, Green, New York.
14. Osborne, T. B., and Leavenworth, C. S. (1913). Do gliadin and zein yield lysine on hydrolysis? *J. Biol. Chem.* 14:481-487.
15. Osborne, T. B., and Mendel, L. (1914). Nutritive properties of proteins of the maize kernel. *J. Biol. Chem.* 18:1-6.
16. Osborne, T. B., and Mendel, L. (1916). The amino-acid minimum for maintenance and growth as exemplified by further experiments with lysine and tryptophane. *J. Biol. Chem.* 25:1-12.
17. Sodek, L., and Wilson, C. M. (1970). Incorporation of leucine-^{14}C and lysine-^{14}C into protein in the developing endosperm of normal and *opaque-2* corn. *Arch. Biochem. Biophys.* 140:29-38.
18. Widholm, J. M. (1972). Cultured *Nicotiana tabacum* cells with an altered anthranilate synthetase which is less sensitive to feedback inhibition. *Biochim. Biophys. Acta* 261:52-58.
19. Wolf, M. J., Cutler, H. C., Zuber, M. S., and Khoo, U. (1972). Maize with multilayer aleurone of high protein content. *Crop. Sci.* 12:440-442.

21

Genetic Manipulation of Plant Protein Quality and Its Value in Human Nutrition

Alberto Pradilla and C. A. Francis

Centro Internacional de Agricultura Tropical (CIAT)
and
Unidad Metabólica
Universidad del Valle
Cali, Colombia

The "green revolution" is causing an increase in production of major cereal crops in the developing tropics and in some cases may contribute to a reduction in quality of the consumer's diet due to better availability of cereal grains and fewer legumes and other crops. This may be aggravated as well by changes in the relative prices of alternative food sources as a result of increased cereal production and diversion of land and resources from the more protein-rich legume species. A new "quality revolution" is the next frontier for improving cereal grain crops.

Changes in human dietary habits are relatively simple in developed countries where communications and advertising systems are competing for an educated audience. This communication process is practically unknown for rural and subsistence-level families in the developing tropics. Technological advances are slow to come to the pueblo. Therefore, genetic improvement of cereal protein quality must be associated with two essential factors: equal or better yield of the crop relative to existing varieties and a kernel color and grain type essentially equal to that of the existing varieties. This resemblance to the commonly accepted maize in terms of endosperm and/or other phenotypic traits in a specific zone or region is critical to immediate acceptance of the new product.

The improvement of nutritional quality of cereals was given a new impulse when Mertz *et al.* (1) described the amino acid changes caused by the *opaque-2*

Table I. Chemical Analysis of Different Phenotypic Combinations

Variety	Color	Phenotype	Lys.	Tript	Nitrogen	Fractions					Recovery
						1	2	3	4	5	
1. H. 208	Yellow	Soft	4.13	0.95	1.44	23.63	15.89	22.77	18.47	15.45	96.21
2. Calca	Yellow	Soft	1.90	0.38	1.10	7.24	41.89	20.17	9.21	18.10	96.61
3. H.208 Pinzon	Yellow	Hard	3.24	0.80	1.36	13.02	26.57	8.89	25.55	25.55	97.71
4. H.207	Yellow	Hard	1.84	0.37	1.67	17.14	39.35	10.20	10.14	22.70	99.53
5. H.255 Pinzon	White	Soft	3.24	0.78	1.33	22.33	14.40	13.78	10.33	33.93	94.77
6. PMC 561	White	Soft	1.97	0.36	1.02	11.86	40.54	20.34	11.43	10.09	94.26
7. H.253	White	Hard	2.75	0.77	1.78	15.32	24.95	18.32	8.82	30.55	98.46
8. H.253	White	Hard	1.63	0.38	1.30	5.74	44.31	23.90	9.24	16.26	99.72

and *floury-2* genes in maize. The incorporation of these genes in tropical varieties produces a similar effect (2). There are enough essential amino acids in 155 mg of *opaque-2* maize protein for maintenance of children 24–36 months old, if total nitrogen intake is not the first limiting factor (3).

In spite of the improved nutritional quality of this maize, the associated soft endosperm characteristics have limited its wider utilization. Since 1968 in the first crops of H208 and H255 in Colombia there were segregant kernels with floury, semifloury, and dent phenotypes. The yellow H208 segregated a higher number of modified kernels, and its quality was more consistently high than that of the white hybrid maize, H255 (4). Protein quality evaluation of both phenotypes was very similar in soft and hard types in one early trial in Colombia (5). By analysis and selection of segregating kernels with good quality, genetic selection and inbreeding are being carried out. There is also an awakening interest in determining the gene action and biochemical processes responsible for phenotypic characteristics and the quality of the protein in maize, thus facilitating the screening for both.

In the latest phase of this research, different maize hybrids and varieties with both high and low protein quality and both hard and soft phenotypes are being analyzed. Results from white *vs.* yellow, hard *vs.* soft, and poor *vs.* high quality (based on lysine-tryptophan content) in all combinations are presented here.

METHODS

Five grams of endosperm from each sample was analyzed for lysine, tryptophan, and protein content, and a complete aminogram was made. Protein fractionation of albumins, globulins, zeins, and glutelins (fractions 1, 2, and 3) was performed following the Laudry–Moureaux method.

For microscopic examination of the endosperm, frozen sections of the whole grain were cut and stained with hematoxylin. Slides were prepared for use under high resolution in a light microscope to study the fine structure of the endosperm.

RESULTS

Preliminary results from these evaluations are presented in Table I. Protein levels are usually slightly higher in hard phenotypes. Lysine and tryptophan have different levels among the several samples, with highest values found in varieties 1, 3, 5, and 7. These are assumed to be the genotypes with the best-quality protein, at least among the types tested. Among these samples, this quality level does not appear to have any direct relationship with either a soft or a hard endosperm phenotype. Fraction 2 (zein) has high values in all samples with very low lysine content (samples 2, 4, 6, and 8). The other fractions, however, are not consistent with either quality or type, except for the increased proportion of non-zein protein when summed together over fractions in those varieties with good quality.

Microscopic examination of the stained sections very clearly showed the large number of zein granules in kernels of those genotypes with poor protein quality. Four independent observers, none with any experience in maize, were able to classify by quality and by endosperm type each one of the genotypes included in the test. This separation was entirely made by visually noting the amount of these deeply staining granules in the endosperm. Reports of this screening method are found in the literature for sorghum and wheat. However, the system is not used widely to our knowledge and requires more elaborate starch removal procedures (6, 7). It appears to be a valuable tool for rough screening of maize for zein content and quality differences. From these preliminary observations, it is apparent that one may select any type of final combination of color, endosperm type, and protein quality for maize. It is also clear that hardness of the endosperm is not dependent on the zein concentration.

Frozen sections and a simple method of selection for protein quality in individual kernels will be particularly valuable for conversion of the floury highland varieties (usually soft) in which no genetic markers have been detected. This method will also permit the remainder of the kernel to be planted for future crossing.

CONCLUSION

Preliminary data presented suggest that (a) Phenotypic characteristics of the endosperm in maize are not dependent on zein concentration or protein quality. (b) Other fractions could be controlled by independent genes, either related to endosperm type or not. (c) Frozen hematoxylin-stained sections can be used as an inexpensive, rapid test method which may be accurate for preliminary screening for zein content and thus protein quality in kernels of maize.

REFERENCES

1. Mertz, E., Nelson, O., and Bates, L. S. (1964). Mutant gene that changes composition and increases lysine content of maize endosperm. *Science* 154:279.
2. Pradilla, A., Linares, F., Francis, C., and Fajardo, L. (1971). El Maíz de alta lisina en nutrición humana. *Acta. Méd. del Valle* 2:91.
3. Pradilla, A., Linares, F., Harpstead, D., Francis, C., and Sarria, D. (1972). Quality protein maize in human nutrition. International Symposium on Production and Utilization of Quality Protein Maize, Mexico.
4. Harpstead, D., and Pradilla, A. (1970). Improving acceptability of o_2 maize. Eighth Nutrition Congress, Prague.
5. Pradilla, A., Linares, F., and Francis, C. (1973). Studies on protein quality of flint phenotypes of o_2 maize. *Arch. Lat. Nutr.* 23:217, 1973.
6. Wolf, M. J., Khow, U., and Seckinger, N. L. (1967). Subcellular structure of endosperm protein in high lysine and normal corn. *Science* 157:556.
7. Wolf, M. J., and Kwoleh, N. (1970). Mature cereal grain endosperm, rapid glass knife sectioning for examination of proteins. *Stain Technol.* 45:277.

22

Solanum tuberosum X S. andigena Hybrids and Their Importance in Potato Breeding

Nelson Estrada Ramos
Instituto Colombiano Agropecuario
Bogotá, Colombia

After a brief review of the pertinent literature, this chapter provides examples of hybrid varieties of the potato derived in Colombia after crossing clones of *Solanum tuberosum* with clones of *S. andigena* obtained from several countries. The varieties display hybrid vigor that is expressed in high yield and greater disease resistance, frost tolerance, and uniformity, and in other attributes. The vigor remains relatively high after one generation of selfing of the hybrids. The vigor is accounted for on the basis of gene complementation or interaction of combinations of genes selected under quite different environmental conditions. The chromosome duplication of these hybrids ($2n = 96$) appears promising as a basis for further improvement of certain clones, but the effects of chromosome doubling are still under evaluation.

INTRODUCTION

The narrow genetic base of *Solanum tuberosum* in contrast to that of *S. andigena* has been indicated by several investigators both in the United States and in Europe. Hawkes (3) states that "cultivated potatoes in South America, besides being much more varied in shape, size and color than the European type, vary much more also in their physiological attributes." This situation has been reflected in the rather slow progress in producing newer and better varieties. Good examples are the Dutch potato variety Bintje, the English variety Majestic, and the American varieties Russet Burbank and Katahdin. They are the products of crosses made more than 40 years ago.

Tuberosum potato varieties are adapted to long days and high average temperatures (18°C). *Andigena* potato varieties are short-day (11–12 hr) plants and are adapted to cooler temperatures (12°C as an average).

The purpose of work reported here was to combine the genes of *tuberosum* with those of *andigena* in order to obtain varieties with higher yield, better characters for disease resistance, and wider adaptation for conditions of light and temperature.

LITERATURE REVIEW

Heterosis

Bukasov (1) indicated that striking data could be presented to show how hybrids of *andigena* and *tuberosum* excel intervarietal hybrids (of *tuberosum*) in yield. Kameraz (6) claimed also that hybrids between domestic varieties of *tuberosum* and *andigena* proved to be superior in yield to the best domestic varieties. Estrada (2) said that, in general, after crossing *tuberosum* to *andigena* varieties higher yield was obtained as compared with either of the parents. R. L. Plaisted at Cornell University (personal communication) has also been deeply interested in the potential of *andigena* for improving many characters in *S. tuberosum*. These opinions are supported by Howard (4), who considered that potatoes are outbreeding species and that on inbreeding they lose vigor.

Kostina (6) evaluated manifestations of significant hybrid vigor when making crosses among several wild potato species. Quantitative characters such as stem length, branching, and number and size of leaves were affected.

Moreno (7) studied two varieties of *S. tuberosum,* four varieties of *S. andigena,* and 24 hybrids of *tuberosum* × *andigena.* The yield and number of tubers in the seedlings were more than doubled in the hybrids as compared to the *tuberosum* or *andigena* varieties. Tuber size was similar in the three groups.

In relation to disease resistance, Thurston (10) stated that the commercial Colombian variety Monserrate has maintained its resistance to late blight since 1954 and has shown a high level of field resistance to blight when grown at Toluca Valley in Mexico. This variety is a *tuberosum* × *andigena* hybrid.

Effect of Chromosome Duplication

Rowe (9) indicated that no difference was detected in total number of tubers or weight when the yield of diploids was compared with that of tetraploids. He had reported previously, however, that in some trials the diploid clones outyielded the doubled clones and that the response to doubling varied according to genotypes (8).

MATERIALS AND METHODS

A collection of about 50 varieties of *S. tuberosum* was obtained from the Netherlands, England, Germany, Brazil, USA, and USSR and has been used in crosses to nearly 100 varieties of *S. andigena* from Colombia, Ecuador, Peru, Bolivia, and Venezuela. Observations on the behavior of parents and hybrids have been carried out for about 20 years. During this time, more than 500,000 potato seedlings have been planted and observed as a basis for selecting new potato varieties. A heterotic effect was readily observed in many characters. With the exception of a few genomic combinations, the hybrid effect is so striking that no statistical analysis is necessary to demonstrate hybrid vigor. The selection of these new varieties or hybrids has been carried out under conditions of high elevation in Colombia (Bogotá Savanna 2,600 m, Pasto, Narino 2800 m, Department of Boyaca 2900 m). A smaller number of hybrids of *tuberosum* × *tuberosum* and *andigena* × *andigena* has been obtained.

More recently, vegetative duplication of chromosomes has been made for some hybrids to obtain clones with $2n = 96$ chromosomes and to observe their preliminary behavior.

RESULTS AND DISCUSSION

Heterosis

Several potato varieties have been released in Colombia as a result of the crosses described in materials and methods. The following outstanding varieties can be mentioned: Monserrate, Cumbal, Capiro, Quindio, Tenerife, and Purace. They outyielded any of the parents by at least 50%. In addition, heterotic effects have been observed in characters such as tuber size, frost tolerance, disease tolerance, and vine growth. Other characters in the hybrids appear intermediate between the parental attributes. Examples are specific gravity of tubers, keeping quality on storage, and earliness. The hybrids cannot be cultivated at very high elevations (3500 m), since the *tuberosum* parent is quite sensitive to the reduced light of Colombian cloudy *paramos* and the low temperature (8°C) prevailing in these regions.

Transgressive inheritance or complementary genetic action has been observed in cases like that of late blight (*P. infestans*) field resistance observed in Monserrate and Cumbal varieties and in frost tolerance observed in Monserrate and Purace varities.

Our current general explanation of the high hybrid vigor, especially for yield, is based on complementation or interaction of combinations of genes selected under quite different environmental conditions.

Chromosome Duplication

Chromosome duplication (to $2n = 96$) appears promising as a means of improving earliness, tuber size, and tuber uniformity in certain hybrids or clones. Response to doubling differs according to genotype, and not all clones treated behave superiorly to the nontreated ones.

A striking and beneficial effect has been observed in the variety Quindio, where doubling improved the earliness from 180 days to almost 100 days. It also increased tuber size and uniformity to a better market type (grade A), in contrast with the untreated clone, which has numerous, rather small tubers (grades B and C).

The yield of the duplicated clone decreased about 15%, but on the whole it was 90% commercial *vs.* 60% commercial yield of the nontreated clone.

Adaptation to different elevations (out of 2600 m) is now in the process of testing to measure its capability of wide adaptation.

REFERENCES

1. Bukasov, S. M. (1939). Interspecific hybridization in the potato. *Physis* 18:269-284.
2. Estrada, N. (1955). Los hibridos interespecíficos e intervarietales de papa *tuberosum* X *andigenum,* una forma practica para mejorar las variedades en las zonas andinas. *Agr. Tropical (Bogota)* 11:87-94.
3. Hawkes, J. G. (1945). The story of the potato. *Discovery* 1945:38-45.
4. Howard, H. W. (1961). Potato cytology and genetics. *Bibl. Genet.* 19:87-216.
5. Kameraz, Y. (1949). *Bull. Appl. Bot. Gen. Plant Breed.* 28:57-70.
6. Kostina, L. I. (1968). A contribution to the knowledge of heterosis in potato. *USSR Acad. Sci. Genet.* 8:182-184.
7. Moreno, G. (1969). Efecto de la autofecundación en variedades de *S. tuberosum* L., *S. tuberosum* subsp. *andigena* Juz et Buk e hibridos entre estas dos especies de papa. Thesis, Fac. Agron. Univ. Nal. Bogota, 55 pp.
8. Rowe, P. R. (1967). Performance of diploid and vegetatively doubled clones of *phureja* - haploid *tuberosum* hybrids. *Am. Potato J.* 44:195-203.
9. Rowe, P. R. (1967). Performance and variability of diploid and tetraploid potato families. *Am. Potato J.* 44:263-271.
10. Thurston, H. D. (1971). Relationships of general resistance: Late blight of potato. *Phytopathology* 61:620-626.

23

Plant-*Rhizobium* Interaction
and Its Importance to Agriculture

P. H. Graham

Centro Internacional de Agricultura Tropical
Cali, Colombia

Rhizobia gain entry to leguminous roots, form nodules, and fix atmospheric nitrogen through a complex process, many stages of which may be influenced by host-bacteria interaction. The most common mechanism for nodule formation is described briefly here, and some of the interactions affecting both nodule formation and N_2 fixation are discussed.

a. Nodulation begins when a suitable strain of *Rhizobium* encounters a leguminous root system. The *Rhizobium* multiplies, in the process producing substantial amounts of IAA and other as yet unidentified but specific substances. These substances cause deformation and curling of the plant root hairs (Fig. 1).

b. The root hair invaginates at the apical portion, and some rhizobia pass into the invaginated section. This reaction is very localized and in many plants is also acid sensitive (Fig. 2).

c. A fungus-like infection thread is formed by the plant, and the rhizobia are contained within this thread even as they move down the root hair and into the cortex of the plant (Figs. 3 and 4).

d. When the infection thread penetrates a tetraploid cell, it begins to break up, and the rhizobia, still surrounded by a coating of plant mucilage, are released into the plant cell cytoplasm (Fig. 5). They begin to multiply, and the IAA produced causes multiplication of the tetraploid and surrounding diploid cells. This multiplication leads to the structure we call a "nodule." When released into the plant cell, the rhizobia are still bacil-

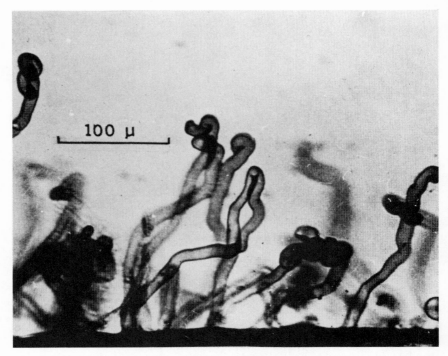

Fig. 1. Distortion in the root hair of Trifolium repens induced by the presence of an infective strain of R. trifolii. Photo by G. Fahraeus.

lary in shape. They quickly lose this cylindrical appearance, becoming "bacteroids," and in this form begin N_2 fixation.

e. During active fixation, there are usually four distinct nodular zones (Fig. 6): an outer cortical tissue uninfected by bacteria, an inner zone where the cells are infected but the rhizobia are still in the bacillary form, the central tissue containing N_2-fixing but generally nonviable *Rhizobium* "bacteroids," and an area of degenerating nodule tissue.

Even without human intervention, the nodule symbiosis has many specificities. Thus we recognize at least six species of *Rhizobium,* bacteria from each species nodulating a completely different group of legumes (Table I). Soybean rhizobia, for example, do not nodulate clovers and *vice versa.* There are numerous legumes, mostly primitive, which do not form nodules, and even in those legumes which are normally nodulating, e.g., soybean or clover, there are many instances of non-nodulating mutants. The effects of these mutations vary. Some mutants excrete toxic amino acids which kill the rhizobia before nodulation can occur; with others, the root hair may deform but not invaginate. In some, infection threads form but abort before nodules can be produced. Each mutation gives us a little more information about the mechanism of nodulation. To date, all have had one feature in common: the agronomic yield of the mutants is less than that of their nodulating isolines under most field conditions.

Compatibility of *Rhizobium* and legume can result in nodulation differences. In a recent trial with *Phaseolus vulgaris,* our strains varied markedly in the number and in the weight of nodules produced (Figs. 7 and 8). The reactions

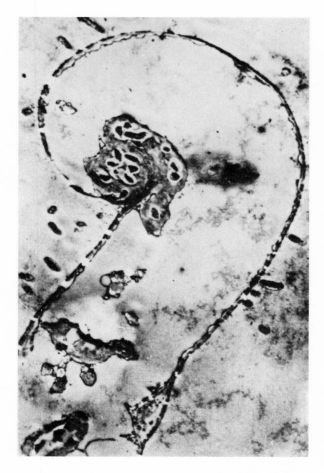

Fig. 2. Initiation of the infection thread in the invaginated root hair. (× 5500.) Photo by P. S. Nutman.

appeared to be compensatory, and net growth as shown by plant development in a nitrogen-free medium was little affected. In one instance, we did get a very strong host-*Rhizobium* interaction that affected all aspects of nodulation and fixation (Figs. 9 and 10).

Such specificity in nitrogen fixation is not uncommon, especially with soybeans. In the experiment reported in Table II, we were testing commercial soybean varieties to determine a suitable inoculant strain. Note the response of CIAT 51, producing excellent growth with one of the varieties but reacting poorly with the others. CIAT 4 would be a better strain for inoculants inasmuch as the results obtained with it are not markedly influenced by variety.

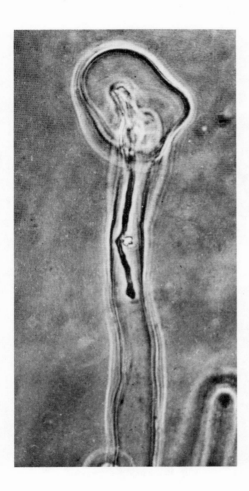

Fig. 3. Formation of the infection thread within a root hair of clover. (×600.) Photo by G. Fahraeus.

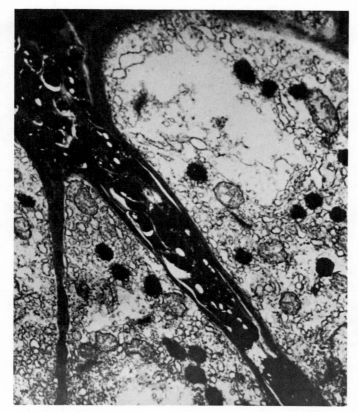

Fig. 4. Passage of the infection thread containing Rhizobium between two cells in the plant root cortex.

Environmental influences may compound host-*Rhizobium* interactions. Figure 11 shows the influence of root temperature on N_2 fixation by Tallarook clover. At 22°C, both strains compared are equal in fixing ability, but at 30°C the strain TA I is markedly superior. In the tropics, we can expect similar interplay between host-*Rhizobium* and temperature, emphasizing the necessity of careful inoculant section.

Soil pH is important. Bean rhizobia are acid sensitive and at low pH (say, pH 4.0–5.0) will be killed before nodulation can occur. Thus in soils from the Carimagua region (pH 4.2) our only hope of obtaining adequate nodulation is to pellet the seed with some neutral substance such as lime or phosphate. The improvement in nodulation, even when soil has been amended with quite high

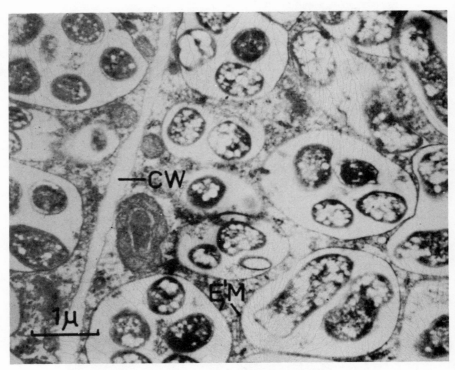

Fig. 5. A cell in the host plant infected with Rhizobium. The bacteria are enclosed in groups of two to six within their membrane envelope (EM). CW is the host cell wall. Photo by D. J. Goodchild and F. J. Bergersen.

Table I. *Rhizobium* Species and Their Appropriate Legumes

Species	Legumes nodulated
R. trifolii	*Trifolium* spp.
R. meliloti	*Medicago, Melilotus* spp.
R. leguminosarum	*Pisum, Vicia, Lens, Cicer*
R. japonicum	*Glycine max*
R. phaseoli	*Phaseolus vulgaris*
R. lupini	*Lupinus*
R. "cowpea"	*Vigna, Desmodium, Centrosema* and many others

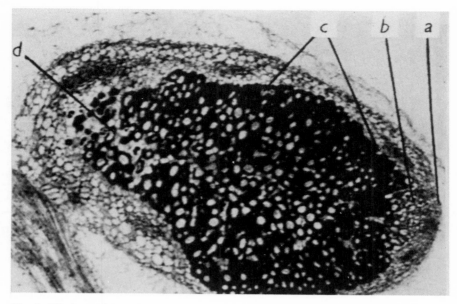

Fig. 5. *The internal organization of an effective root nodule.* (a) Uninfected cortical tissue, (b) inner zone infected by bacillary form of rhizobia, (c) central tissue containing N_2-fixing but generally nonviable "bacteroids," (d) area of degenerating nodule tissue. Photo by F. J. Bergersen.

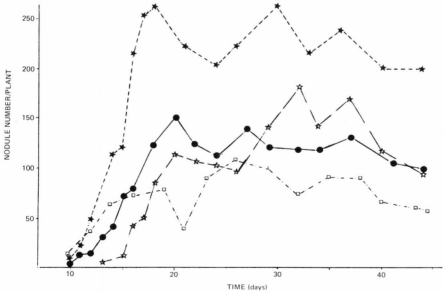

Fig. 7. *Difference in number of nodules produced with time, as influenced by inoculant strain.* Plant: *Phaseolus vulgaris.* ★, CIAT 40; ●, CIAT 57; □, CIAT 15; ☆, CIAT 16.

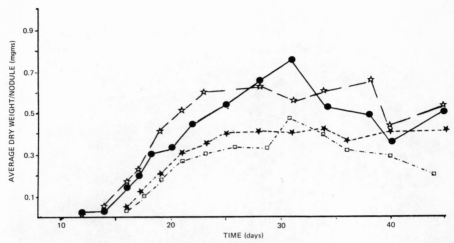

Fig. 8. Difference in nodule dry weight with time, as influenced by inoculant strain. Plant: *Phaseolus vulgaris.* Symbols as in caption of Fig. 7.

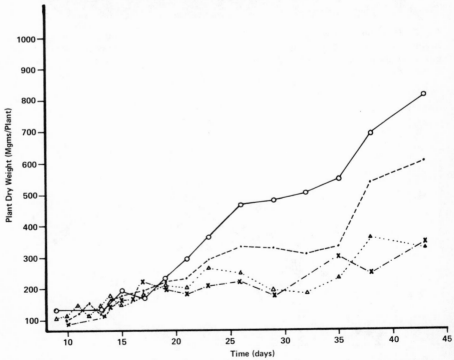

Fig. 9. Increase in dry weight per plant with time, as influenced by inoculant strain. Plant: *Phaseolus vulgaris,* var. 20574. Δ, CIAT 40; ○, CIAT 57; X, CIAT 15; ·, CIAT 16.

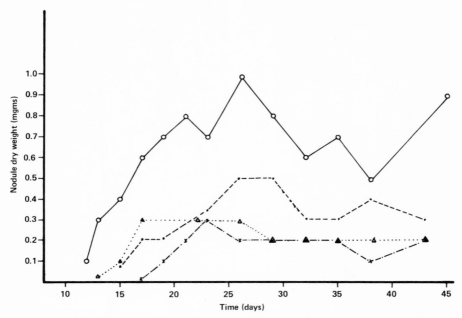

Fig. 10. *Average dry weight per nodule with time, as influenced by inoculant strain.* Plant: *Phaseolus vulgaris,* var. 20574. Symbols as in caption of Fig. 9.

Table II. Influence of Variety and of Strain of Inoculants on the Production of Dry Matter[a] in Soybean

Variety	No Inoculation	Strain 3	Strain 4	Strain 51	Subtotals of varieties
Mandarin	11.90	17.72	20.32	15.31	65.25
Pelikan	11.70	21.30	18.69	12.99	64.68
Americana	16.89	18.96	20.26	14.31	70.42
Lili	9.04	18.97	25.81	27.02	80.84
Subtotals of strains	49.53	76.96	85.08	69.63	

[a] As grams/plant.

dressings of ground lime, is obvious (Fig. 12). For somewhat less acid conditions, we are screening our strains for acid resistance, as has already been found in *Leucaena* and *Pisum* rhizobia.

Nodules containing effective strains of rhizobia are usually red in color due to the presence of hemoglobin. By contrast, nodules produced by particular legume strain combinations are black. Such markers can be extremely useful,

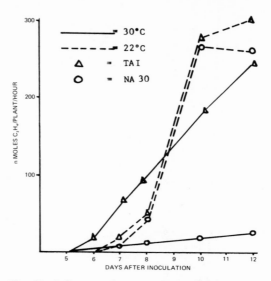

Fig. 11. Influence of temperature and of inoculant strain on reduction of acetylene by nodules of subterranean clover. Data of A. Gibson.

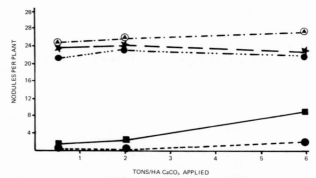

Fig. 12. Influence of method of inoculation and of soil calcium amendment on nodule number per plant in Phaseolus vulgaris, grown in Carimagua soil. F (inoculation) = 256.84, F (lining) = 7.53. •—•, no inoculation; ■, inoculation; ▲, $CaCo_3$, pelleted; ★, Carolina phosphate, pelleted; •····'•, Boyaca phosphate, pelleted.

especially in assessing the performance of an inoculated culture against that of strains that occur naturally in the soil.

Even a brief consideration of the legume-*Rhizobium* symbosis, such as just given, must reveal something of the complexity of the relationship and of the agricultural importance of interactions between the partners.

24

Exploratory Induction of Solid Mutations in Yams by γ-Irradiation

Francis K. S. Koo and Jose Cuevas Ruiz

Tropical Agro-Sciences Division
Puerto Rico Nuclear Center
Mayaguez, Puerto Rico

Yam tubers are consumed widely, particularly in tropical regions of the world, as a source of starchy food. *Dioscorea alata,* one of the edible yams that originated in Southeast Asia, is by far the most economically important yam species. It is grown mainly in Southeast Asia, the Caribbean, and some wet areas of Central and South America (5,6).

Yam production during the 1969-1970 season in Puerto Rico alone reached 30 million pounds with a farm value of nearly 3 million dollars (7). Local demand often exceeds production, and imports must be made to alleviate the shortage.

Selections for better traits in yam cultivars have been made but only haphazardly (5). Virtually no systematic work on varietal improvement has been undertaken to date, particularly on breeding by hybridization. This is mainly due to poor flower production, high pollen sterility, and low seed set inherent in the common cultivars. In some instances, strains of high standing are completely sterile. Under Puerto Rican climatic conditions, flowering has not been observed in a majority of the *D. alata* collections. The cultivars that may flower set no seeds (Martin, personal communication).

In the presence of such recombination barriers, varietal improvement through hybridization in *D. alata* is practically futile if not impossible. To circumvent such difficulties, one may resort to mutation breeding techniques by which traits of agronomic value might be improved. However, the main stumbling block in mutation breeding of vegetatively propagated species is the chimera formation following mutagenic treatment of the multicellular apices. Moreover, a mutated cell in such tissue is most likely subject to diplontic selection at great disadvantage.

One promising technique for mutation induction in such crops which has been well explored recently is that of inducing mutations in single cells of leaves, scales, stolons, etc., that may differentiate into adventitious buds later (1, 2, 4). In such cases, chimera formation is prevented and diplontic selection restricted. The mutant so derived is often a solid mutant; i.e., the whole plant is a mutant of a single type in contrast to a sectorial or periclinal mutant. Successful application of this technique to improve vegetatively propagated crops has been reported in *Saintpaulia* (8), *Streptocarpus* and *Achimenes* (1), and also *Begonia, Peperomia,* and *Lilium* (*cf.* ref. 2). The possible improvement of other crops such as *Chrysanthemum, Endymion, Kalanchoe, Muscari, Ornithogalum,* and *Scilla* is also being investigated with the same technique (*cf.* ref. 2).

The use of tissues capable of regenerating adventitious buds anew appears to be the most nearly ideal technique for mutation induction in the vegetatively propagated crops, but one should not overlook the possibility of employing the plant parts generally having preformed multicellular apices to achieve the same purpose. In such tissues, solid mutations might be induced if the mutagenic treatment is applied at an early stage before the multicellular apices are formed. Broertjes and Ballego (3) irradiated *Dahlia* tubers immediately after harvest and obtained some solid mutants. Mutagenic treatment of stolons from the actively growing young *Alstroemeria* plants also produced solid mutants (2).

Unsuccessful attempts have been made to root yam leaves with petiole but without stem tissue. Therefore, the application of the adventitious bud technique does not seem to be feasible with leaves at the present time. Many varieties of *D. alata* produce aerial tubers on the vines during the maturing stage. These aerial tubers, locally known as *gundas,* are often used as seed pieces for propagation. It has been observed that one to several dominant buds are present in the crown of the tuber, and new buds may be forced to develop in the lower portion of the tuber by cutting off the crown. It is uncertain, however, if these buds are preformed, but in a dormant stage, or if they are newly developed from single cells located most probably in the cambial layer of the tuber. Nevertheless, there seems to exist the possibility of inducing the solid type of mutations in materials such as the aerial tubers of yam. The study as reported here was designed to explore this possibility and at the same time to develop a mutation breeding protocol for yam improvement.

MATERIALS AND METHODS

The material consisted of some 700 aerial tubers from six varieties: Cuello Largo, Purple Lisbon, Hawaii Branched, Brazo Fuerte, Farm Lisbon, and Irene. The tubers were stored for 1–2 months at ambient room temperature (75–85°F) before use. The tubers were each cut into two parts in a proportion of one third for the crown part and two thirds for the lower part. The crown part served as nonirradiated control, and the lower part was treated with 2000 rad of γ-rays at a dose rate of 1000 rad/min. The material was then planted in rows in soil benches in the greenhouse. Seedlings that developed from the first sprouts of the irradiated material were examined for variant types at the three- to four-leaf stage by comparing with their corresponding controls. Then the shoots were cut back above the ground to force the new shoots to develop from the tubers or leaf axils for observation, and this process was repeated until there were no new shoots to emerge from the tubers.

For ease of observation, changes in the leaf color, leaf size, plant gross morphology, etc., were used as indices. When a mutation of solid type was observed, the whole plant together with the tuber was dug out for determining if the mutant was developed independently from any other shoots on the same tuber or from the shoot which had been pruned earlier.

RESULTS

In the first shoots of the irradiated material, the mottlings found most commonly in seedling leaves in numerous seed irradiation studies were not observed. However, crinkled leaves in various degrees were common, particularly in the varieties Purple Lisbon and Hawaii Branched. Also found, but in lower frequency, were deformed or abnormally shaped leaves. The least frequent changes were light green and/or yellow green sectors of various sizes in otherwise normal green leaves, and these were observed once each in Purple Lisbon and Farm Lisbon, and twice in Brazo Fuerte. The first shoots were cut back above the ground soon after the notes were taken. All the shoots from the tubers originated at the cuts or from the areas very close to the cuts. The main purpose of cutting back the shoots was to force new shoots to develop from the tubers, but quite often new shoots were generated from the leaf axils or the base portion of the shoots which had been pruned. The solid mutations were observed as early as in the second shoots, and some occurred after later prunings. The results are presented in Table I.

It is evident that some varieties were more amenable to mutation induction by γ-irradiation than the others. Cuello Largo had a much higher mutation frequency than all other varieties. Irene produced no mutant at all, probably because of the small number of tubers used. The mutant type recovered most abundantly was the light green leaf type. However, only in two cases was the pale green leaf type noted, and in one case the small leaf type (about one-half normal size). All the varieties except Irene produced solid mutants from the tubers, but only one variety, Cuello Largo, produced mutants from the leaf axils of the stems pruned back once or twice.

In the variety Purple Lisbon, four tubers each developed several new shoots

Table I. Frequencies of Various Solid Mutant Types Induced in Aerial Tubers of Six Varieties of *Dioscorea alata* by γ-Irradiation

Variety	Number of tubers studied	Mutants from tubers			Mutants from leaf axils	Total
		Light green leaf	Pale green leaf	Small leaf	Light green leaf	
Cuello Largo	200	5	—	—	12[a]	17
Purple Lisbon	100	1	1	—	—	2
Hawaii Branched	50	—	1	1	—	2
Brazo Fuerte	250	2	—	—	—	2
Farm Lisbon	70	1	—	—	—	1
Irene	13	—	—	—	—	0

[a] In two cases, the light green leaf mutant was developed from the leaf axil of the pruned shoot borne on the first shoot which had been pruned earlier.

after the pruning, and these shoots were completely stunted and twisted, with tightly folded and crinkled vestigial leaves. Most of these shoots either died later or unfolded their deformed leaves of various sizes. In one case, a new shoot was developed with normal-looking stem and leaves from the leaf axil of the stunted shoot. It appears that such a variant type might be chimeric in nature.

DISCUSSION

Our findings suggest that many new shoots in the test material were derived from single cells following prunings. Such capacity of regenerating new shoots from single cells in the tubers or in the leaf axils is of great importance to the yam mutation breeding program because the probability of success is much greater when mutations of solid type can be induced in these vegetative parts. In a practical breeding program, of course, the traits of interest to be induced are not necessarily recognizable without testing. Therefore, special methods for obtaining such desired mutants must be developed. At present, however, only the general technique may be outlined, with the purpose of securing all potential solid mutations instead of any specific type or types. The procedure seems to call for saving all the shoots that are developed from the tubers, including the first shoots. These shoots should be established as individuals by splitting off from the tubers as soon as they have developed two or three leaves. The first shoots may be pruned several times to force out axillary shoots which may be established individually later by rooting. Using appropriate methods, all the established individual plants then can be tested or screened for mutations of interest.

In this study, all the shoots that originated from the tubers were observed to develop at or close to the cuts. This observation might suggest that the wound area is endowed with the capacity of developing dominant shoots. If so, then one may choose to obtain additional breeding material by cutting the tubers into more sections.

Our results also show that some varieties are more amenable to mutation induction or recovery than others. This may indicate that certain varieties might have higher heterozygosity than others.

In the group of light green mutants, many died in a very early stage accompanied by rotting tubers. This leads one to question if these were all true mutants. It is quite possible that some of these plants had light green leaves simply because they were infected by root rot.

ACKNOWLEDGMENT

The authors are indebted to Dr. F. W. Martin of the Federal Experiment Station, U.S. Department of Agriculture, in Mayaguez for supplying the material for the study and his critical review of the paper.

REFERENCES

1. Broertjes, C. (1968). Mutation breeding of vegetatively propagated crops. Proc. Vth Congr. Europ. Ass. Res. Plant Breeding, Milan. *Eucarpia,* pp. 139-165.
2. Broertjes, C. (1972). Improvement of vegetatively propagated plants by ionizing radiation. Proceedings of FAO/IAEA Sponsored Latin-American Study Group Meeting on Induced Mutations and Plant Improvement, Buenos Aires, pp. 293-299.
3. Broertjes, C., and Ballego, J. M. (1967). Mutation breeding of *Dahlia variabilis. Euphytica* 16:171-176.
4. Broertjes, C., Haccius, B., and Weidlich, S. (1968). Adventitious bud formation on isolated leaves and its significance for mutation breeding. *Euphytica* 17:321-344.
5. Coursey, D. G. (1967). *Yams,* Longmans, London, 230 pp.
6. Martin, F. W. (1972). Yam Production Methods, U.S. Department of Agriculture Production Research Report No. 147, 17 pp.
7. Puerto Rico Agricultural Experiment Station (1972). Basic Concepts and Program, UPR-Agricultural Experiment Station, 165 pp.
8. Sparrow, A. H., Sparrow, R. C., and Schairer, L. A. (1960). The use of X-rays to induce somatic mutations in *Saintpaulia. Afr. Violet Mag.* 13:32-37.

NOTE ADDED IN PROOF

We have no way of ascertaining the true nature of the mutants observed in this study except by inference. If the leaf-pigment-deficient mutants arisen from the tubers were developed from the preformed multicellular meristems, then they would have had variegated leaves rather than those in solid mutant colors. Of course there is a possibility that the "solid-looking" mutants might be periclinal in nature if they happened to derive from the meristems with only a single cell in the layer at the time of mutation induction. Unfortunately all the leaf color mutants except one died early. One pale green mutant, extremely spindly and weak, did survive to maturity and produce a few small aerial tubers (ca. 4–5 mm in diameter) but these tubers failed to produce any new plants. The small leaf mutant also reached maturity but bore only the "sterile" aerial tubers.

25

Insect Control with γ-Rays

Juan E. Simon F.

Centro Nacional de Investigaciones Agropecuarias
La Molina, Lima, Perú

The Peruvian entomologist J. E. Wille stated in the late 1940s that "A man can legally own his own land, but biologically he never owns it. . . ." The world is just now beginning to appreciate the meaning of these words. The excessive use of pesticides resulting from the philosophy that a man can do whatever he wishes with his own land is now being recognized as a significant upsetting of the balance of nature. Thus scientists in basic, as well as applied, fields are now working to restore the land to an unpolluted state where pests are managed by means less drastic than complete reliance on chemicals.

Neither pests nor pesticide pollutants respect political borders. Agricultural workers are thus more than ever cognizant of the consequences of pesticide use not only within the borders of the region of application but also on a broader scale.

THE ALTERNATIVES

With the popularization of the use of insecticides and the awareness of the excellent results that can be obtained with them, it is a significant turnabout to announce that, under some circumstances, more damage than benefit results from their use. If we think about the almost complete eradication of malaria, typhus, and bubonic plague, and the good control of Chagas' disease and other diseases transmitted by insects, it is difficult to condemn pesticide use. Furthermore, the losses in agricultural crops and livestock have been tremendously reduced with the use of insecticides. The fact remains that in some places it will be impossible to raise sufficient food without the auxiliary use of insecticides.

The concerned entomologist in the first half of the twentieth century was thus faced with a dilemma: let the people die of malnutrition or permit them to live some years more by consuming adequate food with a potential chemical hazard. There was very little choice in this circumstance. Nevertheless, our social responsibility called our attention to other systems, and Peruvians were among the first, not only because we were so lucky as to have J. E. Wille working with and for the people, but also because our geography provides us with coastal deserts, or what we can call "open greenhouses."

In these deserts, a very small amount of cultivated land ($20-100$ km^2) is spaced along the rivers draining the Andes to the west. These valleys are completely isolated from one another, and in each of them existed a very well-defined and specific fauna. These few species formed a naturally balanced complex of parasites and predators which was broken in a few months after applications of insecticides. There was little possibility of recovery. Peru then faced the problem that the rest of the world was to face within 20 years.

The integrated control idea thus came to Peru when, at the end of the 1940s, Wille wrote: "wait as much as possible and, only when the biological control has been unable to take care of the pest, then refer to the use of the correct insecticide . . . ." Here we find the first option to chemical control, the use of biological control with parasites and predators. Biological control was complemented by a second possibility, cultural measures. Examples of cultural measures include allowing land to lie unplanted for a period; irrigating at minimum rates to make the plants less attractive to insects; growing intercalated crops with corn, as Hambleton had observed in the late 1930s; improving the beneficial fauna; or increasing the population of predators.

With insects for which there are no biological controls, traps with food attractants (e.g., cotton seed for cotton red stainer, sugar for domestic flies) are useful. With the introduction of the pheromones or sexual attractants, a male or female annihilation method can be considered as a third option. More attention is being given to this last system, and some entomologists, after the eradication of the Oriental fruit fly *Dacus dorsalis* from Rota Island in 1963, have begun to think that it is less complex than any other technique that has been used. Others, such as Y. Ito and colleagues, have demonstrated that some biological and genetic complications can arise from the pheromones method. Another option that has been extensively used is light traps with baits or lures combined with a lower number of applications of insecticides to the field where the traps are installed.

All of these systems cause major or minor disturbances in the population dynamics not only of the pest to be controlled but also of other species of insects which may be beneficial. Hence the possibility of using an autocide method, which results in little or no disturbance to the ecological system, is especially appealing.

The sterile insect release method (SIRM) uses the insect pest to control itself. It provides the following advantages:

a. Where a pest insect is able to live or survive, the sterile insect will duplicate its behavior; therefore, there is no haven for the pest.
b. The insect pest need not reach a high population level, as is necessary before a system such as parasites and predators begins to work. The SIRM requires a depressed population level such as occurs seasonally.
c. The sterile insects are able to mate with and decrease the population of only their own kind; thus the system is highly specific.

On the other hand, this method is not as simple as it looks. At the beginning, seven requirements were established for its use:

a. A mass-rearing system must be established or must at least be possible with current knowledge.
b. The female must mate only once or at most twice during its life cycle.
c. The radiation must cause complete sterility of the insects without decreasing their other biological attributes such as competitiveness.
d. The zone where SIRM is going to be applied must be isolated naturally or artificially.
e. The insect must not cause crop injury at the stage in which it is going to be liberated.
f. The insect population must naturally fluctuate, or, if this fluctuation does not occur naturally, it must be possible to depress the population by use of insecticides or other means.
g. An intensive knowledge of the insect's habits and ecology must be available. This knowledge should include its longevity, where and when copulation occurs, the number of generations a year, flight capacity, sex ratio, and reproductive potential.

MASS-REARING SYSTEMS

In some cases, mass-rearing requires that billions of insects be reared in a year, which seems to be possible only when artificial media are used. The costs of using agricultural or animal products for a natural medium may exceed the value of the crop or livestock being protected.

At the present moment, several species of Diptera are being reared by the millions per week. These include screwworm fly (200 million per week), *Ceratitis capita* (Wied.) or medfly (10–40 million per week), and *Culex fatigans* mosquito (5 million per week). Some others have been raised in lesser amounts, including *Glossina morsitans* and *Glossina tachinoides,* two species of tsetse flies; *Stomoxys calcitrans,* or stable fly; the onion fly, *Hylemya antigua;* the Oriental fruit fly, *Dacus dorsalis;* the South American fruit fly, *Anastrepha fraterculus;* the Mexican fruit fly, *Anastrepha ludens;* and the Caribbean fruit fly, *A. suspensa.* Some Lepidoptera are also being reared; these include *Cydia pomonella;* the corn earworm, *Heliothis zea;* the tobacco budworm, *Heliothis virescens;* the tobacco hornworm, *Manduca sexta;* and the pink bollworm, *Pectinophora gossypiella.* Several million of these species are being reared per week, and it is also true with the sugarcane borer, *Diatraea saccharalis.* Representatives of Coleoptera are also raised in this way; the cotton boll weevil, *Anthonomus grandis,* is reared in a factory with a capacity of 15 million insects per week.

Investigators working with all these species are ready to start, or have already started, projects with the SIRM. Most of the insects are sterilized by ionizing radiation; the boll weevil, however, is sterilized chemically.

Since my own work is on medfly, I will describe how these insects are reared at the Centro Nacional de Investigaciones Agropecuarias of the Ministerio de Agriculture of Peru, at La Molina.

The eggs are obtained from flies in cages 2.00 by 0.60 by 0.40 m; one side of each cage is covered by a screen. The front side is covered by a dacron cloth and is used as an oviposition surface. The eggs fall to trays which are partially filled with water and are located on the floor below the cages. Every morning, eggs are collected, measured, and seeded on aluminum trays (0.80 by 0.30 by 0.10 m) with a diet suitable for the growth of larvae. The larval diet is a mixture of sugarcane bagasse, cane sugar, unicellular forage yeast cultured on sugarcane molasses, HCl, sodium benzoate, and water. All of the ingredients are made in Peru to minimize expense. The larval trays are kept for 8 days at 27 ± 2°C, in wood cabinets covered with a very fine mesh screen in order to prevent contamination by *Drosophila* spp. Following this period, the media are turned over on iron frames and held for 3 days at the same temperature in what we call "turnover cabinets," which have incliner sheets of plywood (60° inclination) and a drawer at the bottom which the larvae fall into. Three times a day, the larvae are transferred from the cabinet drawers to smaller pupation drawers sprinkled with sawdust, where after 3 days at 27 ± 2°C the larvae pupate. The pupae are separated from the sawdust in a grain cleaner and transferred to drawers in pupal cabinets where they are held for 7½ days of "physiological aging." The first 3 days of maturation are at 27°C, but the rate of growth may be slowed by holding at 20°C; the requirement for insects varies. Two days at 20°C at the conclusion of maturation is equivalent to 1 earlier day at 27°C.

When the pupae are physiologically mature, they are at the "blue-eye" stage, look dark brown, and are ready for irradiation.

The Irradiation Doses

The doses that are necessary to achieve 99% sterilization vary with the species and with the stage at which the insect is being sterilized. The data

Table I. Irradiation Doses Required for
99% Sterilization

Species	Dose (krad)
Glossina morsitans	19
G. tachinoides	15
G. austni	12
G. fuscipes	10
Hylemya antigua	3
Cydia pomonella	25–40
Argas persicus (soft ticks)	12
Ceratitis capitata	9–13
Anastrepha fraterculus	6
Leucoptera coffeella	90

presented in Table I, mostly from other laboratories, give an idea of the doses required. In most cases, the late pupal stage is irradiated. Currently, the lowest dosage which provides about 97% sterility is used in order to yield the greatest number of flies which are competitive with wild flies.

Transportation and Liberation

Several systems have been developed to transport sterile insects from the factory to the release point. For example, the screwworm fly control program in the southwestern United States uses a fleet of 33 airplanes to dispense the flies over a wide area of the United States and Mexico. Other projects transport insects in refrigerated trucks or ships, and still others simply send the insects by commercial airlines, which is what we do in Peru.

After the pupae are received at the southern valleys in Peru, they are dusted with a dye for identification and packaged in No. 12 paper bags with 150 g of dry-folded reed plants to prevent crushing and to provide a support for emerging insects. About 6000 pupae are packaged in each bag with a piece of 0.10- by 0.10-m absorbent cotton soaked in a solution of 1 part honey, 4 parts sugar, and 10 parts water. The mouths of the bags are closed with staples. The bags are then placed in large paperboard cartons which are held for 60 hr at $27°C$. The cartons are brought to the orchards, and the adult flies are liberated by hanging each bag from a tree and cutting one of the sides of each bag.

The sterile flies disperse to mate with the normal as well as with the sterile flies. Four mating combinations may occur:

Sterile male × sterile female   = no eggs
Normal male × sterile female   = no eggs

Sterile male X normal female   = inviable eggs
Normal male X normal female   = viable eggs

Males mate anywhere from four to 15 times, while females mate only once or twice. Thus the objective is to reduce the probability of females mating with fertile males.

Isolation Conditions for the Experiment

Peru is ideal for carrying out a SIRM project since the 52 coastal valleys are isolated from one another by deserts and small chains of hills running north-south at the end of each valley. In the east are the Andes with mountains of 4000–7000 m elevation, and in the west is the Pacific Ocean.

THE PRERELEASE STUDIES

Our team has studied dosage, competitiveness, and natural population dynamics using Steiner traps, sticky traps, and trimedlure, a sex lure for medfly. The medfly's potential damage to fruit has also been studied using cages covering trees where various combinations of normal and irradiated flies were released. These experiments also gave information about the behavior of the flies in a restricted natural situation. The liberation of several million flies and attempts to recapture them with traps checked the effectiveness of the traps and the range of the flies after release. The different host species of trees and annual plants have been determined in each valley to find the reproductive potential of the pest at different seasons of the year.

Finally, the system for rearing the flies has been improved. We now have a provisional installation for producing 40 million flies a week. A new specially designed factory for rearing 100–250 million medflies a week is nearing completion and will be ready when the equipment is available.

RESULTS

We have now accumulated much experience from the development of our programs and from visiting or working outside of our laboratory. The screwworm project in the southwestern United States is a good example of a SIRM project: the number of reported cases was around 50,000 in 1962, 7000 in 1963, less than 400 in 1964, about 900 in 1965, 1900 in 1966, less than 900 in 1967, about 10,000 in 1968, only 219 in 1969, 153 in 1970, 473 in 1971. In the first 10 months of 1972, however, 89,406 cases were reported. Research must determine why the program failed in that year. Good results with SIRM have also been reported from some islands such as Curaçao Island which had a screwworm project. Other projects have been directed against mosquitoes in

India and Florida; tobacco budworm and corn earworm in Florida (St. Croix Island); medfly in Nicaragua and Procrida Island (Italy); and clothing moth in Canada and the northeastern United States. Finally, I would like to describe our results in Tacna and Moquegua, two southern valleys in Peru.

In Tacna in 1969, we made two aerial sprays of a bait insecticide and during the following 20 weeks liberated 1 million sterile flies per week. The number of flies was not sufficient, and the population of flies increased from one fly per trap per week (f/t/wk) to 40 f/t/wk.

In 1970, we decided to use the upper part of the Tacna valley (3 of almost 7 sq miles) where in May 1970 the population was 30.7 flies per trap per month (f/t/m), in June 23.7 f/t/m, and in July 6.2 f/t/m as a result of natural pressures. From July 1970 until July 1971, the population oscillated from 0.8 to 5.7 f/t/m. We obtained 95% of the healthy fruit at the upper part of the valley and liberated 170 million sterile flies in 14 months. The same amount of healthy fruit was obtained at the lower part of the valley with weekly applications of insecticides. We then decided to extend the releases to the whole valley from October 1971 to June 1972, when we stopped the releases because we could not supply the amount of sterile flies necessary to depress the population of normal flies. The main reason for this failure, we believe, was the short winter with the highest recorded temperatures of the century at Tacna, resulting in a failure of normal winter killing.

In Moquegua, the valley was divided into four parts. In the uppermost part, called Tumilaca and Torata, with about 12,000 host trees we used bait insecticide sprays. None was used next to the uppermost part, which is the main fruit zone with about 70,000 host trees, called Estuquiña, Samegua, and Valley. In this area we released the sterile flies alone, and for this reason we know it was the "release zone." The median part of the valley, a narrow and deep canyon extending about 25 km with no fruit trees, received no treatment. The lowest part of the valley, the delta called Ilo and planted mainly with olives and about 8000 other favorite host trees of medfly, is where we neither released flies nor sprayed insecticides; this was the control area (*testigo*).

The areas of the four zones are shown in Table II. In the uppermost and

Table II. Areas of Study Zones

	Hectares	Square miles
Insecticides zone (Tumilaca–Torata)	996	3.890
Release zone (Estuquiña–Samegua–Valley)	2304	9.000
Canyon	107	0.418
Control zone (Ilo)	361	1.410

upper area of Moquegua from July 1969 to July 10, 1970, 266,771 sprays were applied to host trees with bait insecticide to lower the population of flies from 0.11 to 0.06 flies per trap per day (f/t/d). We began liberating sterile flies on July 11, 1970, and the populations increased in August to 0.8 f/t/d. They receded during September, October, November, and December to a minimum of 0.0003 f/t/d. In January, however, the population increased, showing a monthly average of 0.009 f/t/d. In February the average was 0.017, in March 0.02, in April 0.27, in May 0.38, and in June 0.24 f/t/d. Farmers were, nevertheless, happy because they had obtained the best yields since the introduction of medfly to the valley in the late 1950s. In 1970-1971, we released only 491,310,000 sterile flies and made 28,000 applications of insecticides to the "hot spots." The increment in the fly population was due to the fact that the 25-km-long canyon was not adequately isolated, since several thousand flies flew through the canyon from the control zone (Ilo) to the liberation zone. This was deduced from the fact that the number of flies captured in the canyon was inversely proportional to the population in the control zone.

In August 1971, we began again to liberate sterile flies, but we followed the Steiner formula for the calculation of nativity (3) with a population of 0.36 f/t/d. This population did not stop going up; in September it was 0.38, in October 0.57, November 1.11, December 0.88, January (1972) 1.17, February 4.25, March 13.05, April 28.94, May 16.94, June 7.80, July 3.08, August 3.04, and September 4.30. During those 14 months, we liberated 574,740,000 sterile flies in the 2304 ha (9 sq miles).

It is important to remember that during the 1971-1972 period the weather was very hot, thus providing optimum conditions for medfly reproduction. In addition, our efforts in the 1971-1972 release were badly hampered by a variety of factors which interrupted a continuous flow of good-quality flies in the numbers needed. These factors call attention to the fact that to be successful SIRM needs an organization which plans sufficiently well to anticipate potential problems and to make allowances for these problems.

Despite problems, the farmers got an 80% yield of healthy fruit with 54,000 sprays of baits at the "hottest spots." Twenty-five percent of the sprays were made during the period from February to May.

The expanded medfly factory now has a warehouse with enough capacity for a 12-month supply of necessary materials at full production. We have reduced the irradiation dosage from 10 to 9 krad in order to make the sterile males more competitive and have devised new transport systems using small airplanes and even buses. We have established strict quality control of flies with double checks at La Molina and at Moquegua and have made four applications of malathion bait to reduce the population. Finally, we have reduced our project to the 23 km² of the release zone in Moquegua, making weekly applications of bait along the canyon and the upper zone. The extremely efficient adaptability of the insects may yet surprise us. We do know, however, that we will continue to use integrated control, of which the SIRM will be just one part.

REFERENCES

1. Hambleton, Edson J. (1944). *Heliothis virescens* as a pest of cotton, with notes on host plants in Peru. *J. Econ. Entom.* 37:660-666.
2. Ito, Y., and Iwasaki, O. (1972). Ecology problems associated with attempt to eradicate *Dacus dorsalis* from the islands of the south of Japan with a recommendation on the use of the sterile male technique. Proceedings of a panel originated by the Joint FAO/IAEA Division of Atomic Energy in Food and Agriculture, Vienna.
3. Steiner, L. F. (1967). Methods of estimating the size of populations of sterile pest *Tephritidae* in release programs. Proceedings of a panel organized by the Joint FAO/IAEA Division of Atomic Energy in Food and Agriculture, Vienna, p. 63.

26

Social and Economic Orientation of Crop Improvement: An Approach to Maize Breeding

Fidel Marquez-Sanchez
Departamento de Genética
Colegio de Postgraduados
Escuela Nacional de Agricultura
Chapingo, México

It is common to consider Mexico the cradle of the "green revolution." It is not so commonly realized that many Mexicans have not received the green revolution's benefits. Wheat bread, for example, is not yet part of many peasant diets. While Fig. 1 shows that agronomists have improved the wheat crop through breeding and proper cultural practices, the plant breeder should maintain goals that agree with the social and economic reality of the people he is working for. In the case of Mexico, a great percentage of our peasants still practice subsistence agriculture.

Nobody denies the excellence of improved wheat varieties or maize hybrids. These cultivars, together with adequate cultural practices, increase the unitary yields by significant amounts. It is not well known, however, that these benefits cannot be obtained by most peasants in countries such as Mexico where the peasants are not the favorite children of the green revolution—or for that matter of any type of revolution. Very little account is taken of this group of people in planning plant breeding research.

A comparison of some of the huge and well-cultivated areas of some of the Latin American countries with the less favorable lands (which are, unfortunately, the most extensive parts of the agricultural areas) makes it apparent that the orientation of the plant breeding programs should and must be revised. This problem, however, should not be approached emotionally. The solution is not to

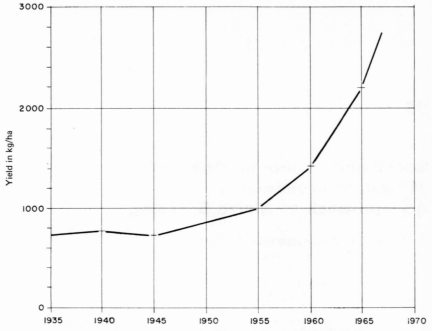

Fig. 1. Average wheat yields in Mexico from 1935 to 1967 (6).

transfer the technology from the rich agricultural areas, or countries, to the underdeveloped ones; for whatever technology is used should accord with both the environmental and the social conditions. Furthermore, this technology should undergo constant and dynamic revision. It is expected that as the peasants adopt new technology their economic status will be modified; these changes will require the modification of the previous technology so as to surpass the previously established goals.

One of the main causes of the lack of development of many Mexican agricultural regions is an unfavorable environment, especially erratic and insufficient rainfall. It should be taken into account, also, that in order to increase the possibilities of a certain margin of profit it is necessary to invest some minimum amount of inputs; it is not possible to expect high production from a crop established by digging holes, throwing seeds in them, and waiting for the harvest.

With these ideas in mind, the plant breeder must first define the environmental, social, and economic situation and then define the type of variety most favorable to real economic development. Of necessity, this process requires the formulation of a theoretical model designed to select out of a population of genotypes the ones most suitable for such a model. Fundamental aspects should be taken into account with regard to subsistence agriculture: First, the peasant cannot buy first-generation hybrid seed every year. Second, the varieties which are to be recommended should have a wide geographical adaptability, because in the first stages of the process it will not be economically possible to obtain as many varieties as there are ecological subdivisions, and should be widely adapted in growing time, because of the erratic amount and distribution of the precipitation from year to year. Third, it is more important for the farmer to have secure yields than excellent yields in good and exceptional years and mediocre or no yields during bad years. The average yield of the improved variety, of course, should be higher than the average yield of the native variety. The qualitative characteristics such as the type of plant, of ear, and of grain that the farmer is willing to adopt should be considered.

It is not enough to demonstrate to the farmer that an improved variety is superior to his variety in yield; the new variety should have the same qualities as or better qualities than the one he has. It should be kept in mind that in some of these matters we are dealing with very conservative people. A new variety has often been rejected or the native variety gradually reaccepted because of, for example, lack of consideration of the type of *tortilla* obtained from the grain or of the facility of hand shelling or of the quality of the plant for fodder. Obviously, a static situation is not desirable. For example, when a social stage has been overcome (either by the change produced by the technology adopted or by the establishment of different social structures, specifically socialism, or by a combination of these two forces), new approaches have to be applied by the breeder. If, for instance, there are surpluses after satisfying the family needs, future varieties will have to have other characteristics, perhaps more in accordance with commercial requirements.

With these premises in mind, we can define the desired model for the initial stages of the breeding program as follows: *An open pollinated variety of wide adaptability which will show a secure yield under the ecological variants of the area and which is of local origin.*

Test and selection of such a variety can be carried out with the technology of theoretical and applied research used in the postgraduate College of the National School of Agriculture at Chapingo, Mexico. The statistical technique known as "stability parameters" (3), which has been studied by several research agronomists, is a very useful tool once the underlying principles of genotype-environment interaction are understood. It consists, in essence, of sowing the group of populations being tested in regionally uniform trials during several years at several locations within the ecological area of interest. In this way, each of the varieties can be described not only by its average yield but also by its behavior in the various environments. Each environment is defined as a particular combination of one location during 1 year. The statistical model for a given variety follows:

$$Y = M + V + BI + D$$

where Y is the average yield of the variety in a given environment, M is the average yield of all varieties in all environments, V is the genetic effect of the variety (therefore its genetic mean is given by the point where the regression line cuts the ordinate at the origin), I is the mean of all varieties in a given environment minus M (known as the environmental index), and B and D are the stability parameters. It is important to note that I measures the productivity potential of the involved environment; thus through regression analysis it is possible to estimate B, the regression coefficient of the yields of the variety in the environments on the respective Is, and D, the mean squares deviations from regression. When B equals 1 and D equals 0 (see Fig. 2), the variety has a response that exactly equals the environmental change. When this is not the situation, the response of the variety is greater or smaller than the environmental change (1, 5) and is not exact.

Figure 3 shows the behavior of two maize hybrids, H129 and H309, included in uniform trials during several years at several locations in the transitional area between El Bajio and the Central Plateau in Mexico (2). Although both hybrids have very similar overall means, H129, with B almost equal to 1, is a variety whose responses are almost equal to the respective environmental changes: either favorable $(+I)$ or unfavorable $(-I)$. This situation is not so for H309, whose B is less than 1. H309 does not respond as well as H129 to environmental changes.

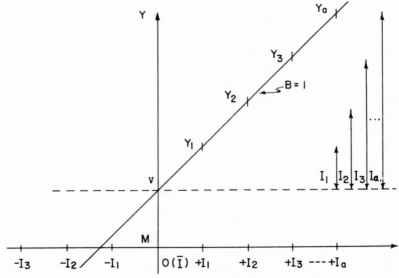

Fig. 2. A variety with stability parameters B = 1 and D = 0.

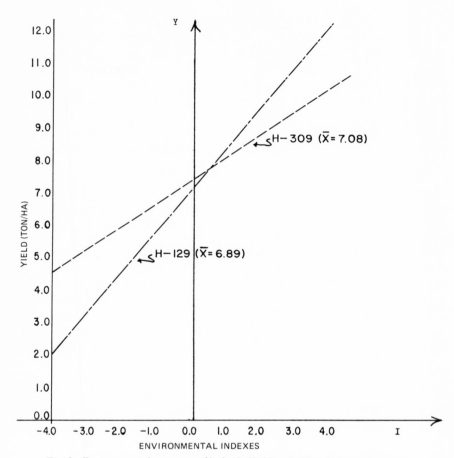

Fig. 3. Environmental response of hybrids H129 and H309 in transition zones.

Moreover, H129 takes more efficient advantage of the favorable conditions of good environments (+I) than does H309. On the other hand, in bad environments (−I) H309 makes better use of the prevailing situation than does H129.

It should be clear that "environments" refers to both the ecological environment and the agronomic one; in other words, we are considering all those agricultural practices such as fertilization, plant population density, insect and disease control, and irrigation that determine as a whole the goodness of a given year or locality. This analysis is thus important in that it permits a decision to be made regarding the variety to be used that accords with the environmental indexes that predominate in a region. It would not be wise to recommend H129 in areas with unfavorable environmental indexes where H309 would do better.

The concept of adaptability can now be transferred to our problem if the years are considered environments, that is, environmental conditions determined mainly by precipitation. There will be good and bad years in variable proportions, and, under the assumption that precipitation of a given year is unpredictable, the farmer is interested in a variety which will give him fair yields year after year rather than one which will give him high yields in good years and poor yields during bad years. The first type of variety would have a B coefficient of less than 1 (its regression line would tend to be horizontal), whereas the second type of variety would tend to have its B value close to 1 or at least greater than that of the first variety.

In order to obtain the type of variety sought, selection must from the beginning consider the characteristics of the model described. The procedure should not be to obtain "many" varieties at random and to postpone the test of adaptability to the final steps; both phases should be combined in their application. The method under study at the Postgraduate College at Chapingo (4) is illustrated in Fig. 4. While the researcher uses a local variety or a composite of local varieties, modern mass selection is carried out in each location. With the germ plasm so selected, a balanced composite is made. This composite is then subjected to genetic recombination (R) in the experimental station. Recombination favors the widening of the genetic diversity, thus increasing the possibilities of selection. Adaptability of the selected individuals will be high since they have been under the selection pressure of all localities. The material selected and recombined in the manner indicated is distributed again to the localities, and a new selection cycle is initiated. The number of selection cycles needed will depend on the velocity at which genetic variability is exhausted, the selection response obtained, and the necessity of change of the prevailing variety, which in turn depends on the rate of social change.

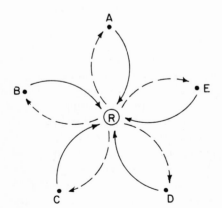

Fig. 4. Mass selection for adaptability at several locations. Solid arrows, genotypes selected at each location are recombined in *R.* Broken arrows, recombined genotypes are allocated to locations for selection.

If a 5% progress per cycle is obtained, for example, it will be possible to release a variety after 4–5 years of selection. The farmers using this variety will not have to buy seed every year since they will be able to produce their own seed through the application of certain elementary techniques. If after several years the social situation demands a change of variety, then other breeding methods will have to be used to produce from the improved variety other improved populations such as synthetics, double-cross hybrids, three-way hybrids, and, finally, single-cross hybrids characterized by a maximum expression of heterosis. As already mentioned, these better populations will need greater inputs to reveal their full potential.

In conclusion, plant breeding, if it is to play a significant role in the social change that our underdeveloped countries desperately need, should be scientifically based and should consider both the biological and the social sciences. Often the solutions to problems are missed, not because of their complex nature, but because of a lack of scientific knowledge and a lack of clear objectives.

ACKNOWLEDGMENT

The author is deeply indebted to Professor Efraim Hernandex X. for his generous help in the revision of the manuscript.

REFERENCES

1. Bucio-Alanis, L. (1966). Environmental and genotype-environmental components of variability. I. Inbred lines. *Heredity* 21(3):387-397.
2. Carballo-Carballo, A., and Marquez-Sanchez, F. (1970). Comparacion de variedades de maiz del El Bajio y la Mesa Central por su rendimiento y estabilidad. *Agrociencia* 1(5):129-146.
3. Eberhart, S. A., and Russell, W. A. (1966). Stability parameters for comparing varieties. *Crop. Sci.* 6:36-40.
4. Marquez-Sanchez, F. (1970). El problema de la interaccion genetico-ambiental en genotécnia vegetal. Postgraduate College, Escuela Nacional de Agricultura, Chapingo, Mexico.
5. Marquez-Sanchez, F. (1971). Analysis of adaptability of cultivated crops. Proceedings of the First Maize Workshop, CIMMYT, El Batan, Mexico.
6. Moreno-Galvez, R. (1968). Aspectos del mejoramiento de los cereales en Mexico. *Memoria del tercer Congreso de Fitogenetica,* Chapingo, México.

Index